PEPTIDES
Design, Synthesis, and
Biological Activity

PEPTIDES
Design, Synthesis, and Biological Activity

Channa Basava
G. M. Anantharamaiah
Editors

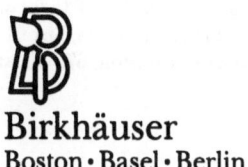

Birkhäuser
Boston • Basel • Berlin

Channa Basava
Novabiochem USA
10394 Pacific Center Court
San Diego, CA 92127
USA

G. M. Anantharamaiah
Atherosclerosis Research Unit
Department of Medicine
The University of Alabama at Birmingham
University Station, DREB 640
Birmingham, AL 35924-0012
USA

Library of Congress Cataloging-in-Publication Data

Peptides: design, synthesis, and biological activity / Channa Basava, G. M.
   Ananthamaiah, editors.
      p.   cm.
   Includes bibliographical references.
   ISBN-13: 978-1-4615-8178-9   e-ISBN-13: 978-1-4615-8176-5
   DOI: 10.1007/978-1-4615-8176-5
      1. Peptides–Synthesis.   2. Protein engineering.   I. Basava, Channa, 1949– .
   II. Anantharamaiah, G. M. (Gattadahalli Manjunath), 1947– .
   QP552.P4P476   1994
   574.19'2456–dc20
                                                                93-36761
                                                                CIP

Printed on acid-free paper.   *Birkhäuser* ®

©1994 Birkhäuser Boston
Softcover reprint of the hardcover 1st edition 1994

Typeset by S. Lekowicz, Boston, MA

9 8 7 6 5 4 3 2 1

CONTENTS

Preface ix

Contributors x

1   K. M. Sivanandaiah: Twenty-Five Years of Peptide Research in
    Central College, Bangalore University, Bangalore, India
    V. V. Suresh Babu and M. N. Palgunachari 1

I PEPTIDE SYNTHESIS AND METHODOLOGY

2   Catalytic Transfer Hydrogenation and Hydrogenolysis by
    Formic Acid and Its Salts
    S. Rajagopal, M. K. Anwer, and A. F. Spatola 11

3   Syntheses of Natriuretic Peptides Using a New S-Protecting
    Group, S-Trimethylacetamidomethyl (Tacm) Group
    *Yoshiaki Kiso, Makoto Yoshida, Yoichi Fujiwara, Tooru Kimura,
    Kenichi Akaji, and Haruaki Yajima* 27

4   Solid-Phase Synthesis of Cyclic Peptides
    *Steven A. Kates, Núria A. Solé, Fernando Albericio,
    and George Barany* 39

5   Enzymatic Semisynthesis of Growth Hormone-Releasing
    Factor and Potent Analogs
    Jacob Bongers, Arthur M. Felix, and Edgar P. Heimer 59

6   Recent Developments in the Synthesis of Glycopeptides
    Horst Kunz 69

II PEPTIDE DESIGN AND APPLICATIONS

7   Synthesis, Characterizations, and Medical Applications
    of Bioelastic Materials
    D. Channe Gowda, Timothy M. Parker, R. Dean Harris,
    and Dan W. Urry 81

8   Synthetic Peptides in the Study of Viral Fusion,
    Inflammation, and Atherosclerosis
    Ewan M. Tytler, Jere P. Segrest, and G. M. Anantharamaiah 113

9   "De Novo" Engineering of Peptide Immunogenic and
    Antigenic Determinants as Potential Vaccines
    Pravin T. P. Kaumaya, Susan Kobs-Conrad, Ann M. DiGeorge,
    and Vernon C. Stevens 133

10 Complementary Peptides: Applications of the Molecular
    Recognition Theory to Peptide and Protein Purification
    and Design
    Michael A. Jarpe and J. Edwin Blalock 165

11 Conformational Studies on Model Peptides and
    Peptidomimetics
    Shashidhar N. Rao, K. Ramnarayan, and V. N. Balaji 181

III STUDIES OF PEPTIDE HORMONES

12 The Design and Synthesis of Long-Acting Oxytocin
    Antagonists Substituted in Positions 2, 7, and 8
    Victor J. Hruby, W. Y. Chan, Todd W. Rockway, Jan Hlavacek,
    and James Ormberg 199

13 Calcitonin: A Minireview
    Channa Basava 209

14 Importance of Ca^{2+}-Hormone Interaction in
    Conformation–Activity Correlations
    Vettai S. Ananthanarayanan 223

IV OTHER BIOLOGICALLY ACTIVE PEPTIDES

15   The Binding of Peptides and Proteins to Membranes
     Containing Anionic Lipid
          Marian Mosior and Richard M. Epand 237

16   Synthetic Peptides Mimic the Active Sites of Fibronectin
     Receptors from Gram-Positive Bacteria
          Sivashankarappa Gurusiddappa and Magnus Höök 251

17   Analyses of Various Folding Patterns of the HIV-1 Loop
          Goutam Gupta and Gerald Myers 259

18   Regulation of Human Immunodeficiency Virus Gene
     Expression by the Tat and Rev Proteins
          Shabbir A. Khan 279

Index 301

PREFACE

A successful scientific career requires constant effort on the part of the scientist. If such a career is to be achieved by scientists in developing countries where the facilities are not easily available, even more dedication is required. Dr. K. M. Sivanandaiah, having completed a successful career in the field of peptide chemistry, is such a scientist. Being well aware of the limited research facilities available in India, we are extraordinarily appreciative of Professor Sivanandaiah's dedication to the advancement of science. As a Professor of Chemistry and, until his retirement in 1992, the Head of the Department of Studies in Chemistry at Bangalore University, India, he not only devoted much of his time to his students, teaching basic organic chemistry, but was also able to contribute to the field of peptide chemistry.

After completing 25 years of service at Central College, Bangalore, where he was admired as an outstanding teacher, Professor Sivanandaiah is still active in research. He is now Professor Emeritus and continues to contribute to the field of peptides. As former students of Professor Sivanandaiah, we felt that publishing a book containing articles related to the design, synthesis, conformation, and biological activity of peptides and written by eminent scientists in the field of peptide research would be a fitting tribute to his role in the field of bioorganic chemistry.

We are pleased with the response from these outstanding scientists and are particularly grateful to the authors for providing current perspectives of their research for inclusion in this volume.

Channa Basava
G. M. Anantharamaiah
January 1994

CONTRIBUTORS

Kenichi Akaji, Department of Medicinal Chemistry, Kyoto Pharmaceutical University, Yamashina-ku, Kyoto 607, Japan

Fernando Albericio, Millipore Corporation, 75A Wiggins Avenue, Bedford, Massachusetts 01730, USA.

Vettai S. Ananthanarayanan, Department of Biochemistry, Health Sciences Center, McMaster University, 1200 Main Street West, Hamilton, Ontario, Canada L8N 3Z5

G. M. Anantharamaiah, Artherosclerosis Research Unit, Department of Medicine, The University of Alabama at Birmingham, University Station, DREB 640, Birmingham, Alabama 35924-0012, USA

Mohmed K. Anwer, Telios Pharmaceuticals Inc., San Diego, California 92121, USA

V. V. Suresh Babu, Department of Studies in Chemistry, Bangalore University, Bangalore 560001, India

V. N. Balaji, ImmunoPharmaceutics Inc., 11011 Via Frontera, San Diego, California 92127, USA

George Barany, Department of Chemistry, University of Minnesota, Minneapolis, Minnesota 55455, USA

Channa Basava, Novabiochem USA, 10394 Pacific Center Court, San Diego, California 92121, USA

J. Edwin Blalock, Department of Physiology and Biophysics, Center for Neuroimmunology, The University of Alabama at Birmingham, 896 Basic Health Sciences Building, 1918 University Boulevard, Birmingham, Alabama 35294-0005, USA

Jacob Bongers, Department of Peptide Research, Roche Research Center, 340 Kingsland Street, Nutley, New Jersey 07110, USA

W. Y. Chan, Department of Pharmacology, Cornell University Medical College, New York, New York 10021, USA

Ann M. DiGeorge, The Comprehensive Cancer Center, College of Medicine and Biological Sciences, The Ohio State University, 410 West 12th Avenue, Columbus, Ohio 43210, USA

Richard M. Epand, Department of Biochemistry, McMaster University, Health Sciences Centre, 1200 Main Street West, Hamilton, Ontario, Canada L8N 3Z5

Arthur M. Felix, Department of Peptide Research, Roche Research Center, 340 Kingsland Street, Nutley, New Jersey 07110, USA

Yoichi Fujiwara, Department of Medicinal Chemistry, Kyoto Pharmaceutical University, Yamashina-ku, Kyoto 607, Japan

D. Channe Gowda, Laboratory of Molecular Biophysics, The University of Alabama at Birmingham, VH300, Birmingham, Alabama 35294-0019, USA OR Bioelastics Research, Ltd., 1075 South 13th Street, Birmingham, Alabama 35205, USA

Goutam Gupta, Los Alamos National Laboratory, Biomedical Sciences Division, Los Alamos, New Mexico 87545, USA

Sivashankarappa Gurusiddappa, Institute of Biosciences and Technology, Center for Extracellular Matrix Biology, Texas A&M University, 2121 West Holcombe Boulevard, Houston, Texas 77030, USA

R. Dean Harris, Bioelastics Research, Ltd., 1075 South 13th Street, Birmingham, Alabama 35205, USA

Edgar P. Heimer, Department of Peptide Research, Roche Research Center, 340 Kingsland Street, Nutley, New Jersey 07110, USA

Jan Hlavacek, Department of Chemistry, University of Arizona, Tuscon, Arizona 85721, USA

Magnus Höök, Institute of Biosciences and Technology, Center for Extracellular Matrix Biology, Texas A&M University, 2121 West Holcombe Boulevard, Houston, Texas 77030, USA

Victor J. Hruby, Department of Chemistry, University of Arizona, Tucson, Arizona 85721, USA

Michael A. Jarpe, Department of Physiology and Biophysics, Center for Neuroimmunology, University of Alabama at Birmingham, 896 Basic Health Sciences Building, 1918 University Boulevard, Birmingham, Alabama 35294-0005, USA

Steven A. Kates, Millipore Corporation, 75A Wiggins Avenue, Bedford, Massachusetts 01730, USA

Pravin T. P. Kaumaya, The Comprehensive Cancer Center, Suite 302, College of Medicine and Biological Sciences, The Ohio State University, 410 West 12th Avenue, Columbus, Ohio 43210, USA

Shabbir A. Khan, The Wistar Institute, 3601 Spruce Street, Philadelphia, Pennsylvania 19104, USA

Tooru Kimura, Department of Medicinal Chemistry, Kyoto Pharmaceutical University, Yamashina-ku, Kyoto 607, Japan

Yoshiaki Kiso, Department of Medicinal Chemistry, Kyoto Pharmaceutical University, Yamashina-ku, Kyoto 607, Japan

Susan Kobs-Conrad, The Comprehensive Cancer Center, College of Medicine and Biological Sciences, The Ohio State University, 410 West 12th Avenue, Columbus, Ohio 43210, USA

Horst Kunz, Institut für Organische Chemie, Universität Mainz, Becherweg 18-20, D-55099 Mainz, Germany

Marian Mosior, Department of Chemistry, Indiana University, Bloomington, Indiana 47405-4001, USA

Gerald Myers, Los Alamos National Laboratory, Biomedical Sciences Division, Los Alamos, New Mexico, 87545 USA

James Ormberg, Department of Chemistry, University of Arizona, Tucson, Arizona 85721, USA

Mayakonda N. Palgunachari, Department of Medicine, Artherosclerosis Unit, University of Alabama at Birmingham Medical Center, 1808 7th Avenue South, DREB 630, Birmingham, Alabama 35294, USA

Timothy M. Parker, The University of Alabama at Birmingham, Laboratory of Molecular Biophysics, VH300, Birmingham, Alabama 35294-0019, USA

S. Rajagopal, Department of Chemistry, University of Louisville, Louisville, Kentucky 40292, USA

K. Ramnarayan, ImmunoPharmaceutics, Inc., 11011 Via Frontera, San Diego, California 92127, USA

Shashidhar N. Rao, Searle Research and Development, 4901 Searle Parkway, Skokie, Illinois 60077, USA

Todd W. Rockway, Department of Chemistry, University of Arizona, Tucson, Arizona 85721, USA

Jere P. Segrest, Arherosclerosis Research Unit, Department of Medicine, The University of Alabama at Birmingham, University Station, DREB 630, Birmingham, Alabama 35294-0012, USA

Núria A. Solé, Department of Chemistry, University of Minnesota, Minneapolis, Minnesota 55455, USA

A. F. Spatola, Peptide Research Laboratory, Department of Chemistry, University of Louisville, Louisville, Kentucky 40292, USA

Vernon C. Stevens, The Comprehensive Cancer Center, College of Medicine and Biological Sciences, The Ohio State University, 410 West 12th Avenue, Columbus, Ohio 43210, USA

Ewan M. Tytler, Atherosclerosis Research Unit, Department of Medicine, The University of Alabama at Birmingham, University Station, DREB 648, Birmingham, Alabama 35294-0012, USA

Dan W. Urry, Laboratory of Molecular Biophysics, The University of Alabama at Birmingham, VH300, Birmingham, Alabama 35294-0019, USA

Haruaki Yajima, Niigata College of Pharmacy, Niigata 950-21, Japan

Makoto Yoshida, Department of Medicinal Chemistry, Kyoto Pharmaceutical University, Yamashina-ku, Kyoto 607, Japan

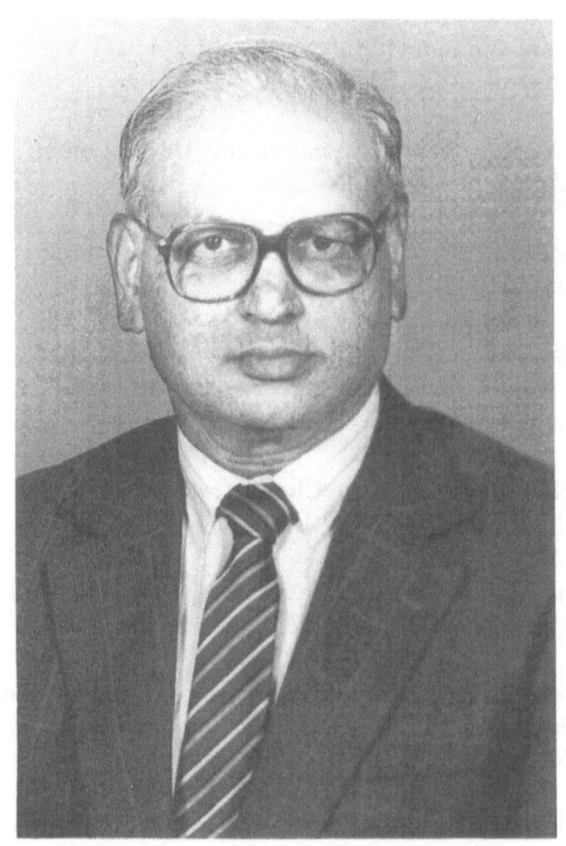

K. M. Sivanandaiah

1

K. M. SIVANANDAIAH: TWENTY-FIVE YEARS OF PEPTIDE RESEARCH IN CENTRAL COLLEGE, BANGALORE UNIVERSITY, BANGALORE, INDIA

V. V. Suresh Babu and M. N. Palgunachari

Scientific research in developing countries is, in general, considerably hampered by a lack of resources and infrastructure. These problems become far more acute if one decides to work in an area such as peptides, because a variety of amino acid derivatives, reagents, and chemicals are needed to synthesize them. The synthesized peptides must then be purified to homogeneity using chromatographic or other techniques and characterized by analytical and spectroscopic methods. Biological testing and physicochemical studies of synthetic peptides are also essential to correlate structure–activity relationships with the design of new analogs. While such resources are readily available in technologically advanced countries, conditions for research in countries like India are quite different. Many reagents and amino acid derivatives may have to be prepared in house because of limited funds or import restrictions. Further, it may be necessary to develop alternative, simplified methodologies to overcome the lack of modern instrumentation and techniques. Being well aware of these limitations, Professor K. M. Sivanandaiah took a bold step in initiating this field of research in Banga-

Peptides: Design, Synthesis, and Biological Activity
Channa Basava and G. M. Anantharamaiah, Editors
©1994 *Birkhäuser Boston*

lore, India, in 1967. He successfully turned these challenges into opportunities, and discovered a number of simple techniques for peptide synthesis adaptable to any laboratory.

Professor Sivanandaiah received his Ph.D degree in 1961 for his research in the area of steroid synthesis (Banerjee and Sivanandaiah, 1960, 1961a, 1961b). He continued work in this area for 2 more years (1961–1963) as a postdoctoral fellow at Clark University, Worcester, Massachusetts, in the United States (Sivanandaiah and Nes, 1965). In 1963, he was invited to join the laboratories of Dr. F. M. Bumpus at Cleveland Clinic Foundation, Cleveland, Ohio, and to carry out research in the area of angiotensin analogs. During his tenure at Cleveland Clinic, he synthesized analogs of angiotensin using the solution-phase method of peptide synthesis (Sivanandaiah et al., 1966). During this period he also conducted some preliminary experiments in the newly emerging field of solid-phase synthesis.

After his return to India, Professor Sivanandaiah joined the faculty of the newly created Bangalore University and decided to establish a center for the study of peptide chemistry and biology. When this research was initiated in Central College, Bangalore, in 1967, he found himself to be all alone in the vast country of India with virtually no one with whom he could interact and with only one or two L-amino acids available at the College. He had to build this area of research from scratch. It was not always easy to import chemicals from more advanced countries because of the tight foreign exchange regulations in existence at that time. With these conditions as a background, he began work in this research area.

At the beginning, he continued to synthesize analogs of angiotensin II by the solution-phase method (Khan and Sivanandaiah, 1971). As might be expected, initial synthesis of the first biologically active analog was slow. The next couple of years were fruitful, and included the synthesis of biologically active peptides such as those related to fibrinopeptide A (the 15-peptide active site sequence of triose phosphate isomerase), fibrinopeptide B of the green monkey, and physalamien (Anantharamaiah and Sivanandaiah, 1974; Baligidad and Sivanandaiah, 1974; Channabasabaiah and Sivanandaiah, 1973, 1975, 1976; Khan and Sivanandaiah, 1972).

By this time, the solid-phase method of peptide synthesis (Merrifield, 1963; Stewart and Young, 1969) was increasingly coming into usage all over the world, and this naturally prompted Dr. Sivanandaiah to use this approach. However, the basic hurdle was the cost involved. The method as practiced elsewhere required using an excess of amino acids [as much as 6 equivalents (equiv)] at each stage of coupling in a multistep synthesis; compared to the solution-phase method, the cost was exorbitant. Funding for such an expensive exercise, in which 5 equiv of amino acids was wasted, was simply not available in India. About this time, Konig and Geiger (1973) introduced 1-hydroxybenzotriazole (HOBt); this accelerated the moderately reactive amino acid active ester. The significance of this reaction was that this enhanced reactivity could also be observed on the solid phase, permitting recovery of the excess protected active esters of amino acids used at each stage of peptide synthesis. The very first biologically active peptide synthesized in Central College using active esters throughout the synthesis was oxytocin (Khan and Sivanandaiah, 1976a). This peptide was selected because the biological activity was standardized and thus the identity of the synthesized peptide could be readily established. Subsequently, [desamino]oxytocin and [Thr^4]oxytocin were also synthesized (Khan and Sivanandaiah, 1978a).

Although the synthesis of peptides by stepwise elongation in solid-phase peptide synthesis was very common, fragment condensation was only rarely practiced in solid phase. The largest peptide synthesized in this laboratory was an analog of adrenocorticotropic hormone. [β-Ala^1,Glu^5,Lys^{17,18}]ACTH (1–18)NH$_2$ was synthesized by fragment condensation in the solid phase, thus reducing the presence of truncated peptides in the final product. This peptide was as potent as the naturally occurring ACTH, a 39-peptide chain. Another feature of this synthesis was that some of the bifunctional amino acids such as Arg were used without side-chain protection (Anantharamaiah and Sivanandaiah, 1978). In recent years, 9-fluorenylmethoxy carbonyl (Fmoc) amino acid active esters have been used almost exclusively because the Fmoc group can be cleaved by a mild base treatment.

Many biologically active peptides were studied by Sivanandaiah and his co-workers to determine their structure–activity relationships (Sivanandaiah and Rangaraju, 1986; Sivanandaiah et al., 1985, 1988a, 1988b, 1991a). Noteworthy among these studies was the observation that [Thr^7]dermorphin has pronounced opiate agonistic activity, being nearly twice as potent as dermorphin in the guinea pig ileum assay. This peptide is one of the most potent dermorphin analogs reported to date (Sivanandaiah et al., 1989a, 1989b).

Development of Methods for Peptide Synthesis

Catalytic Transfer Hydrogenation

As mentioned earlier, in this laboratory virtually all the starting protected amino acid derivatives are made by the students themselves. Efforts are constantly being made to improve existing methodology. While it is frustrating to find that some of the common reagents required for peptide synthesis are not available, at times this spurs the development of alternative methodologies. One such experience during the deprotection of the nitro group present in an Arg-containing peptide stimulated the discovery that catalytic transfer hydrogenation can be advantageously used in the synthesis of peptides. Deprotection of the nitro group from peptide Boc-Phe-Arg(NO2)-Trp-Gly, an intermediate required for the synthesis of an ACTH analog, did not go to completion even with prolonged hydrogenation. This nagging difficulty, which is usually faced by a peptide chemist when removal of the protecting groups is incomplete in the final step after a careful assembly of the required peptide sequence, was solved by the application of catalytic transfer hydrogenation to peptide synthesis. Review of the literature revealed that cyclohexene can be used to cleave a nitro group from dinitrobenzene. This was appealing, but the reagent cyclohexene was not available because chemical suppliers such as Sigma and Aldrich do not exist in India. Such limitations are not a problem for a good organic chemistry laboratory, however; Dr. Sivanandaiah and his student Anantharamaiah prepared the required cyclohexene by the sulfuric acid-mediated dehydration of cyclohexanol, purified it for use in peptide synthesis, and used it successfully in the deprotection of the nitro group from the intermediate. This procedure marked the beginning of catalytic transfer hydrogenation in peptide synthesis (Anantharamaiah and Sivanandaiah, 1977).

Although deprotection of almost all benzyl-based protection groups could be achieved, including cleavage of the peptide from the peptide resin (Khan and Sivanandaiah, 1978b), this method suffered from two limitations: (1) the reaction had to be carried out at the boiling point of cyclohexene (80°C), which is not suitable for many biologically active peptides, and (2) many peptides are not soluble in cyclohexene or the resulting by-products of disproportionation of cyclohexene (benzene and cyclohexane). Felix and co-workers (1978) from Hoffman–La Roche were able to solve the first problem by using cyclohexadiene as a hydrogen donor that can undergo disproportionation reaction at room temperature.

Cyclohexene and cyclohexadiene, in the presence of catalysts, are converted into benzene and toluene in the disproportionation reaction. Introduction to this reaction mixture of a compound to be reduced yields the product. However, for peptide synthesis neither the starting materials nor the products are good solvents for peptides. Being thus well aware of the shortcomings of cyclohexene and cyclohexadiene as hydrogen donors in catalytic transfer hydrogenation, Sivanandaiah and co-workers continued their investigations to improve the method and thus introduced formic acid as a hydrogen donor (Sivanandaiah and Gurusiddappa, 1979). In addition to solving the problems inherent in using cyclohexene as the hydrogen donor, introduction of formic acid enabled the refinement of this method in other laboratories as well as that of Dr. Sivanandaiah (Allen et al., 1992; Anwer and Spatola, 1980; Anwer et al., 1978; Elamin et al., 1979; Kumari et al., 1979; Overman and Sugai, 1985; Ram and Spicer, 1987; Sivanandaiah and Rangaraju, 1986). Because it involves mild reaction conditions, easy accessibility of needed reagents, and facile removal of the protecting groups, this technique is now used by peptide chemists to synthesize not only oligopeptides and unusual amino acid derivatives (Anantharamaiah and Roeske, 1981; Anantharamaiah et al., 1985) but also glycopeptides (Ekborg et al., 1987). Some of these investigations have been reviewed by Johnstone and Wilby (1985).

Active Esters in Solid-Phase Peptide Synthesis

Active esters have several advantages as coupling agents in peptide synthesis. They can be readily prepared, purified, and stored, but their usefulness in solid-phase peptide synthesis was limited by their moderate reactivity. Khan and Sivanandaiah (1976b) largely solved this problem, however, by the addition of HOBt during active ester coupling on the solid phase, which provides considerable acceleration in the coupling rate. Oxytocin was thus synthesized on solid phase by employing Boc-amino acid 2,4,5-trichlorophenyl esters. One equivalent of HOBt provided completion of coupling within 60–80 min, with the exception of Boc-iLeu-OPCP (pentachlorophenyl ester), which required 210 min. Further, because of the high degree of coupling efficiency 3 equiv of active ester suffices, compared to the usual practice of adding 3–6 equiv when using the N,N'-dicyclohexylcarbodiimide (DCC) method of coupling of protected amino acids. Incidentally, this was the first synthesis of a biologically active peptide using the solid-phase method in India.

During these investigations, it also became apparent that toluene can also serve as a satisfactory medium for these syntheses (Khan and Sivanandaiah, 1976b). While these may appear to be only moderate improvements, the yield and purity of biologically active peptides synthesized is very significant. Use of Fmoc-amino acid active esters on the solid support resulted in a dramatic improvement in the overall yield of protected oxytoceine to 70% (Sivanandaiah and Gurusiddappa, 1981, 1982).

The use of minimal side-chain protection using the active esters in the solid-phase method of peptide synthesis was demonstrated by the synthesis of LH–RH analogs (Sivanandaiah et al., 1989c). The utility of this approach was also demonstrated by the synthesis of the acyl carrier protein 65–74 sequence, Val-Glu-Ala-Ala-Ala-Asp-Tyr-Ala-Asp-Gly, which is known to pose several difficulties in its chemical synthesis (Sivanandaiah et al., 1991b). It may be recalled here that assembly of the same molecule using either Fmoc-amino acid-p-nitrophenyl or N-hydroxysuccinimide esters has been reported to be unsuccessful.

Acid Chlorides as Coupling Agents

The use of acid chlorides in peptide synthesis had long been considered obsolete because of various side reactions. In recent years, optically pure, shelf-stable Fmoc-amino acid chlorides have been prepared and used successfully for peptide bond formation. Carpino and co-workers (1986, 1991) have employed them in the solution-phase as well as the solid-phase method for synthesis of [Leu]enkephalin, peptides related to tachykinin, and other peptides.

Acid chlorides significantly enhance the rate of acylation reactions leading to rapid incorporation of the amino acid moiety. An amine such as triethylamine or diethylisopropylamine is necessary for acylation, because no reaction takes place in its absence. In solid-phase peptide synthesis, however, coupling with Fmoc-amino acid chloride/base does not go to completion even after a prolonged reaction period unless a catalyst such as HOBt or pivalic acid is also present. Thus, the solid-phase synthesis of [Leu]enkephalin, dermorphin, and deltotrophin have been accomplished using the conventional Merrifield or Wang resins (Sivanandaiah et al., 1992a, 1993).

It has been demonstrated in this laboratory that condensations involving Fmoc-amino acid chlorides can be conveniently carried out in the presence of the potassium salt of HOBt (KOBt); no additional base is needed (Sivanandaiah et al., 1992b). Further, for solution-phase synthesis an organic solvent can be used instead of the biphasic solvent system, and the coupling is free from racemization. Employing this methodology (Fmoc-amino acid chloride/KOBt), many peptides such as [Leu]enkephalin and cyclosporin A fragments have been synthesized (Sivanandaiah et al., personal communication). This method is also suited for solid-phase synthesis, as is demonstrated by the synthesis of peptides such as β-casomorphin (Sivanandaiah et al., in manuscript).

To avoid acidolysis and the occurrence of impurities, the reagent trichloroiodosilane has been used for deprotection of Boc groups. Although these investigations must be elaborated and compared to the existing methodologies for advantages and disadvantages, preliminary studies have shown that this reagent can be used successfully for solution-phase as well as solid-phase peptide synthesis (Sivanandaiah and Palgunachari, unpublished data).

As mentioned, improvements in the methods appear simple but have significantly enhanced the rate of synthesis of biologically active peptides. Despite scarcity of resources for his research, Professor Sivanandaiah has been able to publish quite extensively; many of his publications have appeared in international journals. As evidenced by the wide use of the catalytic transfer hydrogenation technique in many laboratories around the world, his methodology development has often been used successfully. More than 10 students have obtained their Ph.D under his guidance. It is noteworthy that many of his students are established in a number of laboratories in the United States. Professor Sivanandaiah believes that a new student learning the techniques of peptide synthesis should first be exposed to the solution-phase method. This belief has allowed his students to obtain an outstanding training in peptide synthesis techniques. Their success abroad can be attributed mainly to the complete understanding of peptide synthesis methodology they obtained at Central College in Bangalore, India.

It is important to recognize that in addition to a successful research career, Dr. Sivanandaiah was also very much appreciated for his teaching ability. Indeed, it was his ability to teach students at the Master's level that attracted students to continue to learn under his guidance. Thus, he had a constant supply of students eager to work with him toward their Ph.D programs. In addition, he served as the Principal of Central College and as Head of the Department of Studies in Chemistry at Bangalore University. In spite of his administrative responsibilities, he was constantly in touch with research and with his students.

Acknowledgments

A felicitation was arranged by his students and colleagues to show appreciation of Professor Sivanandaiah's services to the Institution and its students. We take this opportunity to thank Professor M. Shadaksharaswamy, President of the Felicitation Committee, and the Committee members, for their unstinting efforts in organizing this function.

Dr. Sivanandaiah's research was supported financially by the Department of Science and Technology, Government of India, New Delhi.

REFERENCES

Allen MS, Skolniek P, Cook JM (1992): *J Med Chem* 35:368.
Anwer MK, Spatola AF (1980): *Synthesis* 929.
Anwer MK, Khan SA, Sivanandaiah KM (1978): *Synthesis* 10:751.
Anantharamaiah GM, Roeske RW (1981): In P*eptides, Chemistry and Biology,* Proceedings of the 9th American Peptide Symposium. Pierce Chemical Co., Rockford, IL
Anantharamaiah GM, Sivanandaiah KM (1974): *Int J Pept Protein Res* 6:51.
Anantharamaiah GM, Sivanandaiah KM (1977): *J Chem Soc Perkins Trans I* 490
Anantharamaiah GM, Sivanandaiah KM (1978): *Indian J Chem* 168:797.
Anantharamaiah GM, Jones JL, Brouillette CG, Schmidt CF, Chung BH, Bhown AS, Segrest JP (1985): *J Biol Chem* 260:10248-10253.
Baligidad SK, Sivanandaiah KM (1974): *Curr Sci (Bangalore)* 43:373.
Banerjee DK, Sivanandaiah KM (1960): *Tetrahedron Lett* 5:20.
Banerjee DK, Sivanandaiah KM (1961a): *J Org Chem* 26:1634.

Banerjee DK, Sivanandaiah KM (1961b): *J Indian Chem Soc* 38:652.

Carpino LA, Chao HG, Beyermann M, Bienert M (1991): *J Org Chem* 56:2635.

Carpino LA, Cohen BJ, Stephens KE, Sadat Aalaee SY, Tien J-H, Langridge DC 1986): *J Org Chem* 51:3732.

Channabasabaiah K, Sivanandaiah KM (1973): *Indian J Chem* 11:641.

Channabasabaiah K, Sivanandaiah KM (1975): *Int J Pept Protein Res* 7:281.

Channabasabaiah K, Sivanandaiah KM (1976): *Int J Pept Protein Res* 8:323.

Ekborg G, Klinger M, Roden L, Anantharamaiah GM (1987): *Glycoconjugate* 4:255-266.

Elamin B, Anantharamaiah GM, Royer GP, Means GE (1979): *J Org Chem* 44:3442.

Felix AM, Heimer EP, Lambros TJ, Tzougraki C, Meinhofer J (1978): *J Org Chem* 43:4196.

Johnstone RAW, Wilby AH (1985): *Chem Rev* 85:129.

Khan SA, Sivanandaiah KM (1971): *Indian J Chem* 9:1984.

Khan SA, Sivanandaiah KM (1972): *Indian J Chem* 10:382.

Khan SA, Sivanandaiah KM (1976a): *Tetrahedron Lett* 3:199.

Khan SA, Sivanandaiah KM (1976b): *Synthesis* 9:614.

Khan SA, Sivanandaiah KM (1978a): *Int J Pept Protein Res* 12:164.

Khan SA, Sivanandaiah KM (1978b): *Synthesis* 10:750.

Konig W, Geiger R (1973): *Chem Ber* 106:3626.

Kumari NSS, Khan SA, Sivanandaiah KM (1979): *Indian J Chem* 17B:152.

Merrifield RB (1963): *J Am Chem Soc* 85:2149.

Overman LE, Sugai S (1985): *Helv Chim Acta* 681:745.

Ram S, Spicer LD (1987): *Tetrahedron Lett* 28:515.

Sivanandaiah KM, Gurusiddappa S (1979): *Indian J Chem Res* 108

Sivanandaiah KM, Gurusiddappa S (1981): *Synthesis* 7:565.

Sivanandaiah KM, Gurusiddappa S (1982): *Indian J Chem* 21B:139.

Sivanandaiah KM, Nes WR (1965): *Steroids* 539

Sivanandaiah KM, Rangaraju NS (1986): *Indian J Chem* 168:797.

Sivanandaiah KM, Smeby RR, Bumpus FM (1966): *Biochemistry* 5:1224.

Sivanandaiah KM, Gurusiddappa S, Rangaraju NS (1985): *J Biosci (Bangalore)* 8:263.

Sivanandaiah KM, Gurusiddappa S, Gowda DC (1988a): *J Biosci (Bangalore)* 13:181.

Sivanandaiah KM, Gurusiddappa S, Babu VVS (1988b): *Indian J Chem* 278:645.

Sivanandaiah KM, Gurusiddappa S, Babu VVS (1989a): *Int J Pept Protein Res* 33:463.

Sivanandaiah KM, Gurusiddappa S, Babu VVS (1989b): *Indian J Chem* 288:338.

Sivanandaiah KM, Gurusiddappa S, Channegowda D, Babu VVS (1989c): *J Biosci (Bangalore)* 14:311.

Sivanandaiah KM, Gurusiddappa S, Palgunachari (1991a): *Indian J Chem* 308:201.

Sivanandaiah KM, Gurusiddappa S, Babu VVS (1991b): *Indian J Chem* 30B:302.

Sivanandaiah KM, Babu VVS, Renukeshwar HC (1992a): *Int J Pept Protein Res* 39:201.

Sivanandaiah KM, Babu VVS, Shankaramma SC (1992b): *Indian J Chem* 31B:379.

Sivanandaiah KM, Babu VVS, Renukeshwar HC, Gangadhar BP (1993): *Indian J Chem* 32B:465.

Sivanandaiah KM, Babu VVS, Gangadhar BP: (in manuscript).

Stewart JM, Young JD (1969): *Solid Phase Peptide Synthesis*. San Francisco: Freeman.

I

PEPTIDE SYNTHESIS AND METHODOLOGY

2

CATALYTIC TRANSFER HYDROGENATION AND HYDROGENOLYSIS BY FORMIC ACID AND ITS SALTS

S. Rajagopal, M. K. Anwer, and A. F. Spatola

Introduction

Catalytic transfer hydrogenation and related reactions are widely employed in organic chemistry. Although numerous laboratories have contributed to the success of this procedure, much of its success can be attributed to pioneering work by Professor K. M. Sivanandaiah, his former students, and his associates.

Transfer hydrogenation catalyzed by both homogeneous and heterogeneous catalysts has been reviewed extensively (Brieger and Nestrick, 1974; Johnstone et al., 1985; Ram and Ehrenkaufer, 1988; Zassinovich et al., 1992). Catalytic reduction can broadly be divided into (i) hydrogenation (addition of hydrogen to unsaturated groups such as olefins) and (ii) hydrogenolysis (addition of hydrogen across single bonds leading to cleavage of functional groups, e.g., $PhCH_2OR$ to $PhCH_3 + ROH$). Hydrodehalogenation (a typical substitution reaction) is closely related to hydrogenolysis; here, the carbon-bound halogen is replaced by hydrogen. This chapter emphasizes the importance of formic acid and its salts as hydrogen donors for the catalytic reduction of various functional groups. A plausible mechanism of transfer hydrogenation/hydrogenolysis is also proposed.

Peptides: Design, Synthesis, and Biological Activity
Channa Basava and G. M. Anantharamaiah, Editors
©1994 *Birkhäuser Boston*

Transfer Hydrogenation Reaction

Hydrogenation is traditionally performed using molecular hydrogen in the presence of a catalyst. The catalyst is usually a transition metal such as palladium, which is employed in either a bulk or supported form. Transfer hydrogenation employs a compound that contains active hydrogens (hydrogen donor) instead of molecular hydrogen. In contrast to conventional hydrogenation, catalytic transfer hydrogenation possesses several advantages: (1) the reaction conditions are mild; (2) the procedure employs simple apparatus such as an open flask instead of high-pressure vessels; and (3) the nature of the hydrogen donor also influences the selectivity and activity of reduction.

The transfer hydrogenation reaction can be generalized as follows:

$$DH_2 + A \rightarrow AH_2 + D \tag{1}$$

where DH_2 = hydrogen donor and A = hydrogen acceptor.

The nature of the hydrogen donors, substrates (hydrogen acceptors), catalysts, and reaction variables encountered in catalytic transfer hydrogenation are described next.

Hydrogen Donors

Virtually any compound (organic or inorganic) with a low oxidation potential can serve as a useful hydrogen donor; the low oxidation potential enables the transfer of hydrogen(s) from the donor to the substrate under mild reaction conditions. The choice of donor is based on the nature of the reaction, its availability, and solubility in the reaction medium. Alcohols, hydrazine, cyclic olefins, and hydroaromatics have been employed as hydrogen donors for the transfer hydrogenation of various functional groups. Formic acid and its salts occupy a special place as hydrogen donors because the ease of hydrogen donation is higher than with the donors listed above. This results from the fact that a stable molecule such as CO_2, which has a very large negative enthalpy of formation ($\Delta H°_{f,298} = -393.51$ kJ/mol), is released from the hydrogen donor during the transfer hydrogenation reaction. Simply stated, the hydrogen donation is irreversible. This is one of the major driving forces for the high reactivity of formates.

Useful hydrogen donors have a common property: the stability of their dehydrogenation product prevents the reverse reaction (formation of the donor). For instance, CO_2, N_2, and benzene, which are the dehydrogenated products of ammonium formate, hydrazine, and cyclohexadiene, respectively, are among the most stable compounds known.

Recent studies have demonstrated that formate salts are superior to formic acid as hydrogen donors. For example, Anwer and Spatola (1980) first reported that numerous benzyl-protecting groups are rapidly and efficiently cleaved using ammonium formate-catalytic transfer hydrogenation (AF-CTH). Under similar conditions, the rate of debenzylation is negligible in HCOOH. Wiener et al. (1991) also observed that potassium formate is better than formic acid as a donor for nitrotoluene reduction.

The formate salts can be classified into two categories based on the source of H^+ that is needed to complete the reduction process: (i) salts of alkali metals (or possibly any metal), and (ii) salts of NH_3 or organic bases such as Et_3N, piperidine. In the case of metal formates, the H^+ is derived from the solvent (usually water or alcohol); in the latter instance, the conjugate acid (NH_4^+ or $NHEt_3^+$) serves as the H^+ source. The parent, formic acid, can be classified in the second set.

In contrast to formic acid, ammonium formate ($HCOONH_4$) and triethylammonium formate ($HCOONHEt_3$) are preferred as hydrogen donors for hydrogenation and hydrogenolysis reactions because they can furnish $HCOO^-$ ion to the Pd surface to undergo activation and dissociative chemisorption generating H^- and CO_2. In addition to this essential feature, the H^+ required to complete the hydrogenolysis reaction is readily and more efficiently supplied by NH_4^+ or $NHEt_3^+$ at virtual neutral conditions.

By the same token, alkali metal formate salts are not recommended for hydrogenation or hydrogenolysis reactions (e.g., C–O, C–N, and C–S bonds). These reactions require two hydrogen atoms; one comes from formate (H^-) and the other from water or alcohol (H^+). As a consequence, hydroxide or alkoxide, generated during the reaction, combines with CO_2 to form a bicarbonate. The bicarbonate might increase the basicity of the medium and also reduce the activity by physically blocking the catalytic sites because the solubility of these bicarbonates is generally low in common organic solvents. However, for reactions such as hydrodechlorination, all formate salts behave alike because proton addition is not essential. The hydride formed from formate displaces halide ion leading to the formation of a salt (e.g., NaCl, NH_4Cl). It should be mentioned that formic acid under these conditions generates HX (X = halogen), which has a dramatic negative influence on the overall reaction.

As previously stated, the nature of the hydrogen donor influences the selectivity and activity of the reduction. This additional flexibility can be illustrated with an aromatic substrate possessing nitro and halo functionalities. While the palladium coupled with a formate salt is a remarkably effective reagent to remove halogens from an aromatic nucleus and to reduce a nitro function to an amino group, the same catalyst with phosphinic acid as hydrogen donor can reduce the nitro group without affecting halogen (Entwistle et al., 1977).

Hydrogen Acceptors

Practically any organic compound that can be hydrogenated can be transfer hydrogenated using a suitable hydrogen donor and a catalyst. This representative list consists of alkenes, dienes, alkynes, aldehydes, ketones, and
compounds containing nitro, halo, benzylic, and allylic functions.

Catalysts

Both homogeneous and heterogeneous catalysts have been employed for
transfer hydrogenation reactions. The homogeneous catalysts are more
selective and active under moderate reaction conditions. In other words,
the turnover number (TON) is higher as the entire metal ions are available
for catalytic activity. Heterogeneous catalysts, on the other hand, are less
selective and not all the catalytic material participates in the reaction. In
spite of this, the ease of separation of the catalyst from the reaction products favors the use of heterogeneous catalysts. However, homogeneous catalysts are preferred for reactions such as asymmetric hydrogenation or
transfer hydrogenation.

Homogeneous Catalysts

Most homogeneous hydrogenation catalysts are soluble complexes of
platinum metals. Those which are active for hydrogenation are equally active for transfer hydrogenation. Literature abounds with the applications
of $RuCl_2(PPh_3)_3$, $RhCl(PPh_3)_3$, $PdCl_2(PPh_3)_2$, and $IrCl(PPh_3)_3$. As most of
these complexes are insoluble in water, these reactions are carried out in
nonaqueous media. Metal complexes having water-soluble ligands (m-
sulphophenylbiphenylphosphine, for example) have been designed for reactions that demand an aqueous or a biphasic medium. The homogeneous
catalysts are often anchored to an insoluble polymer to surmount the product isolation difficulty while retaining the advantages of homogeneous catalysts.

Heterogeneous Catalysts

Heterogeneous hydrogenation catalysts, similar to their homogeneous
counterparts, are transition metal elements but in their zero oxidation state.
Sometimes, the catalyst is used in the bulk form, for example, Raney nickel.
While this is possible in the case of base metals, the use of platinum metals
in the bulk form is not cost effective. For this reason, supported catalysts
are preferred because they are economical and are also more efficient on a
metal weight basis as they increase the availability of metal atoms for the
catalysis. Catalyst supports commonly employed are activated carbon, alu-
mina, silica, amorphous silica-aluminas, zeolites, $BaSO_4$, and $CaCO_3$. The

crystallite size and hence dispersion of the supported metal depends on the method of preparation and subsequent treatments. For 10% Pd/C, the Pd crystallite size is estimated to be 3.5–5 nm (Pope et al., 1971).

Activated carbon is the most widely used catalyst carrier for liquid-phase hydrogenation reactions. This preference is for the following reasons: (1) activated carbon can be synthesized with high purity and possesses large surface areas (≈ 1000 m²/g); (2) the metal support interaction is the least among the various common catalyst carriers and thus the electronic properties of the active material are not modified; and (3) activated carbon, being a good adsorbent for organic compounds, can facilitate the reaction by aiding the migration of the adsorbate to the active sites of the catalyst.

Although palladium is an excellent metal of choice for most of the common reactions, platinum, ruthenium, and rhodium are useful complementary candidates when selectivity is crucial. For instance, a ruthenium complex can be used to selectively transfer hydrogenate the carbonyl group to a carbinol in α,β-unsaturated carbonyl compounds (Khai and Arcelli, 1985), while Pd/C is used to selectively reduce the C=C double bond (Cortese and Heck, 1978). Similarly, in halonitro aromatics, Pt/C can be employed to reduce nitro groups without eliminating halogen functionality while Pd/C may be utilized to remove halogens with simultaneous reduction of nitro groups to amines (Cortese and Heck, 1977).

Reaction Conditions

Since most transfer hydrogenation reactions are performed at room temperature and atmospheric pressure, they are simple to accomplish. The most common solvents for these reactions are alcohols, particularly methyl or ethyl alcohol. Dimethylformamide and dimethylacetamide are useful for reactants that are less soluble in alcoholic solvents. Acetic acid is very effective as a solvent medium when acidic conditions are demanded.

The efficiency of heterogeneously catalyzed reactions is influenced by the rate of mixing. Increased mixing improves the contact between the catalyst and the reactants and therefore has a beneficial effect on the reaction rate. Surfactants have been used to effect transfer hydrogenation under phase-transfer conditions. In addition to the familiar process parameters such as temperature and pressure, ultrasound is found to promote the Pd-catalyzed reduction of olefins using HCOOH in alcohols (Boudjouk and Han, 1984).

Reactions Involving Various Functional Groups

The list of reactions that can be accomplished by transfer hydrogenation or hydrogenolysis is proliferating at a remarkable pace. In all cases, the advantages of transfer hydrogenation over conventional hydrogenation are obvious.

Halo Compounds

Because a halogen atom is often introduced to mask the reactivity at a given position, hydrodehalogenation is an important reaction in complex organic synthesis. The ease of removal of halogen from organic compounds decreases with the increase in electronegativity: I > Br > Cl > F. Also, the carbon–halogen bond strength follows the same order: 53, 67, 81, and 108 kcal/mol (Pinder, 1980). The order of reactivity is also determined by the nature of the hydrocarbon segment bearing the halogen and follows the order: benzyl, allylic >> aryl, vinyl, acyl > alkyl (Kieboom and van Rantwijk, 1977).

Whether the hydrodehalogenation is a substitution (nucleophilic displacement by the hydride ion) or hydrogenolysis reaction may depend on the type of hydrogen donor used. If the hydrogen donor is an alkali metal formate or ammonium formate, then the reaction pathway is probably of the substitution type, that is, Cl⁻ is replaced by H⁻. Other donors such as cyclohexene seem to favor the hydrogenolysis route. Partial evidence to support this claim comes from the fact that HX is formed during these reactions.

Hydrogen donors such as HCOOH are not suitable for dehalogenation unless a base is included in the reaction medium to scavenge the liberated HX. In the absence of a base, the initially formed HX suppresses the formic acid dissociation, resulting in the depletion of formate ion concentration. The formate ion is critical for the reaction to proceed.

Recently, HCOOH has been successfully utilized for dechlorination of several chloro compounds in boiling dimethylformamide (Pandey and Purkayastha, 1982). The removal of HCl at the reaction temperature of 153°C or the likely presence of dimethylammonium formate (formed from dimethylamine, a decomposition product of DMF) may have contributed to this success. In another example, HCOOH in DMF and Pd/C were successfully used for hydrodechlorination at 50–60°C; here, the substrate had two amine functionalities which served as scavengers for HCl (Mitsui, 1985).

Ammonium formate and Pd/C combination is an effective system for the dechlorination of aromatic chlorides. Anwer and Spatola (1985) used this reagent for 2,4,6-trichlorophenol and polychlorobiphenyls and achieved complete conversion in 4 minutes. This was followed by a detailed study that examined the effect of solvents, temperature, donor concentration, and catalyst support on the dechlorination reaction (Anwer et al., 1989). Debromination of aryl bromides has also been achieved using HCOONa in the presence of $Pd(PPh_3)_4$ at 100°C in DMF (Helquist, 1978) or $CH_3CN:DMSO$ (Pri-Bar and Buchman, 1986).

Nitro Compounds

Davies and Hodgson (1943) used copper to catalyze the transfer hydrogenation of nitrobenzene in the presence of HCOOH at 200°C. In contrast to this, in liquid-phase, aromatic nitro compounds are reduced with ammonium formate or triethylammonium formate in the presence of Pd/C at ambient conditions. Further, these studies suggest that the vapor- and liquid-phase hydrogenation reactions may be occurring via different mechanistic pathways.

A facile liquid-phase reduction of nitro compounds with HCOOH/Et$_3$N in the presence of Pd/C was reported by Cortese and Heck (1977). They mentioned that PhNO$_2$ did not undergo reduction in the presence of HCOOH. This observation is surprising in the context of literature reports. Our inference is that the order of addition of reagents may also play an important role. In this particular case, formic acid was added at the end, preventing the activation of the catalyst; thus, not a trace of aniline was formed to initiate autocatalysis. The formation of aniline would result in an increase in the formation of HCOO$^-$ ions, which demand very low activation energy for dissociation into H$^-$ and CO$_2$, thus propagating the reaction. Unlike dehalogenation of haloaromatics where the HCOOH liberates H$^+$ ions (HCl), nitrobenzene yields aniline, CO$_2$, and H$_2$O as products according to the equation:

$$Ar-NO_2 + 3HCOOH \rightarrow Ar-NH_2 + 3CO_2 + 2H_2O \qquad (2)$$

Therefore, one should not be tempted to conclude that formic acid is a poor hydrogen donor for nitro compounds.

Entwistle and co-workers (1977) have used formic acid as a hydrogen donor and 10% Pd/C as the catalyst for the reduction of 1,3-dinitrobenzene to 1,3-diaminobenzene. They reported that the reaction ceased immediately on addition of either HCl or chlorobenzene. The authors interpreted these results by proposing that the chloride ion present in HCl poisons the catalyst. From our experience, we concluded that the proton, not the chloride, is the culprit in these reactions. As mentioned earlier, H$^+$ ion prevents the dissociation of formic acid, thus suppressing the activation of the donor completely.

Partial reduction of dinitro compounds has been achieved by catalytic transfer hydrogenation using Pd/C and triethylammonium formate (Terpko and Heck, 1980). This particular system hydrogenated the less hindered *para*-nitro group in 2,4-dinitrotoluene to 2-nitro-4-aminotoluene (yield, 92%). However, the reduction of the more hindered *ortho*-nitro group in the following compounds was modest: 2,4-dinitrophenol (57%), 2,4-dinitroanisole (24%), 2,4-dinitroaniline (49%), and 2,4-dinitroacetanilide (56%).

Other formate salts such as alkali metal formates are also useful but result in the formation of bicarbonate. Water-soluble organic nitro compounds (e.g., disodium salt of $3,6,8,1\text{-}(HO_3S)_3C_{10}H_4NO_2$) were reduced to the corresponding amines in aqueous HCOOH or its salts in the presence of Pd/C (Bamfield et al., 1976).

Reductive cyclization of 2-nitro-β-nitrostyrene to indole is achieved using ammonium formate and 10% Pd/C in fair yields (60%) (Rajeswari et al., 1989). Barrett and Spilling (1988) demonstrated that the aliphatic nitro group can be reduced to the amine function with retention of configuration. Ram and Ehrenkaufer (1986) synthesized amino acid derivatives from α-nitro esters using ammonium formate and Pd/C at room temperature. They also described the transfer hydrogenation of a wide variety of both aliphatic and aromatic nitro compounds using ammonium formate at room temperature with conversions ranging from 31% to 98% (Ram and Ehrenkaufer, 1984).

O-Benzyl Compounds

Benzyl alcohol and its derivatives undergo ready hydrogenolysis under catalytic transfer hydrogenation conditions, especially with palladium as catalyst. In benzyl derivatives ($PhCH_2OR$), the rate of cleavage depends on the ability of the leaving groups (OR) to carry a negative charge; that is, the rate decreased in the order $OCOCF_3 > OCOCH_3 > OH_2^+ > OHR^+ > OAr > OR > OH$ (Khan et al., 1967). For this reason, acidic solvents favor hydrogenolysis reactions.

The reactivity of –OH groups in phenols, alcohols, and acids is commonly masked by converting them to benzyl derivatives. Among the numerous methods developed for their deprotection, catalytic hydrogenation has proved to be highly useful.

In the past decade, ammonium formate-mediated catalytic transfer hydrogenation has been demonstrated to be superior to conventional hydrogenation for effecting the removal of benzyl-based protecting groups in peptide synthesis. The ease, simplicity, speed (activity), selectivity, and economy of this AF-CTH process has been established.

Reduction of sensitive compounds such as peptides must be carried out under mild reaction conditions (ambient temperature, atmospheric pressure, and neutral pH). It may be essential to keep the reaction time as short as possible to avoid any side reactions. Short reaction times are also desirable when dealing with compounds containing radioactive nucleides with short half-lives (for example, synthesis of ^{11}C-labeled α-amino acids from α-nitro acids). Ammonium formate–catalytic transfer hydrogenation fulfills these criteria.

The first report of the rapid nature of AF-CTH processes was illustrated in the synthesis of leucine-enkephalin (Anwer and Spatola, 1980). Here, the N^α-benzyloxycarbonyl protecting group was cleaved in minutes. The rapid, quantitative AF-CTH cleavage of the pentapeptide leucine-enkephalin from its Merrifield resin support under ambient conditions in the presence of Pd(OAc)$_2$ is another example that demonstrates the rapid and clean nature of these reactions (Anwer and Spatola, 1981).

In carbohydrate chemistry, the –OH group is often protected as its benzyl ether. The benzyl ethers are stable to both acids and bases but can be cleaved under mild conditions using either conventional or transfer hydrogenation techniques. Bieg and Szeja (1985) reported O-debenzylation of protected sugars using HCOONH$_4$, 10% Pd/C in boiling methanol with very high yields (91–98%). Araki et al. (1989) reported debenzylation of benzyl-protected ribofuranosyl derivatives with HCOOH, Pd/C at room temperature.

The removal of the benzyl-protecting group of 1-benzyloxyaminoalkyl phosphonic and phosphinic acids and their N-acetylated derivatives was affected by catalytic transfer hydrogenation with ammonium formate and 10% Pd/C (Elhaddadi et al., 1991). Sodium formate/formic acid and 10% Pd/C has been used for the conversion of hydroxyflavanones (Krishnamurty and Sathyanarayana, 1989).

N-Benzyl Compounds

In contrast to O-benzyl groups, the N-benzyl groups are difficult to cleave because the nitrogen is less electronegative than oxygen. ElAmin et al. (1979) observed that N-debenzylation required 10 h (yield, 81%), whereas O-debenzylation was completed in 10 min (yield, 98%) under similar experimental conditions.

Ram and Spicer (1987) reported N-debenzylation of various compounds using ammonium formate and Pd/C in refluxing methanol. Hydrogenolytic cleavage of a benzyl group attached to quaternary nitrogen has also been used in the synthesis of pyrazoloisoquinoline derivatives (Allen et al., 1992). Overman and Sugai (1985) utilized Pd/C and ammonium formate to remove N-benzyl groups during the total synthesis of crinine.

S-Benzyl Compounds

Elimination of benzyl groups from sulfur-containing compounds (e.g., cysteine and methionine) introduced a special type of obstacle. The sulfur in the divalent state is a definite poison to the commonly employed catalysts such as platinum metals in transfer hydrogenolysis. For this reason, only a few catalytic methods have been reported so far, and with limited success.

Instead of catalytic hydrogenation, a traditional sodium in liquid ammonia reagent has been used for the removal of the S-benzyl group.

Kuromizu and Meienhofer (1974) circumvented the problem of catalyst poisoning by carrying out the catalytic hydrogenation experiments in liquid ammonia. Obviously, divalent sulfur is not inhibiting the catalytic sites in liquid ammonia. Using this method, the N-benzyloxycarbonyl group has been quantitatively cleaved from S-benzylcysteine derivatives. Nevertheless, S-benzyl was refractive under these conditions. While 1,4-cyclohexadiene removed the benzyloxycarbonyl group from methionine, it failed to cleave the S-benzyl group of S-benzylcysteine in glacial acetic acid at elevated temperatures. However, 1,4-cyclohexadiene in liquid ammonia effected N-debenzyloxycarbonylation from methionine and partial S-debenzylation from S-benzylcysteine (Felix et al., 1978).

The ease of accessibility of the sulfur atom to the catalyst surface appears to be an important factor in the inhibition of the catalyst. When the protecting group is attached to sulfur, its removal is difficult. When the functional group to be hydrogenolyzed is situated far from the divalent sulfur, it is easier to remove. This is evident from the successful application of cyclohexene (Anantharamaiah and Sivanandaiah, 1977), 1,4-cyclohexadiene (Felix et al., 1978), and formic acid (ElAmin et al, 1979; Sivanandaiah and Gurusiddappa, 1979) in the presence of Pd/C for the removal of benzyl-protecting groups from methionine-containing peptides.

Allyl Compounds (Allyl–X; X = Cl, Br, I, O, N)

Ammonium formate catalytic transfer hydrogenolysis of allylic compounds in the presence of a Pd-tributylphosphine catalyst has been shown to regioselectively furnish 1-alkenes (Tsuji et al., 1984). The terminal alkenes are also obtained when $PdCl_2(PPh_3)_2$ is used as the catalyst (Tsuji and Yamakawa, 1979). N-Allyl compounds have been hydrogenolyzed to olefins and amine with $HCOONHEt_3$ and Pd/C at 100°C (Weir et al., 1980). Sodium formate in the presence of a water-soluble Pd complex affected the dechlorination of allyl chlorides in the counter phase-transfer mode (Okano et al., 1986).

Olefins, Diolefins, and Acetylenes

Alkenes are also reduced to alkanes by catalytic transfer hydrogenation. Thus, HCOOH in the presence of 10% Pd/C at 110°C converts cycloheptene to cycloheptane (Nishiguchi et al., 1976). Formic acid or a mixture with lithium formate in the presence of Ru, Os, Ir, Rh, or Pt complexes has been employed for the transfer hydrogenation of alkenes and alkynes (Vol'pin et al., 1971). Activated olefins are reduced employing formate salts and [Rh(cod)Cl]₂ and chiral sulphonated phosphines (Sinou et al., 1991). Enantiomeric excesses up to 43% are obtained in the reduction of αacetamidocinnamic acid. Indoles are converted to indolines by HCOOH and Pd/C at 70°C. α,β-Unsaturated compounds are readily transfer hydrogenated by HCOOH (Azran et al., 1984) or triethylammonium formate (Cortese and Heck, 1978).

Dienes and acetylenes were selectively reduced by triethylammonium formate and Pd/C (Weir et al., 1980). In the presence of 5% Pd/C, formic acid reduced methyl linoleate under mild conditions (Nishiguchi et al., 1979). Hydrogen transfer reduction of isoflavones using ammonium formate and Pd/C provides an easy access to polyoxyisoflavanones and also to isoflava-4-ols without the need for protection of the hydroxy groups (Wähälä and Hase, 1989).

Aldehydes and Ketones

Aryl alkyl ketones are reduced to alcohols under ambient conditions in high yield. For example, acetophenone is converted to 1-phenylethanol in the presence of ammonium formate and 10% Pd/C at room temperature in 4 h with 90% yield (Radhakrishna et al., 1989). Under these conditions, AF-CTH failed to reduce aromatic aldehydes. However, in glacial acetic acid at 110°C, anhydrous ammonium formate in the presence of Pd/C reduced aromatic aldehydes and ketones to their corresponding $-CH_3$ or $-CH_2-$ analogs (Ram and Spicer, 1988).

Triethylammonium formate and $RuCl_2(PPh_3)_3$ at room temperature reduced various aldehydes to alcohols in excellent yields. The halogen, nitro, and olefinic double bonds are not affected by this reagent (Khai and Arcelli, 1985). Similarly, α,β-unsaturated aldehydes were transfer hydrogenated to α,β-unsaturated alcohols at 80°C in very high yields (93–98%) using HCOONa and $RuCl_2(m\text{-}SPPh_2)_2$ where S is a sulphophenyl group (Joó and Bényei, 1989).

The vapor-phase transfer reduction of benzaldehyde using HCOOH and Cu at 200°C yielded 56% $PhCH_2OH$ and 18% $PhCH_3$ (Davies and Hodgson, 1943). Formic acid reduces aldehydes to alcohols in the presence of Ir, Pt, Ru, or Os complexes. For instance, HCOOH and $IrH_3(PPh_3)_3$ reduced 1-butanal to a mixture of BuOH and BuOAc in AcOH at 50°C (Coffey, 1967).

Deoxygenation of Phenolic Compounds

Catalytic hydrogenolysis of phenols to arenes is difficult unless the phenolic group is converted to its tetrazolyl ether derivative. Formic acid in the presence of Pd/C has been used for the conversion of phenyl tetrazolyl ethers to arenes (Hussey et al., 1982). Alternatively, phenols are first converted to aryl triflates ($ArOSO_2CF_3$) followed by transfer hydrogenolysis using $Pd(OAc)_2/PPh_3$ and $HCOOH/Et_3N$ (Cacchi et al., 1986). Unsaturated functional groups such as nitro, ketones, esters, and olefins are found to tolerate the reaction conditions.

Aromatic Nitriles

Hydrogenation of an aromatic nitrile to benzylamine is a commonly known reaction. However, the direct conversion of Ar–C≡N to Ar–CH₃ is only recently gaining importance. This reaction can be achieved in very good yield with the help of $HCOONH_4$ and Pd/C at room temperature (Brown and Foubister, 1982). Using H_2, this reaction is performed in the vapor-phase at 150°C using 30% Ni/Al_2O_3 as catalyst (Andrade et al., 1980). This contrast serves to illustrate the hydrogenolytic potential of ammonium formate.

Coupling Reactions: Synthesis of Biaryls

Under dehalogenation conditions, if a strong base such as NaOH is introduced into the reaction system, halogen is eliminated and coupling of aromatic rings in the positions formerly occupied by halogen occurs. The ready availability of the starting material together with the low cost of the reagents make this a useful method for the preparation of biaryl compounds.

Biphenyls can be made in good yields by the reductive coupling of bromobenzenes with HCOONa in the presence of Pd/C (Bamfield and Quan, 1978). The yields are generally low (about 50%), but the unreacted starting material can be recycled so that the overall conversions are high. A surfactant is generally used as a phase-transfer reagent in these coupling reactions. Some authors have attributed the coupling selectivity to the presence of surfactant. Cetyltrimethylammonium bromide is found to be an excellent surface active agent for this purpose. Recently, cyclodextrins have been used as a phase-transfer agent for coupling reactions of 2-methoxybromobenzene using HCOONa, NaOH, and Pd/C at 60°C (Shimizu et al., 1990).

Mechanism of Transfer Hydrogenation

Pd/C emerges as the catalyst of choice in most of the transfer reduction reactions in this review. It is also apparent that the formate anion is a prerequisite for the reaction. The following postulate is advanced to rationalize the various literature observations that have been made.

The first step in these reactions is the chemisorption of formate salts that may decompose into CO_2 and H^- ions on the metal surface. The adsorbed hydrogen can exhibit H^-, H, or H^+ behavior depending on the environment. There is some evidence that hydrogen exhibits either H^- or H^+ character on palladium in the liquid-phase. For example, in the case of dehalogenation, it is most likely that the hydride-like behavior is predominant. In the case of coupling reactions performed in the presence of a strong base such as NaOH, the chemisorbed hydrogen on palladium may exhibit H^+ character; the abstraction of this H^+ by OH^- would leave two electrons on the surface of the metal cluster. These electrons may be responsible for the radical chemistry witnessed in the coupling reaction of bromobenzene to biphenyls. The H–D exchange reactions also support the H^+ nature of PdH^- species. For example, the deuterium of PdD^- can exchange freely with H_2O, alcohols, benzylic protons, organic acids, and NH_4^+.

Hydrodehalogenation Mechanism

A number of studies have been carried out on the mechanism of catalytic hydrogenation. However, few experimental studies have succeeded in elucidating the mechanism of transfer hydrogenation. Recent results obtained in our lab on the mechanism of hydrodehalogenation are given below. From the kinetic data, the following mechanism has been proposed for the dechlorination of 2-chlorotoluene by HCOONa under the catalytic influence of 10% Pd/C. For convenience, Pd/c is designated as $Pd°$.

$$HCOONa \overset{K_1}{\rightleftharpoons} HCOO^- + Na^+ \tag{3}$$

$$Pd° + HCOO^- \overset{K_2}{\rightleftharpoons} Pd(HCOO^-)_{ad} \tag{4}$$

$$Pd(HCOO^-)_{ad} \overset{slow}{\underset{k}{\rightarrow}} PdH^- + CO_2 \tag{5}$$

$$PdH^- + Cl-C_6H_4-CH_3 \overset{fast}{\rightarrow} PdH^-(Cl-C_6H_4-CH_3)_{ad} \tag{6}$$

$$PdH^-(Cl-C_6H_4-CH_3)_{ad} \overset{fast}{\rightarrow} Pd° + C_6H_5-CH_3 + Cl^- \tag{7}$$

A rate expression has been derived based on this mechanism. HCOONa, being a strong electrolyte, dissociates completely and hence K_1 is considered large.

$$Rate = k \, [Pd(HCOO^-)_{ad}] \tag{8}$$

$$[Pd(HCOO^-)_{ad}] = K_2 \, [Pd°] \, [HCOO^-] \tag{9}$$

$$\therefore Rate = k\,K_2\,[\text{Pd}^\circ]\,[\text{HCOO}^-] = k\,K_2\,[\text{Pd}^\circ]\,[\text{HCOONa}] \qquad (10)$$

Mechanism of Hydrogenolysis

From the similarity of the time-conversion plots for hydrogenolysis of O-benzyl groups, we assume that the mechanism may be similar but not identical to hydrodehalogenation. A detailed kinetic study is in progress.

Mechanism of Coupling

Although detailed mechanistic studies for coupling reactions are lacking in the literature, a mechanism is proposed based on known information on this subject. The palladium hydride in the presence of a strong base loses a proton, retaining two electrons. These two electrons are momentarily accommodated in the catalyst via delocalization (the Pd metal cluster size is 3.5–5 nm for 10% metal loading). These electrons may then react with aryl halide to yield two phenyl radicals and halide ions. A biaryl is formed from these radicals in a fast step. The rate-limiting step may be any one of the following first three stages:

$$\text{Pd}^\circ + \text{HCOO}^- \rightarrow \text{PdH}^- + \text{CO}_2 \qquad (11)$$

$$\text{PdH}^- + \text{OH}^- \rightarrow \text{Pd}^{2-} + \text{H}_2\text{O} \qquad (12)$$

$$\text{Pd}^{2-} + 2\text{Ph–Br} \rightarrow \text{Pd}^\circ + 2\text{Ph·} + 2\text{Br}^- \qquad (13)$$

$$2\text{Ph·} \rightarrow \text{Ph–Ph} \qquad (14)$$

Conclusions

Until recently, transfer hydrogenation reactions were mostly used on the laboratory scale. Because of their simplicity of operation and cost-effectiveness, they are now widely used in industry. Further gains in the mechanistic knowledge of transfer reduction reactions by systematic kinetic and spectral studies directed toward characterization of the reactive intermediates are anticipated. Asymmetric synthesis using transfer hydrogenation is also now possible. Further augmentation of asymmetric induction by using formate salts of chiral bases in the presence of chiral catalysts is another promising area for future investigations.

REFERENCES

Allen MS, Skolnick P, Cook JM (1992): *J Med Chem* 35:368.
Anantharamaiah GM, Sivanandaiah KM (1977): *J Chem Soc Perkin Trans I* 490.
Andrade JG, Maier WF, Zapf L, Schleyer PvR (1980): *Synthesis* 802.
Anwer MK, Spatola AF (1980): *Synthesis* 929.
Anwer MK, Spatola AF (1985): *Tetrahedron Lett* 26:1381.
Anwer MK, Spatola AF (1981): *Tetrahedron Lett* 22:4369.
Anwer MK, Sherman DB, Roney JG, Spatola AF (1989): *J Org Chem* 54:1284.
Araki Y, Mokubo E, Kobayashi N, Nagasawa J, Ishido Y (1989): *Tetrahedron Lett* 30:1115.
Azran J, Buchman O, Orchin M, Blum J (1984): *J Org Chem* 49:1327.
Bamfield P, Quan PM (1978): *Synthesis* 537.
Bamfield P, Quan PM, Smoth TJ (1976): *Ger Offen* 2,536,914.
Barrett AGM, Spilling CD (1988): *Tetrahedron Lett* 29:5733.
Bieg T, Szeja W (1985): *Synthesis* 76.
Boudjouk PR, Han BH (1984): *U.S. Patent* 4,466,870.
Brieger G, Nestrick T (1974): *Chem Rev* 74:567.
Brown GR, Foubister AJ (1982): *Synthesis* 1036.
Cacchi S, Ciattini PG, Morera E, Ortar G (1986): *Tetrahedron Lett* 27:5541.
Coffey RS (1967): *British Patent* 1,227,601.
Cortese NA, Heck RF (1977): *J Org Chem* 42:3491.
Cortese NA, Heck RF (1978): *J Org Chem* 43:3985.
Davies R, Hodgson HH (1943): *J Chem Soc* 281.
ElAmin B, Anantharamaiah GM, Royer GP, Means GE (1979): *J Org Chem* 44:3442.
Elhaddadi M, Jacquier R, Petrus C, Petrus F (1991): *Phosphorus Sulfur Silicon* 57:119.
Entwistle ID, Jackson AE, Johnstone RAW, Telford RP (1977): *J Chem Soc Perkins Trans I* 443.
Felix AM, Heimer EP, Lambros TJ, Tzougraki C, Meienhofer J (1978): *J Org Chem* 43:4194.
Helquist P (1978): *Tetrahedron Lett* 1913.
Hussey BJ, Johnstone RAW, Entwistle ID (1982): *Tetrahedron* 38:3775.
Johnstone RAW, Wilby AH, Entwistle ID (1985): *Chem Rev* 85:129.
Joó F, Bényei A (1989): *J Organomet Chem* 363:C19.
Khai BT, Arcelli A (1985): *Tetrahedron Lett* 26:3365.
Khan AM, McQuillin FJ, Jardine I (1967): *J Chem Soc* 136.
Kieboom APG, van Rantwijk R (1977): *Hydrogenation and Hydrogenolysis in Synthetic Organic Chemistry.* The Netherlands: Delft University Press.
Krishnamurty HG, Sathyanarayana S (1989): *Synth Commun* 19:119.
Kuromizu K, Meienhofer J (1974): *J Am Chem Soc* 96:4978.
Mitsui Toatsu Chemicals, Inc. (1985): *Jpn Kokai Tokkyo Koho JP* 60 16,956 [85 16,956].
Nishiguchi T, Tagawa T, Fukuzumi K (1979): *Yukagaku* 28:174.
Nishiguchi T, Imai H, Hirose Y, Fukuzumi K (1976): *J Catal* 41:249.
Okano T, Moriyama Y, Konishi H, Kiji J (1986): *Chem Lett* 1463.
Overman LE, Sugai S (1985): *Helv Chim Acta* 68:745.
Pandey PN, Purkayastha ML (1982): *Synthesis* 876.
Pinder AR (1980): *Synthesis* 425.
Pope D, Smith WL, Eastlake MJ, Moss RL (1971): *J Catal* 22:72.
Pri-Bar I, Buchman O (1986): *J Org Chem* 51:734.

Radhakrishna AS, Prasad Rao KRK, Nigam SC, Bakthavatchalam R, Singh BB (1989): *Org Prep Proced Int* 21:373.

Rajeswari S, Drost KJ, Cava MP (1989): *Heterocycles* 29:415.

Ram S, Ehrenkaufer RE (1984): *Tetrahedron Lett* 25:3415.

Ram S, Ehrenkaufer RE (1986): *Synthesis* 133.

Ram S, Ehrenkaufer RE (1988): *Synthesis* 91.

Ram S, Spicer LD (1987): *Tetrahedron Lett* 28:515.

Ram S, Spicer LD (1988): *Tetrahedron Lett* 29:3741.

Shimizu S, Sasaki Y, Hirai C (1990): *Bull Chem Soc Jpn* 63:176.

Sinou D, Safi M, Claver C, Masdeu A (1991): *J Mol Catal* 68:L9.

Sivanandaiah KM, Gurusiddappa S (1979): *J Chem Res (Synop)* 108.

Terpko MO, Heck RF (1980): *J Org Chem* 45:4992.

Tsuji J, Yamakawa T (1979): *Tetrahedron Lett* 613.

Tsuji J, Shimizu I, Minami I (1984): *Chem Lett* 1017.

Vol'pin ME, Kukolev VP, Chernyshev VO, Kolomnikov IS (1971): *Tetrahedron Lett* 4435.

Wähälä K, Hase TA (1989): *Heterocycles* 28:183.

Weir JR, Patel BA, Heck RF (1980): *J Org Chem* 45:4926.

Wiener H, Blum J, Sasson Y (1991): *J Org Chem* 56:4481.

Zassinovich G, Mestroni G, Gladiali S (1992): *Chem Rev* 92:1051.

3

SYNTHESES OF NATRIURETIC PEPTIDES USING A NEW S-PROTECTING GROUP, S-TRIMETHYLACETAMIDOMETHYL (TACM) GROUP

Yoshiaki Kiso, Makoto Yoshida, Yoichi Fujiwara,
Tooru Kimura, Kenichi Akaji, and Haruaki Yajima

Introduction

Protection of the thiol function of cysteine is required during peptide synthesis (Hiskey, 1981). One of the widely used protecting groups is S-acetamidomethyl (Acm), which is stable in acidic conditions such as trifluoroacetic acid (TFA) and hydrogen fluoride (HF) but can be removed with Hg(OAc)$_2$ in TFA (Veber et al., 1972) or I$_2$ in aqueous AcOH (Kamber et al., 1980; Sieber et al., 1980). However, during the preparation of Cys(Acm), thiazolidine-2-carboxylic acid was formed as a by-product. The activation of Boc-Cys(Acm)-OH using the N,N'-dicyclohexylcarbodiimide (DCC) and 1-hydroxy-benzotriazole (HOBt) method was also accompanied by a side reaction. When the S-benzamido-methyl (Bam) group (Chakravaty and Olsen, 1978) is used, these side reactions are greatly reduced, but it is slightly unstable during HF cleavage condition (0°C, 1 h) and alkaline conditions. We describe here the preparation and characterization of a new S-protecting group, the S-trimethylacetamidomethyl (Tacm) group, and its application to the syntheses of natriuretic peptides.

Peptides: Design, Synthesis, and Biological Activity
Channa Basava and G. M. Anantharamaiah, Editors
©1994 *Birkhäuser Boston*

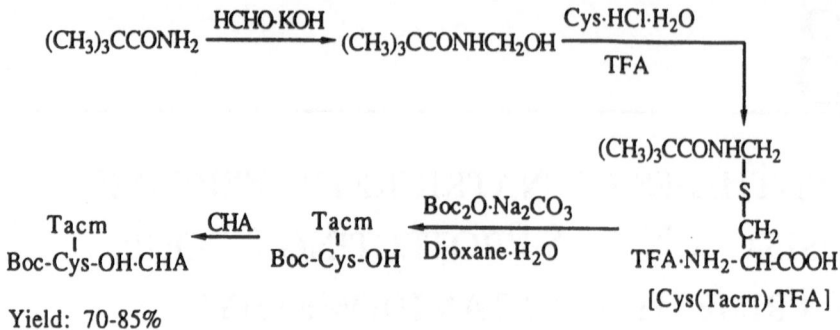

Figure 3–1. Preparation of Boc-Cys(Tacm)-OH-CHA.

Preparation and Characterization of Cys(Tacm) Derivative

The S-Tacm group was conveniently introduced into cysteine without any serious side reaction (Figure 3–1). N-Hydroxymethyl trimethylacetamide was obtained nearly quantitatively from trimethylacetamide (1 equivalent, equiv) in a solution of formaldehyde:water (7:13; 0.7 equiv) in the presence of KOH (0.1 equiv) (Albercio et al., 1987; Einhorn, 1905). Subsequently, the Tacm group was incorporated into cysteine by treatment with N-hydroxymethyl trimethylacetamide (1.1 equiv) in TFA at room temperature for 1 h. The N-Boc derivative, Boc-Cys(Tacm)-OH, was prepared with di-*tert*-butyl dicarbonate (1.4 equiv) in the presence of sodium carbonate and then isolated as the cyclohexylamine salt in 70%–85% yield.

The S-Tacm group was stable to acidic and basic conditions, such as HF (0°C, 1 h), 1 M trifluoromethanesulfonic acid (TFMSA)-thioanisole/TFA (0°C, 2 h) (Kiso et al., 1980; Yajima et al., 1974) or 1 N NaOH/MeOH (0°C, 1 h), while it could be readily converted to cystine by 20% I_2/EtOH (10 equiv) in 90% AcOH (25°C, 1 h), and also removed by Hg(OAc)$_2$ (1 equiv) in TFA (0°C, 30 min) (Table 3–1). This protecting group had stability simi-

Table 3-1. Stability of Tacm Group to Various Conditions

Reagents (Temp., Time)	Stability
TFA(r.t., 24 h.)	stable
0.5M MSA/CH$_2$CL$_2$: dioxane(9:1) (r.t., 24 h.)	stable
1M TFMSA-thioanisole/TFA(0°C, 1 h.)	stable
HF-m-cresol (0°C, 1 h.)	stable
Zn-90% AcOH (r.t., 3 h.)	stable
6N HCl (110°C, 20 h.)	unstable
NH$_2$NH$_2$/MeOH (r.t., 24 h.)	stable
1N NaOH (0°C, 1 h.)	stable

Removal of Tacm Group			
Reagents	Conditions	Cysteine	Cystine
Hg(OAc)$_2$/TFA(1 eq.)	0°C, 30 min.	98%	– –
I$_2$(10 eq.)/90% AcOH	r.t., 1 h	– –	100%

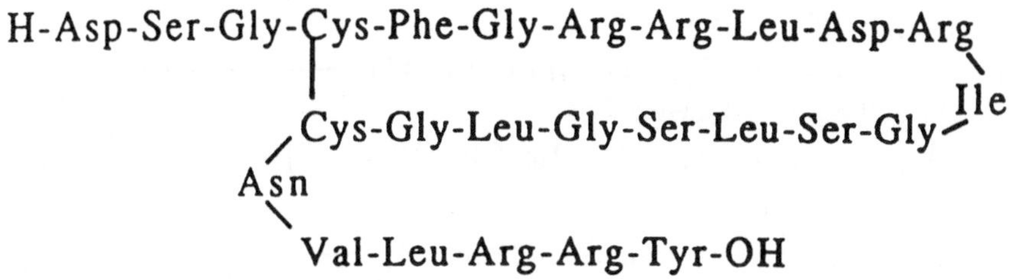

H-Asp-Ser-Gly-Cys-Phe-Gly-Arg-Arg-Leu-Asp-Arg
                    | \
                    | Cys-Gly-Leu-Gly-Ser-Leu-Ser-Gly⟋   Ile
                   ⟋Asn
                  Asn
                    \
                     Val-Leu-Arg-Arg-Tyr-OH

Figure 3-2. Structure of pBNP.

lar to that of the S-Acm group, but we observed that Boc-Cys(Tacm)-OH had less tendency to sulfoxide formation than Boc-Cys(Acm)-OH. The results indicated that Cys(Tacm) is less susceptible to air oxidation than Cys(Acm), presumably because of the steric hindrance of the bulky side chain.

Solution-Phase Synthesis of Porcine Brain Natriuretic Peptide

In 1988, Sudoh et al. isolated a 26-amino-acid-residue peptide that included a disulfide bridge, "brain natriuretic peptide" (BNP), from porcine brain (Sudoh et al., 1988). As shown in Figure 3-2, the structure of porcine BNP is remarkably similar to but definitely distinct from that of alpha (α-) human atrial natriuretic peptide (α-hANP). We applied this new cysteine derivative to the synthesis of porcine BNP (pBNP) by the conventional solution method.

The synthetic route to pBNP is illustrated in Figure 3-3. The entire sequence was divided into four fragments, 1–4, at Gly residues because no racemization was involved in the coupling reaction, using a water-soluble carbodiimide (WSC), 1-ethyl-3-(3'-dimethylaminopropyl)-carbodiimide in the presence of HOBt as an additive (Kimura et al., 1981). In combination with a TFA-labile Boc group for N^α-protection, amino acid derivatives bearing protecting groups removable with HF were employed: Asp(OcHex), Ser(Bzl), Arg(Tos), and Tyr(BrZ), except for Cys(Tacm). To suppress the succinimide formation at the Asp–Ser sequence, Asp(OcHex) was employed.

Every fragment was synthesized by the known amide-forming reactions. In the synthesis of the fragments containing Cys(Tacm), fragments 1 and 4, no side reaction was observed during activation using the DCC-HOBt procedure. After removal of the C-terminal phenacyl ester (OPac) by Zn in AcOH, each fragment was successively assembled by the WSC-HOBt procedure. Each protected peptide was purified by precipitation from DMF with EtOH. The homogeneity of each product was ascertained by thin-

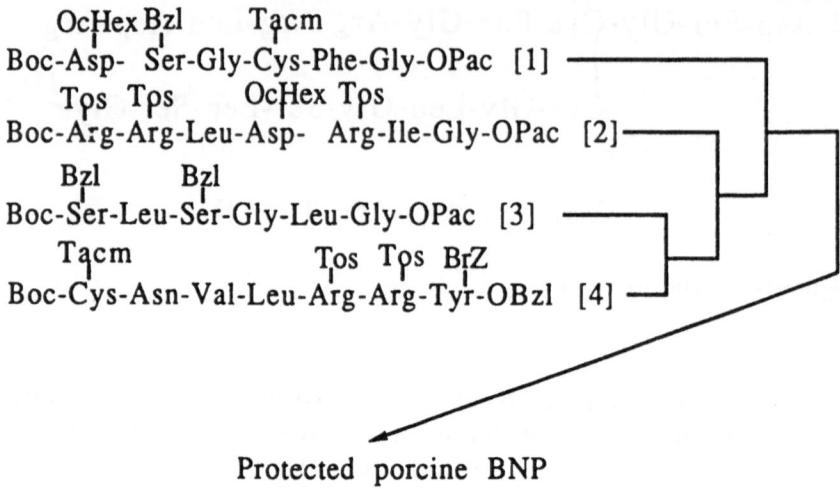

Protected porcine BNP

Figure 3–3. Synthetic route to porcine BNP.

layer chromatography (TLC) and amino acid analysis after acid hydrolysis. Throughout this synthesis, Leu was used as a diagnostic amino acid. The fully protected peptide was treated with HF in the presence of m-cresol and dimethylsulfide (0°C, 1 h) to remove all protecting groups except the Tacm groups. The di-Tacm peptide was purified by gel filtration on Sephadex G-25 (1 N AcOH) and ion-exchange chromatography on CM-cellulose using gradient elution with 0.25 M AcONH$_4$, followed by fast protein liquid chromatography (FPLC) on a YMC-gel AQ120 ODS column. The purity of this peptide was ascertained by amino acid analysis, analytical HPLC, and fast atom bombardment mass spectrometry (FAB-MS).

The observed mass value (3098) of the base peak in molecular ion regions on the FAB-MS spectrum agreed well with the theoretical value (3097.634) corresponding to [Cys(Tacm)[4,20]]-pBNP. The product thus obtained was diluted with 90% AcOH and oxidized with 20% I$_2$/EtOH (10 equiv). After stirring for 1 h at 25°C, this solution was evaporated under reduced pressure and purified by gel filtration on Sephadex G-25 (1 N AcOH). The crude oxidized peptide was further purified by HPLC on a YMC-gel D-ODS-5 column to give a homogeneous peptide (overall yield from the deprotection and purification steps, 12%) (Figure 3–4). The purity of synthetic pBNP was confirmed by TLC, amino acid analysis after acid hydrolysis, analytical HPLC on a cosmosil 5C$_{18}$ column (Figure 3–5), and FAB-MS. The observed mass value (2869) of the base peak in molecular regions on the FAB-MS spectrum agreed well with the theoretical value (2869.458) corresponding to pBNP.

Protected porcine BNP

1. HF-*m*-cresol-Me$_2$S (0°C, 1h)

2. Sephadex G-25 (1N AcOH)

3. CM-cellulose (0.01-0.25M AcONH$_4$)

4. Preparative FPLC on YMC-gel ODS AQ-120

[Cys(Tacm)[4,20]]-porcine BNP

5. Oxidation using I$_2$ in 90% AcOH

6. Sephadex G-25 (1N AcOH)

7. Preparative HPLC on YMC-gel D-ODS-5

Synthetic porcine BNP

Figure 3–4. Deprotection and purification.

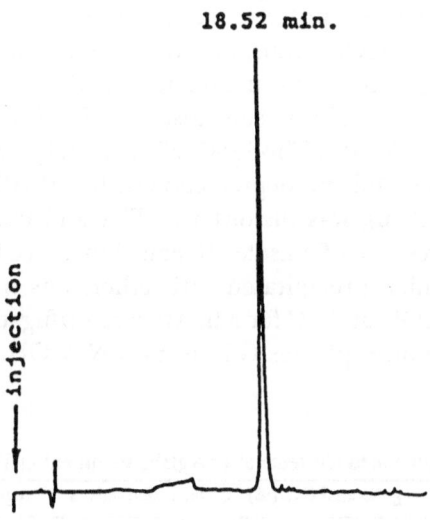

Figure 3–5. HPLC pattern of synthetic pBNP.

Introduction of Silver Tetrafluoroborate (AgBF$_4$) as a New Deprotecting Reagent for the S-Tacm Group

In the course of our investigation of the S-Tacm group (Kiso et al., 1989, 1990a, 1990b), we have observed that partial oxidation of Met to Met(O) occurs during the removal of the S-Tacm group with I$_2$ in 90% aqueous AcOH. We therefore sought a milder method for removal of the S-Tacm group and found that silver tetrafluoroborate (AgBF$_4$) in TFA can remove the S-Tacm group without affecting other functional groups in a peptide chain. In the deprotection of an S-protecting group with monovalent silver ion, anion counterparts play an important role because silver ion can remove several S-protecting groups in the form of nitrate (Guttmann, 1966; Storey et al., 1972) or trifluoromethanesulfonate (Fujii et al., 1989), but its acetate form does not (Nishimura et al., 1978). We have employed silver ion in the form of tetrafluoroborate and examined its usefulness as a deprotecting reagent of S-protecting group. Boc-Cys(Tacm)-OH in TFA was treated with AgBF$_4$ (10 equiv) in the presence of anisole (2 equiv) in an ice bath for 1 h. After treatment with dithiothreitol (DTT) (20 equiv) at 25°C, the regenerated cysteine was quantified by an amino acid analyzer. Quantitative recovery of cysteine from this derivative was observed (Table 3–2). Under identical conditions, Acm was also cleaved quantitatively, but two other S-protecting groups, 4-methoxybenzyl (MBzl) and 2,4,6-trimethylbenzyl (Tmb) (Brtnik et al., 1981; Kiso et al., 1987) were cleaved incompletely (87% and 73%, respectively). tert-Butyl (Bu) and 4-methylbenzyl (MeBzl) were not affected. The results indicated that AgBF$_4$ in TFA is a suitable reagent for peptide synthesis using Cys(Tacm) or Cys(Acm) derivatives.

Trp is known to be susceptible to modification during the I$_2$ oxidation procedure in aqueous AcOH. Thus, we have compared the amounts of this side reaction during AgBF$_4$ and I$_2$ treatments on HPLC using somatostatin as a model peptide. The di-Tacm somatostatin [H-Ala-Gly-Cys (Tacm)-Lys-Asn-Phe-Phe-Trp-Lys-Thr-Phe-Thr-Ser-Cys(Tacm)-OH], prepared by Fmoc-based solid-phase method and deprotection with 1 M HBF$_4$-thioanisole in TFA (Akaji et al., 1990), was dissolved in TFA and treated with AgBF$_4$ (20 equiv) in the presence of anisole (10 equiv) in an ice bath for 1 h. The peptide-Ag salt, which precipitated with ether, was treated with DTT (40 equiv) in 1 N AcOH at 25°C for 3 h. After centrifugation, the supernatant was gel filtered on Sephadex G-15 using 1 N AcOH. The desired elu-

Table 3-2. Regenerated Cysteine after AgBF$_4$ treatment in TFA(4°C, 1h)

cysteine derivatives	regenerated Cys (%)	cysteine derivatives	regenerated Cys (%)
Boc-Cys(Tacm)-OH	107	Boc-Cys(Tmb)-OH	73
Boc-Cys(Acm)-OH	93	Boc-Cys(Bu)-OH	0
Boc-Cys(MBzl)-OH	87	Boc-Cys(MeBzl)-OH	0

a)   b)

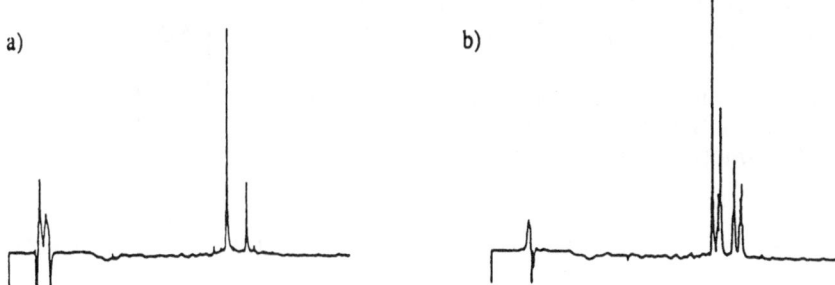

Figure 3-6. HPLC pattern of crude somatostatin. Column, YMC AM-302 (4.6 × 150 mm); eluant, 0.1% aqueous TFA with MeCN (10%–60% in 30 min); flow rate, 0 .7 ml/min; retention time, 19.7 min (same as authentic sample from Peptide Institute, Osaka, Japan). **A.** Air oxidation after Ag treatment. **B.** I$_2$ oxidation in 50% aqueous AcOH.

ate, after being diluted with water, was subjected to air oxidation at pH 7.5. Oxidative cleavage of the S-Tacm group with I$_2$ in aqueous AcOH was carried out in essentially the same manner as described for the S-Acm group. The crude product obtained using I$_2$-aqueous AcOH gave a more complex elution pattern on HPLC than that obtained using AgBF$_4$ (Figure 3–6). The same results were obtained in the comparison of the deprotecting reagents using S-Acm somatostatin as a starting derivative.

Solution-Phase Synthesis of pBNP32

To demonstrate the usefulness of this new S-deprotecting reagent, we have synthesized a newly isolated Met-containing peptide pBNP32 (Figure 3-7) (Sudoh et al., 1988) that consists of 32 amino acids extending from the N terminus of pBNP (26 amino acid residues). The di-Tacm pBNP32 was prepared using an intermediate in the previous pBNP synthesis (Kiso et al., 1989, 1990a, 1990b) in solution, followed by deprotection with HF-m-cresol-dimethylsulfide (0°C, 1 h). After gel filtration on Sephadex G-25, the product was purified by FPLC on a YMC-gel ODS AQ300 (S-50) column and then treated with AgBF$_4$ (40 equiv) in the presence of anisole (10 equiv), followed by DTT (80 equiv) as previously. After air oxidation at pH 7.5, the product was purified by HPLC on a cosmosil 5C18 P-300 to give a homogeneous peptide (Figure 3–8A); the yield was 10.5% (calculated from the protected peptide). The purity of synthetic pBNP32 was confirmed by analytical HPLC (Figure 3–8B) and amino acid analysis after acid hydrolysis with 6 N HCl. The purified product was proved to be a monomer by FAB-MS [the observed mass value, 3569.9 (MH$^+$), agreed well with the theoretical value,

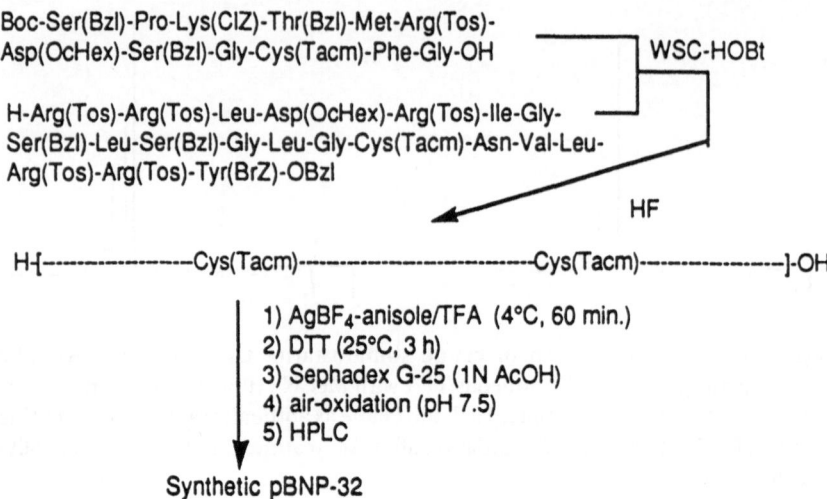

Figure 3–7. Synthetic route to pBNP32.

3569.819]. In an alternative oxidative cleavage of di-Tacm pBNP32 using I_2 in aqueous AcOH, we observed a remarkable amount of Met(O) derivative on HPLC (retention time, 17.2 min; Figure 3–8C); the yield of the purified peptide was 2.1%.

Solid-Phase Synthesis of hBNP32

We also applied this *S*-deprotecting reagent (Yoshida et al., 1990a, 1990b) and *S*-Tacm group to the solid-phase synthesis of human brain natriuretic peptide 32 (hBNP32). The structure of hBNP32 has been deduced from the nucleotide sequence of the hBNP precursor and shown to be highly

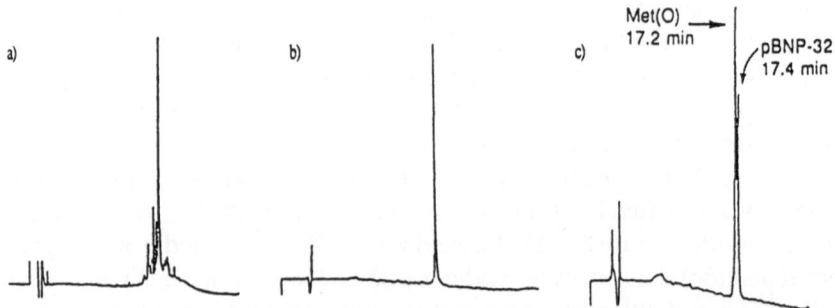

Figure 3–8. HPLC pattern of synthetic pBNP32. **A.** Air oxidation after AgBF$_4$ treatment. **B.** HPLC-purified sample. **C.** I$_2$ oxidation in 90% aqueous AcOH.

Fmoc-Ser(Bu)-Pro-Lys(Boc)-Val-Met-Gln-Gly-Ser(Bu)-Gly-Cys(Tacm)-Phe-Gly-Arg(Mtr)-Lys(Boc)-Met-Asp(OBu)-Arg(Mtr)-Ile-Ser(Bu)-Ser(Bu)-Ser(Bu)-Ser(Bu)-Gly-Leu-Gly-Cys(Tacm)-Lys(Boc)-Val-Leu-Arg(Mtr)-Arg(Mtr)-His(Bum)-O-Wang Resin

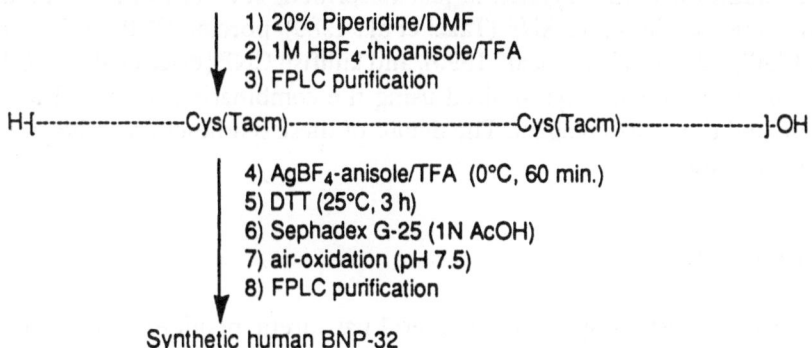

1) 20% Piperidine/DMF
2) 1M HBF₄-thioanisole/TFA
3) FPLC purification

H-[----------------Cys(Tacm)-----------------------Cys(Tacm)-----------------]-OH

4) AgBF₄-anisole/TFA (0°C, 60 min.)
5) DTT (25°C, 3 h)
6) Sephadex G-25 (1N AcOH)
7) air-oxidation (pH 7.5)
8) FPLC purification

Synthetic human BNP-32

Figure 3–9. Solid-phase synthesis of hBNP32.

homologous with that of pBNP32. The 32-peptide form has been assumed to be a minimum endogenous form of hBNP (Sudoh et al., 1989). The di-Tacm hBNP32 was prepared by the Fmoc-based solid-phase method, followed by deprotection with 1 M HBF₄-thioanisole/TFA in the presence of m-cresol and ethanedithiol (0°C, 1 h), and then purified with FPLC as described. The product was treated with AgBF₄ in essentially the same manner. After air oxidation at pH 7.5, purification was similarly carried out (Figure 3–9; the yield was 19%, calculated from the starting resin). The purity of synthetic hBNP32 was confirmed by analytical HPLC (Figure 3–10, A–C) and amino acid analysis after levicine aminopeptidase (LAP) digestion. The purified product was proved to be a monomer by FAB-MS

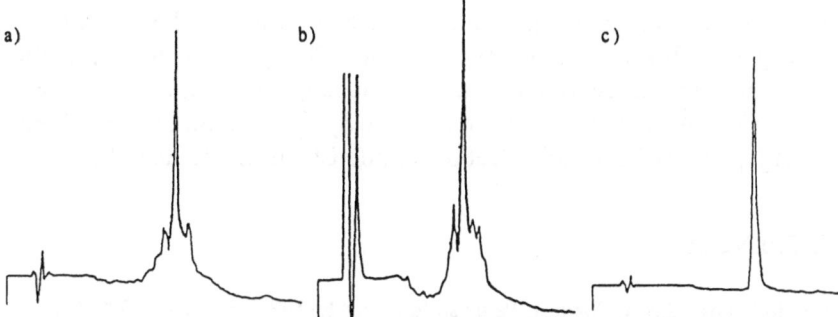

Figure 3–10. HPLC pattern of synthetic hBNP32. Column, YMC AM-302 (4.6 × 150 mm; eluant, 0.1% aqueous TFA with MeCN (10%–60%, 30 min; flow rate, 0.7 ml/min (retention time, 15.7 min, Tacm form; 13.2 min, disulfide form). **A.** FPLC-purified Tacm form. **B.** Crude air-oxidized form. **C.** FPLC-purified nBNP32.

[the observed mass value, 3463.7 (MH⁺), agreed well with the theoretical value, 3463.748].

In addition to the syntheses just described, several newly isolated natriuretic peptides [eel ANP (Takei et al., 1989), porcine CNP (Sudoh et al., 1990), eel CNP (Takei et al., 1990), and killifish CNP (Price et al., 1990)] have been successfully synthesized using the combination of the S-Tacm group and the $AgBF_4$ reagent. The details of these syntheses are to be published elsewhere.

Conclusion

We have successfully synthesized several natriuretic peptides by the solution-phase or solid-phase method using the S-Tacm group in combination with its selective deprotection procedure ($AgBF_4$/TFA). These excellent results show that the S-Tacm group is useful for the synthesis of cystine-containing peptides.

Addendum

After this manuscript had been submitted for publication, we reported a new method for disulfide bond formation using a silyl chloride-sulfoxide system. We have succeeded in the synthesis of natriuretic peptides using the S-Tacm group in combination with this new disulfide bond-forming procedure. For details of the synthetic methods, see Akaji et al. (1991, 1992, 1993a, 1993b).

Acknowledgments

This work was presented in part at the 26th Symposium on Peptide Chemistry of Japan, Tokyo, October 1988, Peptide Chemistry 1988, p. 201; the 27th Symposium on Peptide Chemistry of Japan, Shizuoka, October 1989, Peptide Chemistry 1989, p. 33; and the 28th Symposium on Peptide Chemistry of Japan, Osaka, October 1988, Peptide Chemistry 1990, p. 89.

REFERENCES

Albercio F, Grandas A, Porta A, Pedroso E, Giralt E (1987): *Synthesis* 1987:271.
Akaji K, Yoshida M, Tatsumi T, Kimura T, Fujiwara Y, Kiso Y (1990): *J Chem Soc Chem Commun* 1990:288.
Akaji K, Tatsumi T, Yoshida M, Kimura T, Fujiwara Y, Kiso Y (1991): *J Chem Soc, Chem Commun* 1991:167.

Akaji K, Tatsumi T, Yoshida M, Kimura T, Fujiwara Y, Kiso Y (1992): *J Am Chem Soc* 114:4137.

Akaji K, Nakagawa Y, Fujiwara Y, Fujino K, Kiso Y (1993a): *Chem Pharm Bull* 41:1244.

Akaji K, Fujino K, Tatsumi T, Kiso Y (1993b): *J Am Chem Soc* 115:11384.

Brtnik F, Krojidlo M, Barth T, Jost K (1981): *Collect Czech Chem Commun* 46:286.

Chakravaty PK, Olsen RK (1978): *J Org Chem* 343:1270.

Einhorn A (1905): *Justus Liebig Ann Chem* 343:207.

Fujii N, Otaka A, Watanabe T, Okamachi A, Tamamura H, Yajima H, Inagaki Y, Nomizu M, Asano K (1989): *J Chem Soc Chem Commun* 1989:283.

Guttmann S (1966): *Helv Chim Acta* 49:83.

Hiskey RG (1981): In: *The Peptides*, Vol. 3, Gross E, Meienhofer J, eds., p. 137. New York: Academic Press.

Kamber B, Hartmann A, Eisler K, Riniker B, Rink H, Sieber P, Rittel W (1980): *Helv Chim Acta* 63:899.

Kimura T, Takai M, Masui Y, Morikawa T, Sakakibara S (1981): *Biopolymers* 20:1823.

Kiso Y, Satomi M, Ukawa K, Akita T (1980): *J Chem Soc Chem Commun* 1980:1063.

Kiso Y, Shimokura M, Hosoi S, Fujisaki T, Fujiwara Y, Yoshida M (1987): *J Protein Chem* 6:147.

Kiso Y, Yoshida M, Kimura T, Fujiwara Y, Shimokura M (1989): *Tetrahedron Lett* 30:1979.

Kiso Y, Yoshida M, Fujiwara Y, Kimura T, Shimokura M, Akaji K (1990a): *Chem & Pharm Bull (Tokyo)* 38:673.

Kiso Y, Yoshida M, Kimura T, Fujiwara Y, Shimokura M, Akaji K (1990b): *Chem & Pharm Bull (Tokyo)* 38:1192.

Nishimura O, Kitada C, Fujino M (1978): *Chem & Pharm Bull (Tokyo)* 26:1576.

Price DA, Doble KE, Lee TD, Galli SM, Dunn BM, Parten B, Evans DH (1990): *Biol Bull* 178:279.

Sieber P, Kamber B, Riniker B, Rittel W (1980): *Helv Chim Acta* 63:2358.

Storey HT, Beacham J, Cernosek SF, Finn FM, Yanaihara C, Hofmann K (1972): *J Am Chem Soc* 94:6170.

Sudoh T, Minamino N, Kangawa K, Matsuo H (1988a): *Biochem Biophys Res Commun* 155:762.

Sudoh T, Kangawa K, Minamino N, Matsuo H (1988b): *Nature (London)* 332:78.

Sudoh T, Maekawa K, Kojima M, Minamino N, Kangawa K, Matsuo H (1989): *Biochem Biophys Res Commun* 159:1427.

Sudoh T, Minamino N, Kangawa K, Matsuo H (1990): *Biochem Biophys Res Commun* 168:863.

Takei Y, Takahashi A, Watanabe TX, Nakajima K, Sakakibara S (1989): *Biochem Biophys Res Commun* 164:537.

Takei Y, Takahashi A, Watanabe TX, Nakajima K, Sakakibara S, Takao T, Shimonishi Y (1990): *Biochem Biophys Res Commun* 170:883.

Veber DF, Milkowski JD, Valga SL, Denkewalter RG, Hirschmann R (1972): *J Am Chem Soc* 94:5456.

Yajima H, Fujii N, Ogawa H, Kawatani H (1974): *J Chem Soc Chem Commun* 1974:107.

Yoshida M, Akaji K, Tatsumi T, Iinuma S, Fujiwara Y, Kimura T, Kiso Y (1990a): *Chem & Pharm Bull (Tokyo)* 38:273.

Yoshida M, Tatsumi T, Fujiwara Y, Iinuma S, Kimura T, Akaji K, Kiso Y (1990b): *Chem & Pharm Bull (Tokyo)* 38:1551.

4

SOLID-PHASE SYNTHESIS OF CYCLIC PEPTIDES

Steven A. Kates, Núria A. Solé, Fernando Albericio, and George Barany

Introduction

Interest in cyclic peptides dates back almost half a century to the discovery that the antibiotic gramicidin S is a cyclic decapeptide (Consden et al., 1947). Since then, numerous naturally occurring cyclic antibiotics and toxins have been found. Many of these are *homodetic,* that is, with only peptide (lactam) linkages connecting the constituent amino acid residues, whereas others are *heterodetic,* and include other functions such as disulfide, ester (lactone), ether, or thioether bridges that contribute to the ring(s). Duplication of the natural cycles, and the introduction of unnatural rings, have attracted the attention of chemists because of the extra level of synthetic complexity of such endeavors. Concurrently, a variety of biological studies have suggested that cyclic structures may exhibit improved metabolic stabilities, increased potencies, better receptor selectivities, and more controlled bioavailabilities. Further, the constrained geometries of cyclic peptides are conducive to conformational investigations, and for modeling and/or "locking" key secondary structural elements in protein folding. Early synthetic work focused on peptides with a small ring size, particularly cyclic hexapeptides. With the development of improved methods for peptide synthesis, larger ring sizes and more complex targets have become acces-

Peptides: Design, Synthesis, and Biological Activity
Channa Basava and G. M. Anantharamaiah, Editors
©1994 *Birkhäuser Boston*

sible. The natural occurrence, biological significance, design, and applications of cyclic peptides, as well as synthetic aspects, have been covered in several excellent review articles (Andreu et al., in press; Blout, 1981; Bodanszky, 1984; Hruby, 1982; Hruby et al., 1990a; Kessler, 1982; Kopple, 1972; Mutter et al., 1992; Ovchinnikov and Ivanov, 1982; Rizo and Gierasch, 1992; Schmidt, 1986; Tonelli, 1986).

Cyclic peptides are usually prepared either entirely in solution, or by solid-phase chain assembly of the linear sequence, followed by release from the support and cyclization in solution. Despite the best efforts to develop practical and convenient protocols, classical solution methodologies have limitations. Cyclodimerizations and cyclo-oligomerizations may occur even under high dilution, usually as unwanted side reactions, but occasionally to benefit for certain symmetrical targets (Andreu et al., in press; Hamada et al., 1985; König and Geiger, 1981; Kopple, 1972; Rothe et al., 1977; Schwyzer and Gorup, 1958).

Within the past two decades, numerous examples have shown that cyclizations could be performed while peptides remained anchored to polymeric supports. The solid-phase mode may be advantageous because of *pseudo-dilution*, a kinetic phenomenon that favors intramolecular reactions over intermolecular side reactions (Albericio et al., 1991; Barany and Merrifield, 1979; Mazur and Jayalekshmy, 1979). Additional general advantages of solid-phase synthesis, including the ability to drive reactions to completion with excess soluble reagents, the removal of soluble reactants and by-products by simple filtration and washing without manipulative losses, and the amenability to automation, are also relevant to the specific case of cyclic peptide synthesis.

This chapter surveys the literature on those syntheses of cyclic peptides in which all steps have been carried out in the solid-phase mode. We take as a given efficient assemblies of the linear sequences by standard N^α-*tert*-butyloxycarbonyl (Boc) or N^α-9-fluorenylmethyloxycarbonyl (Fmoc) solid-phase chemistries with appropriate benzyl (Bzl), *tert*-butyl (*t*-Bu), or related side-chain protecting groups, as well as suitable anchoring linkages and optimized conditions for final deprotection/cleavage (Barany and Merrifield, 1979; Barany et al., 1987; Fields et al., 1992); our focus is on optimal procedures for homodetic or heterodetic cyclization(s). An important aspect of this discussion is the requirement for an *extra* level of selectively cleavable protecting groups and/or anchoring linkages, and the benefits of mild *orthogonal* chemistries are emphasized (Barany and Albericio, 1985; Barany and Merrifield, 1977, 1979). The simplest cyclic peptides, that is, 2,5-diketopiperazines (DKPs), are generally encountered as an undesired side reaction to solid-phase peptide synthesis (Barany and Merrifield, 1979; Gisin and Merrifield, 1972) and are not discussed here (however, see Giralt et al., 1985, for intentional DKP synthesis). It should be stressed that the extent to which a cyclization procedure is successful, either in solution or while resin-bound, depends primarily on the conformational preferences of the linear form of the target sequence, as well as on solvent, concentration, and temperature effects.

Homodetic Peptides

Four general topologies of medium- and long-range lactam cyclization of peptides have been demonstrated (Scheme 4–1). A ring may be formed *via* cyclization of the amino and carboxyl groups of the N- and C-termini, that is, head to tail or end to end. Alternatively, side-chain functional groups, usually the ω-amino group of lysine or ornithine together with the ω-carboxylate function of aspartic acid or glutamic acid, can provide a site for lactam formation. This type of cyclization is referred to as "side-chain to side-chain" or "backbone to backbone" cyclization. Third, cyclization can occur through a side-chain to end group (either "head" or "tail"), for example, the ω-amino function of Lys/Orn cyclizing with the C-terminal carboxyl, or the ω-carboxylate of Asp/Glu cyclizing with the N-terminal amino group. For the fourth class, a suitable lactam bridges two chains of a branched peptide, thus forming a ring.

Solid-phase synthesis of **head-to-tail** cyclic peptides was reported initially through intramolecular aminolysis of polymer-bound *o*-nitrophenyl

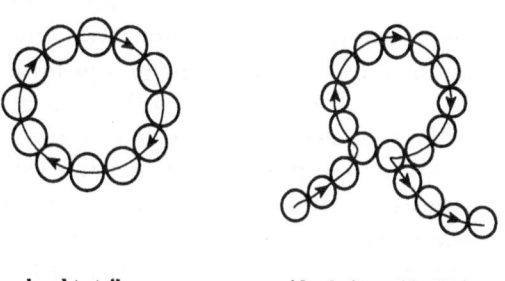

head to tail   side-chain to side-chain

side-chain to head (or tail)   branched

Scheme 4–1. Various topological arrangements of homodetic cyclic peptides. *Arrowheads* are oriented in N → C direction of main chain(s).

esters (Fridkin et al., 1965; see also Mitchell and Merrifield, 1985). After addition, deblocking, and neutralization of the final (N-terminal) amino acid residue, cyclization should proceed concurrent to release of the desired product from the resin. Relatedly, an active ester linkage could be formed, following peptide chain assembly, by "safety-catch" oxidation of a thioether to a sulfone (Flanigan and Marshall, 1970; Rothe et al., 1977). These strategies allowed syntheses of several small peptides lacking hindered side-chains, but failed for an attempted synthesis of the cyclic decapeptide antamanide on an *o*-nitrobenzyl-resin (Giralt et al., 1984). Additional concerns with these methodologies include possible premature loss of chains from the support, racemization, and oligomerization.

The strategy of forming cyclic peptides by intramolecular aminolysis of an electronically activated anchoring linkage was extended independently in two laboratories (Nishino et al., 1992a; Ösapay et al., 1990, 1991), both of which exploited the acid-stable *p*-nitrobenzophenone oxime-resin developed originally by DeGrado and Kaiser (1980, 1982). In Taylor's work (Ösapay et al., 1990), linear chain assembly of the decapeptide tyrocidine A was carried out by Boc/Bzl chemistry, and the N-terminus was exposed by deprotection with trifluoroacetic acid (TFA)–CH_2Cl_2 (1:3) and neutralization with N,N-diisopropylethylamine (DIEA) (1.5 equiv). Simultaneous cyclization/cleavage occurred on 24 h of reaction at 25°C in CH_2Cl_2, with a yield of 55%; the overall yield after final deprotection and purification was 30%. Acetic acid, which usually accelerates cleavage of peptides from oxime-resin, did not affect the cyclization rate. To achieve pseudo-dilution and avoid interchain side reactions, the substitution level of the oxime resin was lowered to 0.11 mmol/g by capping excess groups by acetylation. It should be noted that Boc chemistry is required for this strategy because the secondary amines used for deprotection in Fmoc chemistry are incompatible with oxime linkages. Even so, peptide chain elongation with Boc-amino acids requires the BOP procedure with *in situ* neutralization by DIEA, which is added to avoid premature cleavage of peptide from the resin.

Nishino et al. (1992a) used the oxime-resin to prepare *cyclo*(Arg-Gly-Asp-Phg), a cyclic tetrapeptide with inhibitory activity toward cell adhesion. Following removal of the N-terminal Boc group, the peptide-resin (0.5 mmol/g) was treated with acetic acid (HOAc)–triethylamine (TEA) (2 equiv each) in N,N-dimethylformamide (DMF) at 25°C to effect cyclization of the peptide over a 24-h period (50%–70% cleavage yield). These studies showed that the extent of oligomerization depended significantly on the choice of C-terminal residue. In related work (Xu et al., 1992), the same strategy gave a protected cyclic decapeptide [D-pyrenylalanine[4,4']]gramicidin S. Oxime-resin (0.5 mmol/g) was used to obtain the desired cyclic monomer in 45% overall yield, with only 8% dimerized product. The high overall yield was attributed to the ability of the linear precursor peptide to undergo a β-turn and cyclize rapidly with minimal oligomerization.

Another strategy for the preparation of head to tail cyclic peptides is to anchor the peptide to the support *via* a side-chain. The principle was demonstrated first in an elegant bidirectional synthesis of *cyclo*(Gly-His)$_3$ by Isied et al. (1982). An aminomethyl polystyrene-resin (0.2 mmol/g) was treated successively with 1,5-difluoro-2,4-dinitrobenzene and Boc-His-OH. In this way, a side-chain anchored analog of the N^{im}-2,4-dinitrophenyl (Dnp) histidine protecting group was created. Next, the free C^{α}-carboxyl group was activated with N,N'-dicyclohexylcarbodiimide (DCC)/1-hydroxybenzotriazole (HOBt), and H-Gly-OBzl was added. Further chain elongation in the C → N direction with Boc-Gly-OH and Boc-His(Dnp)-OH gave the linear hexapeptide protected at the C-terminus with a benzyl ester group and at the N-terminus with a Boc group. Removal of the terminal protecting groups was achieved with two 30 min treatments by 40% HBr/HOAc–TFA–CH$_2$Cl$_2$ (2:1:1); under these conditions, the Dnp anchor and His side-chain protecting groups were stable. The peptide-resin was washed with CH$_2$Cl$_2$ and neutralized with pyridine. Cyclization occurred *via* two activations of the C-terminus with 3 equiv of *N*-(ethoxycarbonyl)-2-ethoxy-1,2-dihydroxyquinone (EEDQ) in pyridine–toluene (1:1) at 25°C for 24 h. The peptide was released from the resin (85% cleavage yield) by treatment with deoxygenated 1.5 M thiophenol in DMF for 6 h at 25°C; the overall purified yield was 42%, and there was no evidence for linear or oligomeric peptides.

A more general method for using side-chain anchoring to obtain head to tail cyclic peptides is by attachment of Asp/Glu *via* their ω-carboxyls to hydroxymethyl or benzhydrylamine (BHA)-resins, with the expectation that the corresponding peptides containing Asp/Glu or Asn/Gln, respectively, will be obtained after final cleavage. Rovero et al. (1991) prepared the tachykinin antagonist MEN 10207, *cyclo*(Asp-Tyr-D-Trp-Val-D-Trp-D-Trp-Arg) according to this plan. The linear peptide was assembled on a phenylacetamidomethyl (PAM)-resin (0.35 mmol/g); the α-carboxylate of the anchored Asp residue was protected as its fluorenylmethyl (OFm) ester. Peptide chain elongation was by Boc/Bzl chemistry, following which TFA–CH$_2$Cl$_2$ (1:1) treatment, 5 + 15 min, removed the Boc group at the N-terminus, and piperidine–CH$_2$Cl$_2$ (1:4), 3 + 7 min, removed the OFm group at the C-terminus. The cyclization was accomplished with two separate additions of benzotriazol-1-yloxytris(dimethylamino)phosphonium hexafluorophosphate (BOP) (Castro et al., 1975; Coste et al., 1990) (3 equiv) and DIEA (6 equiv), in DMF for 3 h at 25°C. HF cleavage and purification gave the desired peptide with an estimated overall yield of 46%.

Tromelin et al. (1992) reported the synthesis of a head to tail cyclic peptide by a strategy whereby C-terminal Asp was converted to Asn on cleavage of the support. To prepare a peptide corresponding to a loop involved in the curaremimetic action of a snake toxic protein, *cyclo*(Asn-Tyr-Lys-Lys-Val-Trp-Arg-Asp-His-Arg-Gly-Thr-Ile-Ile-Glu-Arg-Gly-Pro), 0.8 equiv of Boc-Asp-OFm was coupled onto a methylbenzhydryl amine

(MBHA)-resin to achieve a substitution of 0.4 mmol/g. After acetylation of excess MBHA sites, the peptide chain was assembled by Boc/Bzl chemistry. Following removal of the N-terminal Boc and the C-terminal OFm groups by standard methods, cyclization was achieved by two separate additions of BOP (3 equiv) and DIEA (6 equiv) in N-methylpyrrolidone (NMP) for 2 h at 25°C. HF cleavage followed by HPLC purification gave the desired monomeric peptide in 10% overall yield.

The first example of the side-chain anchoring strategy in Fmoc/t-Bu chemistry was reported by McMurray (1991). A 4-hydroxymethylphenoxy-acetylaminomethyl-resin (0.45 mmol/g) was used, and the α-carboxylate of the anchored Glu was protected as a 2,4-dimethoxybenzyl (Dmb) ester. The Dmb group could be removed by 1% TFA in CH_2Cl_2, which will not affect t-Bu and 2,2,5,7,8-pentamethylchroman-6-sulfonyl (Pmc) side-chain protecting groups, although these conditions are still not compatible with triphenylmethyl (trityl or Trt) protection for residues such as Cys and His. As an example, McMurray chose cyclo(Ala-Ala-Arg-D-Phe-Pro-Glu-Asp-Asn-Tyr-Glu), a rearranged sequence derived from the autophosphorylation site of the tyrosine kinase pp60[C-SIC]. The linear sequence was assembled, and the C- and N-termini were exposed, in that order, by respective treatments at 25°C with 1% TFA in CH_2Cl_2, 6 × 5 min, and piperidine–DMF (1:4), 8 min. Next, cyclization was performed with N,N'-diisopropyl-carbodiimide (DIPCDI) and HOBt (3 equiv each) in DMF for 16 h at 25°C. The peptide was cleaved from the resin, and t-Bu side-chain protecting groups were removed by overnight treatment with TFA–phenol (19:1). Gel filtration was carried out to remove oligomers, and the monomeric peptide was obtained in 32% yield (22% after additional purification by DEAE–Sephadex chromatography). The cyclic peptide was also obtained in similar overall yield with a similar level of oligomers after cyclization for 1 h by BOP/HOBt/N-methylmorpholine (NMM) (3 equiv each) in DMF. Thus, it was concluded that the BOP process, although faster, had no advantages in terms of yield or purity.

An ideal strategy to obtain head to tail cyclic peptides is through a three-dimensional orthogonal protection scheme. This has been accomplished independently by Bannwarth, Albericio, and their respective co-workers using an Fmoc/t-Bu/allyl scheme (Albericio et al., 1993; Kates et al., 1993a; Trzeciak and Bannwarth, 1992). Deprotection of allyl derivatives occurs smoothly and quantitatively by mild palladium-catalyzed transfer. Reactive carbocations are not formed and undesired back-alkylation side reactions are avoided. Further, allyl derivatives couple more efficiently than do t-Bu-based derivatives because they have lower steric hindrance and a more hydrophilic character.

Trzeciak and Bannwarth (1992) attached the free β-carboxyl side-chain of Asp either to an amide linker-resin or to Wang's 4-hydroxymethylphenoxy-resin as the starting point for preparation of two cyclic hexapeptides:

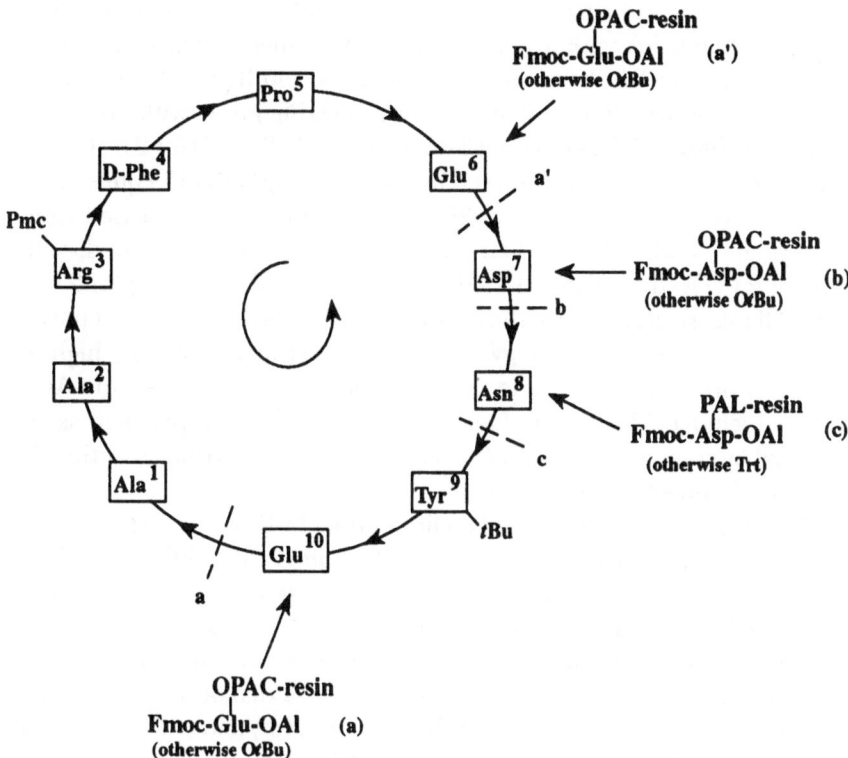

Scheme 4–2. Four synthetic strategies to McMurray's cyclic decapeptide. *Counter-clockwise arrow* in center of diagram shows direction of linear chain growth by Fmoc chemistry. *Arrowheads* between successive residues in sequence are oriented in N → C direction. Starting resins are drawn alongside target structure; final bond that must be formed to achieve cyclization in each strategy is indicated by perpendicular dashed line. (From Kates et al., 1993a.)

cyclo(Lys-Arg-Ser-Lys-Gly-X), where X = Asp or Asn. Chain elongation proceeded with standard Fmoc/*t*-Bu chemistry, with 2-(1H-benzotriazol-1-yl)-1,1,3,3-tetramethyluronium tetrafluoroborate (TBTU) couplings. Following incorporation of the N-terminal amino acid, the allyl ester was cleaved selectively with tetrakistriphenylphosphine palladium (0) [Pd(PPh$_3$)$_4$] and *N*-methylmorpholine in THF–DMSO–0.5 *N* HCl (2:2:1). Cyclization of the head to tail peptide was accomplished with TBTU activation, and final cleavage/deprotection was accomplished with TFA–H$_2$O (9:1).

Kates et al. (1993a) applied this methodology for the preparation of McMurray's sequence according to four different variations (Scheme 4–2). Retrosynthetic analysis revealed that the peptide may be derived from the following starting resins: (a) Fmoc-Glu(OPAC-PEG-PS)-OAl at positions Glu^6 and Glu^{10}; (b) Fmoc-Asp(OPAC-PEG-PS)-OAl at position Asp^7; and (c) Fmoc-Asp(OPAL-PEG-PS)-OAl at position Asn^8. In strategy c, Asn^8 was derived from an aspartic acid with its β-carboxylate bound to the resin *via* the 5-(4-(9-fluorenylmethyloxycarbonyl)aminomethyl-3,5-dimethoxyphenoxy)valeric acid (PAL) handle. Syntheses were carried out on a Millipore 9050 continuous-flow synthesizer. Removal of the allyl-protecting group with Pd(PPh$_3$)$_4$ (3 equiv) in DMSO–THF–0.5 N HCl–morpholine (2:2:1:0.1) for 2 h at 25°C, and N^α-Fmoc removal, was followed by BOP/HOBt/NMM (5 equiv each)-mediated cyclization for 2–5 h at 25°C. The peptides were released from the supports, and t-Bu side-chain protecting groups were removed, with Reagent R (TFA–thioanisole–1,2-ethanedithiol–anisole, 90:5:3:2) for 2 h at 25°C. All four strategies gave the desired peptide; the best yield and purity occurred with the Asn[8] strategy, and the Glu[10] strategy gave the highest level of by-products. The crude peptide product obtained from the Asn[8] strategy included 71% of the desired monomeric cyclized product, as ascertained by comparison of HPLC peak areas with those from an authentic standard of known concentration.

The solid-phase preparation of cyclic peptides by Fmoc/t-Bu/allyl-based methods was automated in a follow-up study (Kates et al., 1993b). Standard allyl removal uses a suspended palladium catalyst. This approach is not feasible on batch and continuous-flow peptide synthesizers because of problems with delivery of insoluble materials. Solvent conditions were required to solubilize the catalyst, prevent undesired Fmoc deblocking, and to be compatible with sensitive amino acids (Trp and Met) and with glyco- and sulfo-peptides. To avoid a biphasic system, HCl was replaced with HOAc, a mild organic acid that is compatible with sensitive functions. CHCl$_3$ was chosen as the solvent because it completely dissolves the palladium catalyst. Last, a weak tertiary base, NMM (which does not remove N^α-Fmoc functions), was added. Thus allyl removal could be achieved with Pd(PPh$_3$)$_4$ (1 equiv) in the optimized solvent of CHCl$_3$–HOAc–NMM (37:2:1), for 2 h at 25°C, followed by washings with a solution of 0.5% DIEA and 0.5% sodium diethyldithiocarbamate in DMF. For the cyclization step, phosphonium or uronium salts were added to an amino acid vial, and a solution of DIEA in DMF was delivered to dissolve the solids. This activation solution was then delivered to the peptide-resin with free end groups for the cyclization to occur; continuous-flow recycling continued until the peptide-resin was ninhydrin negative. The effectiveness of these conditions was demonstrated by the automated synthesis of Rovero's peptide, with results by the automated approach comparable to those from manual cyclization.

The first method for the preparation of **side-chain to side-chain** cyclic lactam peptides was developed by Schiller et al. (1985). Linear peptides could be assembled on BHA-resins (0.4 mmol/g) using N^α-Fmoc-amino acids with Bzl side-chain protecting groups, and using Boc and t-Bu to protect the amino and carboxylate side-chain functions that needed to be joined for the cycle. Boc and t-Bu groups were removed with TFA–CH$_2$Cl$_2$ (1:1) for 30 min, and after neutralization with DIEA–CH$_2$Cl$_2$ (1:9), 2 + 10 min, fresh DCC/HOBt (2.5 equiv each) in DMF was added every 48 h for 5–10 days to cyclize the liberated side-chains. Subsequently, HF treatment for 1 h at 0°C cleaved the peptide from the solid support and removed Bzl side-chain protecting groups. Cyclic peptide opioid analogs including $cyclo^{2,5}$(Tyr-D-Lys-Gly-Phe-Glu), $cyclo^{2,4}$(Tyr-D-Lys-Phe-Glu), $cyclo^{2,4}$(Tyr-D-Orn-Gly-Glu) were obtained in 6%–22% yield by this method.

In a later study, Schiller et al. (1988) reported a generalization of the original strategy, which allowed the preparation of more demanding and larger cyclic peptides, for example, $cyclo^{5,8}$(Tyr-Gly-Gly-Phe-Orn-Arg-Arg-Asp-Arg-Pro-Lys-Leu-Lys-NH$_2$) and $cyclo^{5,10}$(Tyr-Gly-Gly-Phe-Orn-Arg-Arg-Ile-Arg-Asp-Lys-Leu-Lys-NH$_2$), which are cyclic analogs of dynorphin A-(1–13). The linear sequences were assembled on MBHA-resins using Boc/Bzl chemistry for the C-terminal sections and switching to Fmoc/Bzl chemistry for the sections spanning the eventual lactam. The Boc and t-Bu side-chain protecting groups for Orn and Asp, respectively, were then removed as usual, and after neutralization, DCC/HOBt (5 equiv) in DMF at 25°C (fresh DCC/HOBt was added every 2 days for 8 days) was used to close the rings. Subsequently, the N^α-Fmoc group was removed, and Boc/Bzl chemistry was used for the N-terminal sections to complete the synthesis. HF cleavage gave the free side-chain cyclized peptides (for related work, see Schiller et al., 1987, 1991).

The Schiller strategy was applied by Arttamangkul and Aldrich (in press) for the preparation of $cyclo$(D-Asp^2, Dap^5)DynA(1–13)-NH$_2$. The linear sequence was assembled on MBHA-resin (0.27 mmol/g) by Fmoc chemistry. Cyclizations mediated by 2-(1H-benzotriazol-1-yl)-1,1,3,3-tetramethyluronium hexafluorophosphate (HBTU) gave the poorest results, with the tetramethylguanidinium (Tmg) Schiff's base derivative to the ω-amino group of Dap as the major by-product (this side reaction was first described, in another context, by Gausepohl et al., 1992). BOP and DIPCDI/HOBt cyclization procedures were more successful, although 3 days of reaction at 25°C were required. Similarly, Neugebauer and Willick (1993) synthesized side-chain to side-chain lactam analogs of human parathyroid hormone. $Cyclo$(Lys^{26}, Asp^{30}), $cyclo$(Glu^{22}, Lys^{26}), and $cyclo$(Lys^{27}, Asp^{30})-Arg-Val-Glu-Trp-Leu-Arg-Lys-Lys-Leu-Gln-Asp-Val-His-Asn-Phe-NH$_2$, the 20–34 fragment of hPTH, were assembled on an MBHA-resin, using Boc/Bzl chemistry for the first 4 residues and Fmoc/Bzl chemistry for the rest. As in Schiller's later work, side-chain lactamization was achieved at an intermediate stage, after incorporation of the N-terminal component. The Boc and t-Bu-protecting groups were removed with TFA–CH$_2$Cl$_2$ (7:13), and neutralization occurred with DIEA–CH$_2$Cl$_2$ (1:9). Cyclization of those two peptides that did not contain Arg within the lactam occurred with TBTU/HOBt/DIEA (8 equiv each) for 2 h at 25°C. Cyclization for the Arg(Mtr)-containing lactam required a modified protocol because Arg was partially deblocked during the TFA cleavage.

A second general approach for the construction of side-chain to side-chain cyclic peptides was described by Felix et al. (1988a). Linear peptides could be assembled on BHA-resins (0.7 mmol/g) by Boc chemistry with Bzl side-chain protection. For the amino and carboxylate side-chains that must be cyclized, an Fmoc urethane and OFm ester, respectively, could be used. Separate model studies showed that these base-labile functions were sufficiently stable to the DIEA–CH_2Cl_2 (1:19) tertiary amine used to achieve neutralization at each Boc deprotection/coupling cycle. Selective orthogonal removal of Fmoc and OFm was achieved with piperidine–DMF (1:4), 1 + 20 min, followed by cyclization and finally HF cleavage. A significant aspect of Felix's work was the systematic investigation of cyclization agents, including the chronologically first use of Castro's BOP reagent for this purpose. For cyclo[3,12] [Ala[15]]-GRF(1–29)-NH_2, the best cyclization procedures involved BOP (2.5 equiv) in DMF containing an excess of TEA (2.8 equiv), for 4 h at 25°C. After washings, the cyclization was repeated twice for 11 and 3 h, respectively. The reaction also proceeded in CH_2Cl_2 as solvent (without base), and in DMF with lesser amounts of BOP, as judged by quantitative ninhydrin analysis for residual amino sites. On the other hand, cyclizations mediated by DCC/HOBt, bis-(2-oxo-3-oxazolidinyl)phosphinic chloride (BOP-Cl), and diphenylphosphoryl azide (DPPA) revealed low yields and numerous by-products. The best procedures were readily generalized for the syntheses of cyclo[8,12][Asp[8], Ala[15]]-GRF(1–29)-NH_2, stereoisomers of cyclo[8,12][D-Ala[2], Asp[8], Ala[15]]-GRF(1–29)-NH_2 and 1,2-disubstituted analogs of cyclo[8,12][Asp[8], Ala[15]]-GRF(1–29)-NH_2 (Felix et al., 1988b).

Comprehensive applications of both Schiller's and Felix's methods are due to Hruby in the α-melanocyte stimulating hormone (α-MSH), glucagon, and oxytocin systems (Hruby et al., 1990b). An elegant aspect of these studies has been the incorporation of D-amino acids in the analog design, based on the idea that cyclizations might be facilitated by altering conformations of the linear precursors. For these syntheses, chloromethyl or MBHA-resins were loaded in the 0.2 to 0.45 mmol/g range to minimize cyclodimerizations. Hruby confirmed Felix's results on the superiority of the BOP reagent with respect to DIPCDI/HOBt and DPPA. Cyclizations were faster (complete in 2 h, as compared to 12 h–2 days) and provided peptides of higher purity in greater overall yields (e.g., 60% by solid-phase chemistry compared to 35% in solution).

The first report on allyl chemistry for the synthesis of side-chain to side-chain lactams was by Lyttle and Hudson (1992). A human GRF (1–29) sequence, previously made by Felix, was assembled on PAL-PEG-PS-resin using N^α-Fmoc-amino acids with t-Bu side-chain protection, except that Asp[3] and Lys[12] were incorporated into the linear chain as Fmoc-Asp(OAl)-OH and Fmoc-Lys(Aloc)-OH, respectively. Allyl functions were removed by treatment of the fully protected peptide-resin with Pd(PPh$_3$)$_4$, morpholine, and triphenylphosphine in dry THF at 25°C for 24 h, and cyclization was achieved in a yield of greater than 50% by treatment with BOP.

A different orthogonal strategy for side-chain to side-chain cyclic peptides was devised by Taylor and co-workers (Bouvier and Taylor, 1992; Ösapay and Taylor, 1990). In one example, Boc-glutamate was attached to an oxime-resin *via* its γ-carboxyl side chain, while the α-carboxyl was protected by a phenacyl (Pac) function. The linear heptapeptide Boc-Lys(2ClZ)-Leu-Lys(Trt)-Glu(OBzl)-Leu-Lys(2ClZ)-Glu(oxime-resin)-OPac was assembled by fragment condensation. Selective removal of the Trt function from the ε-amino group at Lys[3] with TFA–trifluoroethanol (TFE)–CH$_2$Cl$_2$ (2:19:19), neutralization with DIEA–CH$_2$Cl$_2$ (1:19), and 3 days standing in CH$_2$Cl$_2$ in the presence of HOAc (10 equiv), allowed intramolecular displacement of the anchoring linkage and concomitant cyclization. The resultant cyclic peptide, obtained in 60% yield, retained side-chain protection and was thus a suitable building block for incorporation into a 21-residue tricyclic amphiphilic model peptide by segment condensation in solution.

Side-chain to head cyclic peptides can also be made by solid-phase methodology. A typical application is for the preparation of deaminodicarba analogs of disulfide-containing peptides in which two half-cystine residues are replaced by a single spanning α-aminosuberic acid (Asu) residue. This was carried out by Ho et al. (1990) for the synthesis of (Asu^{1,7})-eel calcitonin by a close variation of Schiller's method. Fmoc chemistry was used to assemble the linear sequence, with side-chain Bzl protection except for the *t*-Bu ester on Asu. The N-terminal Ser was introduced with Boc protection; TFA treatment exposed the functional groups for cyclization, and BOP/HOBt/DIEA (6 equiv each) in DMF for 24 h at 25°C closed the ring in greater than 90% yield. In addition, Nishino et al. (1992b) extended their method of cyclization/cleavage from an oxime-resin (discussed earlier) for the preparation of the cyclic portions of the same eel calcitonin analog, as well as that of (Asu^{1,6})oxytocin.

In a further illustration of solid-phase "side-chain to head" cyclic peptide synthesis, Plaué (1990) synthesized a series of cyclic peptides related to the 139–147 region of the hemagglutinin of influenza virus. Sequences were X-Lys-Arg-Gly-Pro-Gly-Ser-Asp-Phe-Y-Tyr-NH$_2$, where X = Cys, Ser and Y = Asp, Lys(ε-succinyl). The so-called "large-loop" peptides containing the succinyl unit were assembled by Boc/Bzl chemistry on MBHA-resins (0.1–0.6 mmol/g final loading, achieved by limiting the amount of the first residue). Boc-Lys(Fmoc)-OH was incorporated as a precursor for the site of cyclization. Following removal of the N-terminal Boc group, succinic anhydride and DIEA (3 equiv each) were added for 15 min, and the side-chain Fmoc group was subsequently removed with piperidine–DMF (1:1) for 3 + 7 min. Cyclizations were then effected at 25°C by BOP/HOBt/DIEA (3:3:7.5 equiv) in DMF, 2 h, as well as by DIPCDI/HOBt (3 equiv each) in DMF,

3×24 h. With the relatively slow kinetics provided by the DIPCDI reactions, the amount of cyclodimer increased from 8% to 19% over the substitution range investigated. The more rapid activation from BOP caused more oligomerization and thus a less pure product. Plaué's work also described the synthesis of "small-loop" peptides using Fmoc/Bzl chemistry (c-Hex protected Asp[146] to avoid the succinimide side reaction) on the MBHA-resin, and Fmoc-Asp(t-Bu)-OH and N^α-Boc terminal amino acid as the precursor for the site of cyclization. Removal of the N-terminal Boc group and of the t-Bu blocking the Asp side-chain with TFA–CH_2Cl_2 (13:20) for 45 min was followed by DIEA–DMF (1:9) treatment for 2×2 min. Cyclizations with DIPCDI/HOBt (3 equiv each) in DMF were complete in 48 h, indicating more facile folding for the "small" loop.

A **branched** cyclic peptide was prepared by Bloomberg et al. (1993) using Fmoc/t-Bu chemistry and combined allyl and 1-(4,4-dimethyl-2,6-dioxocyclohex-1-ylidine)ethyl (Dde) side-chain protection for glutamic acid and lysine residues, respectively. The first branch was assembled in the $C \rightarrow N$ direction by sequential coupling to a PAL-PEG-PS support of Fmoc-Lys(Dde)-OH, Fmoc-Ala-OH, Fmoc-Glu(OAl)-OH, Fmoc-Cys(Trt)-OH, and N-terminal acetylation. The Dde function was then removed with 1.5% hydrazine in DMF, and a second branch (10 residues) was added by Fmoc chemistry. Removal of the allyl group blocking the Glu side-chain with Pd(PPh$_3$)$_4$, and N^α-Fmoc removal to free the second branch, were followed by HBTU/HOBt/NMM cyclization. Finally, the crude cyclic peptide was deprotected and released from the resin with TFA–1,2-ethanedithiol–phenol–water–tri(iso-butyl)silane (92:3:2:2:1) for 2 h at 25°C.

Heterodetic Peptides

Of the various ways to close rings by covalent bonds other than amide linkages, the most accessible by solid-phase methodology are **disulfide bridges** (see Lebl and Hruby, 1984, for a pioneering approach to solid-phase syntheses of carba analogs of disulfide-containing peptide hormones). The ensuing discussion covers relevant examples that build on an extensive literature covering thiol protection and chemistry for disulfide formation (Andreu et al., in press; Büllesbach, 1992; Cavelier et al., 1989, 1990; Hiskey, 1981; König and Geiger, 1981; Photaki, 1976; Yajima et al., 1988).

One general strategy for resin-bound disulfide cyclization involves selective orthogonal unmasking of a pair of protected cysteine residues, followed by oxidation of the resultant peptide dithiol. Early examples used air or 1,2-diiodoethane as oxidizing agents (Bondi et al., 1968; Buchta et al., 1986; Gray et al., 1984; Inukai et al., 1968). An instructive example with Fmoc chemistry used TFA-labile p-alkoxybenzyl ester (0.3 mmol/g) anchoring as a starting point for synthesis of a decapeptide with S-tert-butylsulfenyl

(S-t-Bu) cysteine protection; orthogonal reduction with β-mercaptoethanol–DMF (1:1) for 5 h at 25°C was followed by overnight oxidation with 1 M aqueous potassium ferricyanide–DMF (1:10), at 25°C, to form an 8-residue cyclic disulfide in 60% overall yield (Eritja et al., 1987). An optimal example from Boc chemistry involves oxytocin, which was prepared on an HF-labile MBHA-resin (0.35 mmol/g) using S-9-fluorenylmethyl (S-Fm) protection for the cysteine residues (Albericio et al., 1991). S-Fm removal under an argon atmosphere with piperidine–DMF–β-mercaptoethanol (10:10:0.7), at 25°C for 3 h, gave the resin-bound dithiol, which was oxidized for 1 h with air or with 5,5-dithiobis(2-nitrobenzoic acid) (DTNB, 0.5 equiv) while the resin was suspended in "buffered" DMF (containing 0.1 M each of HOAc and NMM, with further NMM added to achieve a nominal pH of 7.5 at a glass electrode). The overall solid-phase yield of 60% was considerably better than the yield that resulted when the corresponding chemistry was carried out in solution, and marginally improved over a procedure in which solid-phase S-Fm removal with piperidine–DMF (1:1) at 25°C for 3 h gave *directly* a 6-residue cyclic disulfide (for other examples of the direct deprotection/oxidation protocol, which omits β-mercaptoethanol, see Albericio et al., 1991; García-Echeverría et al., 1989; Ponsati et al., 1990). Results using S-2,4-dinitrophenylethyl (Dnpe) in place of S-Fm were similar (Royo et al., 1992).

Resin-bound dithiols from several sequences could be generated by selective removal of S-2,4,6-trimethoxybenzyl (Tmob) from peptides prepared by Fmoc synthesis on PAL-resins. This was accomplished by treatment with TFA–CH$_2$Cl$_2$–tri(ethyl)silane–water (7:92:1:0.5), 2 × 13 min, at 25°C. Subsequent oxidation occurred with approximately 20 mM CCl$_4$–TEA (2 equiv each) in NMP, at 20°C for 4 h (Munson and Barany, 1993; Munson et al., 1993). These conditions were optimized carefully to maximize intramolecular cyclization and represent a balance between negligible reaction and excessive oligomerization.

A second general approach for solid-phase disulfide formation exploits oxidative reagents that allow concurrent pairwise deblocking/cyclization of suitable S-protected cysteine residues. Conditions optimized in solution can usually be transferred to the solid-phase mode, but it is preferable to use solvents that effectively swell the peptide-resin. DMF is near optimal in this regard for synthetic schemes based on either Boc or Fmoc. Typical conditions, for peptide-resin in the 0.15 to 0.3 mmol/g substitution level range, involve iodine (3–10 equiv = 0.03–0.08 M) at 25°C for 1–2 h, or thallium (III) trifluoroacetate [Tl(tfa)$_3$] (~1.2 equiv = 6 mM) at 0°C for 1–2 h, and peptides protected with S-acetamidomethyl (Acm), S-triphenylmethyl (trityl or Trt), and S-Tmob have been oxidized in this way (Albericio et al., 1991; Albrecht et al., 1992; Canas et al., 1993; Deadman et al., in press; Edwards et al., in press; Funakoshi et al., 1988; Munson and Barany, 1993; Munson et al., 1992; Seidel et al., 1990). S-Acm is compatible with both

Fmoc and Boc chemistry, whereas S-Trt and S-Tmob can only be used with the former. Yields of monomeric intramolecular disulfide-bridged peptides can be as high as 60%–90% by these solid-phase approaches. Everything else being equal, results are generally better using thallium rather than iodine for oxidation (Albericio et al., 1991; Edwards et al., in press; Munson et al., 1992), but it should be noted that Tl is not compatible with S-Trt (Albericio et al., 1991).

When acid-stable anchoring linkages such as MBHA or o-nitrobenzylamide (Nb) are used, TFA (which promotes good swelling) can be a helpful solvent for polymer-supported cyclization (Albericio et al., 1991). Interestingly, the same oxidizing reagents [I_2, Tl(tfa)$_3$, DMSO] in TFA could be applied with acid-labile anchoring linkages such as p-alkoxybenzyl or PAL; in these cases, excellent yields of disulfide-cyclized peptides could be obtained concurrently with deprotection and release of material into solution (Munson et al., 1992). In a different illustration of the general principle, Barlos et al. (1991) reported that iodine could be added to the dilute acid cocktail for cleavage of 2-chlorotritylresins; the resultant peptides included a disulfide bridge from oxidation of Cys(Trt), but other side-chain protecting groups remained intact.

Directed methods of disulfide bond formation can also be adopted to the solid-phase mode. The first example of this concept was provided by Mott et al. (1986) in a synthesis of oxytocin. Boc chemistry was used to assemble a linear octapeptide on a BHA-resin (0.17 mmol/g); Cys[6] was protected by S-Acm. Next, treatment with methoxycarbonylsulfenyl chloride (2 equiv) in CH_2Cl_2 (2×30 min) converted the S-Acm to an S-carbomethoxysulfenyl (Scm) function. The N^α-Boc group was removed from Tyr[2] by TFA–CH_2Cl_2 (3:7), and neutralization was carried out with a mild base, NMM–CH_2Cl_2, (1:19) to ensure the integrity of the base-labile Cys(Scm) residue. Next, Z-Cys(Trt)-OH was added by DCC-mediated coupling, and then a mixture of TFA–anisole–CH_2Cl_2 (15:2:3), 3×10 min, was used to remove the S-Trt group and expose the free β-thiol of Cys[1]. Finally, intramolecular displacement of Scm and concomitant cyclization was achieved by shaking with a solution of NMM–CH_2Cl_2 (1:19) for 16 h at 25°C. HF cleavage followed by reversed-phase MPLC purification provided the desired peptide monomer in an overall isolated yield of 29%.

Ploux et al. (1987) described a directed synthesis of a disulfide-containing analog of Substance P. A Boc/Bzl strategy was used for chain elongation on an MBHA-resin (0.12 mmol/g), with S-3-nitro-2-pyridinesulfenyl (Npys) and S-tBu protection, respectively, for Cys[9] and Cys[5]. Treatment of the protected peptide-resin with HF–anisole (1:3), 0°C for 1 h, removed the S-t-Bu moiety selectively from Cys[5]. This peptide resin was then filtered and washed with DMF; observed discoloration was taken as evidence that a rapid nucleophilic displacement of the S-Npys group by the free thiol had occurred. A further treatment of HF–anisole (9:1), 0°C for 1 h, gave the free cyclic peptide, which was a mixture of monomer and oligomers. After purification, the overall yield was 10%–17%. When methanol or CH_2Cl_2 was used instead of DMF, the amounts of undesired oligomers formed were greater.

An orthogonal synthesis of a parallel dimer of deamino-oxytocin relied on two intermolecular polymer-supported reactions to form disulfide bridges (Munson et al., 1993). The protection scheme involved acid-labile S-Tmob for the N-terminal Cys[1] residue, and S-Acm for the internal Cys[6] residue. Selective removal of S-Tmob and mild oxidation of the free thiols using CCl_4–TEA precluded formation of any intramolecular by-products and thus gave the corresponding pseudo-cyclic intermediate in high yield and purity. This resin-bound intermediate was treated with Tl(tfa)$_3$ to oxidatively remove vicinal S-Acm groups and form the desired target.

Conclusions and Future Challenges

This chapter has described a number of protection strategies and cyclization protocols for the solid-phase preparation of monomeric monocyclic peptides in which the rings have been closed by lactam or disulfide bridges. In many cases the solid-phase mode has proven to be advantageous with regard both to operational convenience and to the yields and purities observed for the desired products. In contrasting solution-phase and solid-phase cyclization approaches, it should be noted that unique to the latter are considerations of optimizing the polymeric support (mobility versus rigidity of network chains; polarity) and compatible solvent milieus that facilitate pseudo-dilution, and the question of how the results are influenced by substitution levels of the peptide-resins. To date, information on these points is fragmentary, and more, carefully controlled studies are required. With the continued development of powerful activating agents (Carpino, 1993) and versatile solid-phase supports (Barany et al., 1993; Eichler et al., 1991; Meldal, 1992; Small and Sherrington, 1989; Zalipsky et al., 1985), there is reason for optimism that further improvements will be forthcoming.

Within the past few years, a number of highly interesting *bicyclic* peptide targets have been described (Brady et al., 1993; Hill et al., 1990; Hruby, in press; Smith et al., 1992; Solé et al., in press; Spinella et al., 1991). These tightly constrained molecules with interlocking rings are based on natural peptides with two disulfides, or have had unnatural disulfide or side-chain lactam bridges "engineered" into their structures; they represent significant synthetic challenges. To the best of our knowledge, the only example in which two rings have both been constructed by orthogonal solid-phase chemistry is in a recent synthesis of α-conotoxin SI by Fmoc chemistry on PAL-PEG-PS, with S-Tmob and S-Acm protection for the two classes of paired

half-cystine residues (Munson and Barany, 1993). The more general expe-
riences from our and other laboratories suggest that solid-phase procedures
of the kind described throughout this chapter often facilitate construction
of the *first* of the two rings in a bicyclic target, but that the second cyclization step is typically conducted best in dilute solution after release of the
monocyclic intermediate from the support. The order in which the lactam
or disulfide bridges of the bicyclic target are formed can be critical in some
cases; it is usually preferable to form the smaller loop first. Systematic investigations on these issues are still at an early stage, and additional developments are awaited with interest.

The usefulness of solid-phase methodology for lactamization and disulfide bridge formation is clear. It is hoped that the general approach can be
extended to the synthesis of natural and engineered peptides with other
ring-forming linkages.

Acknowledgments

We are grateful to the National Institutes of Health (GM 28934, 42722,
43552) for support of some of the experimental work described herein.

Abbreviations

Amino acids and peptides are abbreviated and designated following the
rules of the IUPAC-IUB Commission of Biochemical Nomenclature in *J.
Biol. Chem.* 247:977-983 (1972). The following abbreviations are also used:

Acm, acetamidomethyl; Al, allyl; Aloc, allyloxycarbonyl; Asu, α-aminosuberic
acid; BHA, benzhydrylamine (resin); Boc, *tert*-butyloxycarbonyl; BOP,
benzotriazol-1-yloxytris-(dimethylamino)phosphonium hexafluorophosphate;
BOP-Cl, bis-(2-oxo-3-oxazolidinyl)phosphinic chloride; *t*-Bu, *tert*-butyl; Bzl,
benzyl; Dap, α,β-diaminopropionic acid; DCC, *N,N'*-dicyclohexylcarbodiimide;
Dde, 1-(4,4-dimethyl-2,6-dioxocyclohex-1-ylidine)ethyl; DIEA, *N,N*-diisopropyl-
ethylamine; DIPCDI, *N,N'*-diisopropylcarbodiimide; DKP, diketopiperazine;
Dmb, 2,4-dimethoxybenzyl; DMF, *N,N*-dimethylformamide; DMSO, dimethylsulfoxide; Dnp, 2,4-dinitrophenyl; Dnpe 2-(2,4-dinitrophenyl)ethyl; DPPA,
diphenylphosphoryl azide; DTNB, 5,5'-dithiobis(2-nitrobenzoic acid); EEDQ,
N-(ethoxycarbonyl)-2-ethoxy-1,2-dihydroxyquinone; Fm, 9-fluorenylmethyl;
Fmoc, 9-fluorenylmethyloxycarbonyl; HBTU, 2-(1H-benzotriazol-1-yl)-1,1,3,3-
tetramethyluronium hexafluorophosphate; *c*-Hex, cyclohexyl; HOAc, acetic
acid; HOBt, 1-hydroxybenzotriazole; HPLC, high performance liquid chromatography; MBHA, 4-methylbenzhydrylamine (resin); MPLC, medium pressure liquid chromatography; Mtr, 4-methoxy-2,3,6-trimethylbenzenesulfonyl;
Nb, *o*-nitrobenzyl; NMM, *N*-methylmorpholine; NMP, *N*-methylpyrrolidone;
Npys, 3-nitro-2-pyridinesulfenyl; Pac, phenacyl; PAC, *p*-alkoxybenzyl alcohol
handle; PAL, 5-(4-(9-fluorenylmethyloxycarbonyl)aminomethyl-3,5-

dimethoxyphenoxy)valeric acid handle; PAM, phenylacetamidomethyl (resin); Pd(PPh₃)₄, tetrakistriphenylphosphine palladium (0); PEG-PS, polyethylene glycol-polystyrene graft supports; Phg, phenylglycine; Pmc, 2,2,5,7,8-pentamethylchroman-6-sulfonyl; PS, polystyrene; Scm, methyloxycarbonyl-sulfenyl; S*t*-Bu, *tert*-butylsulfenyl; Reagent R, TFA–thioanisole–1-2 ethanedithiol–anisole (90:5:3:2); TBTU, 2-(1H-benzotriazol-1-yl)-1,1,3,3-tetramethyl-uronium tetrafluoroborate; TEA, triethylamine; Tl(tfa)₃, thallium (III) trifluoroacetate; Tmg, tetramethylguanidinium; Tmob, 2,4,6-trimethoxybenzyl; Trt, triphenylmethyl (trityl) ; TFA, trifluoroacetic acid; TFE, 2,2,2-trifluoroethanol; THF, tetrahydrofuran; Z, benzyloxycarbonyl.

Amino acid symbols denote the L-configuration unless indicated otherwise.

REFERENCES

Albericio F, Hammer RP, García-Echeverría C, Molins MA, Chang JL, Munson MC, Pons M, Giralt E, Barany G (1991): *Int J Pept Protein Res* 37:402–413.

Albericio F, Barany G, Fields GB, Hudson D, Kates SA, Lyttle MH, Solé NA (1993): In: *Peptides 1992*, Proceedings of the 22d European Peptide Symposium, Schneider CH, Eberle AN, eds., pp. 191–193. Leiden: Escom.

Albrecht E, Harada Y, Cooper GJS, Jones H, Lehman de Gaeta LS (1992): In: *Peptides: Chemistry and Biology*, Proceedings of the 12th American Peptide Symposium, Smith JA, Rivier JE, eds., pp. 441–442. Leiden: Escom.

Andreu D, Albericio F, Solé NA, Munson MC, Ferrer M, Barany G: In: *Peptide Synthesis and Purification Protocols*, Pennington MW, Dunn BM, eds. Clifton, New Jersey: Humana Press (in press).

Arttamangkul S, Aldrich JV: In: *Peptides: Chemistry, Structure and Biology*, Proceedings of the 13th American Peptide Symposium, Hodges RS, Smith JA, eds. Leiden: Escom (in press).

Barany G, Albericio F (1985): *J Am Chem Soc* 107:4936–4942.

Barany G, Merrifield RB (1977): *J Am Chem Soc* 99:7363–7365.

Barany G, Merrifield RB (1979): In: *The Peptides*, Gross E, Meienhofer J, eds., pp. 1–284. New York: Academic Press.

Barany G, Kneib-Cordonier N, Mullen DG (1987): *Int J Pept Protein Res* 30:705–739.

Barany G, Albericio F, Solé NA, Griffin GW, Kates SA, Hudson D (1993): In: *Peptides 1992*, Proceedings of the 22d European Peptide Symposium, Schneider CH, Eberle AN, eds., pp. 267–268. Leiden: Escom.

Barlos K, Gatos D, Kutsogianni S, Papaphotiou G, Poulos C, Tsegenidis T (1991): *Int J Pept Protein Res* 38:562–568.

Bloomberg GB, Askin D, Gargaro AR, Tanner MJA (1993): *Tetrahedron Lett* 34:4709–4712.

Blout ER (1981): *Biopolymers* 20:1901–1912.

Bodanszky M (1984): *Principles of Peptide Synthesis*. Berlin: Springer-Verlag.

Bondi E, Fridkin M, Patchornik A (1968): *Isr J Chem* 6:22p.

Bouvier M, Taylor JW (1992): *J Med Chem* 35:1145–1155.

Brady SF, Paleveda WJ, Jr., Arison BH, Saperstein R, Brady EJ, Raynor K, Reisine T, Veber DF, Freidinger RM (1993): *Tetrahedron* 49:3449–3466.

Buchta R, Bondi E, Fridkin M (1986): *Int J Pept Protein Res* 28:289–297.

Büllesbach EE (1992): *Kontakte (Darmstadt)* 1:21–29.

Canas M, Jodas G, Albericio F, Andreu D, García-Antón JM, Parente A, Ponsati B (1993): In: *Peptides 1992*, Proceedings of the 22d European Peptide Symposium, Schneider CH, Eberle AN, eds., pp. 401–402. Leiden: Escom.

Carpino LA (1993): *J Am Chem Soc* 115:4397–4398.

Castro B, Dormoy JR, Evin G, Selve C (1975): *Tetrahedron Lett* 16:1219–1222.

Cavelier F, Daunis J, Jacquier R (1989): *Bull Soc Chim Fr* 788–798.

Cavelier F, Daunis J, Jacquier R (1990): *Bull Soc Chim Fr* 210–225.

Consden RJ, Gordon AH, Martin AJP, Synge RDM (1947): *Biochem J* 41:596–602.

Coste J, Le-Nguyen D, Castro B (1990): *Tetrahedron Lett* 31:205–208.

Deadman U, Lu X, Moreno A, Rahman S, Chino N, Claeson G, Kakkar VV, Williams JA: In: *Peptides: Chemistry, Structure and Biology*, Proceedings of the 13th American Peptide Symposium, Hodges RS, Smith JA, eds. Leiden: Escom (in press).

DeGrado WF, Kaiser ET (1980): *J Org Chem* 45:1295–1300.

DeGrado WF, Kaiser ET (1982): *J Org Chem* 47:3258–3261.

Edwards WB, Anderson CJ, Welch MJ, Fields CG, Fields GB: *J Labelled Compd Radiopharm* (in press).

Eichler J, Bienert M, Stierandova A, Lebl M (1991): *Pept Res* 4:296–307.

Eritja R, Ziehler-Martin JP, Walker PA, Lee TD, Legesse K, Albericio F, Kaplan BE (1987): *Tetrahedron* 43:2675–2680.

Felix AM, Wang C-T, Heimer EP, Fournier A (1988a): *Int J Pept Protein Res* 31:231–238.

Felix AM, Heimer EP, Wang C-T, Lambros TJ, Fournier A, Mowles TF, Maines S, Campbell RM, Wegrzynski BB, Toome V, Fry D, Madison VS (1988b): *Int J Pept Protein Res* 32:441–454.

Fields GB, Tian Z, Barany G (1992): In: *Synthetic Peptides: A User's Guide*, Grant GA, ed., pp. 77–183. New York: Freeman.

Flanigan E, Marshall GR (1970): *Tetrahedron Lett* 2403–2406.

Freidinger RM, Veber DF, Hirschmann R, Paege LM (1980): *Int J Pept Protein Res* 16:464–470.

Fridkin M, Patchornik A, Katchalski E (1965): *J Am Chem Soc* 87:4646–4648.

Funakoshi S, Murayama E, Guo L, Fujii N, Yajima H (1988): *J Chem Soc Chem Commun*:382–384.

García-Echeverría C, Albericio F, Pons M, Barany G, Giralt E (1989): *Tetrahedron Lett* 30:2441–2444.

Gausepohl H, Pieles U, Frank RW (1992): In: *Peptides: Chemistry and Biology*, Proceedings of the 12th American Peptide Symposium, Smith JA, Rivier JE, eds., pp. 523–524. Leiden: Escom.

Giralt E, Eritja R, Navalpotro C, Pedroso E (1984): *An Quim* 80:118–122.

Giralt E, Eritja R, Josa J, Kuklinski C, Pedroso E (1985): *Synthesis* 181–184.

Gisin BF, Merrifield RB (1972): *J Am Chem Soc* 94:3102–3106.

Gray WR, Luque FA, Galyean R, Atherton E, Sheppard RC, Stone BL, Reyes A, Alford J, McIntosh M, Olivera BM, Cruz LJ, Rivier J (1984): *Biochemistry* 23:2796–2802.

Hamada Y, Kato S, Shiori T (1985): *Tetrahedron Lett* 27:3223–3226.

Hill PS, Smith DD, Slaninova J, Hruby VJ (1990): *J Am Chem Soc* 112:3110–3113.

Hiskey RG (1981): In: *The Peptides: Analysis, Synthesis, Biology*, Gross E, Meienhofer J, eds., Vol. 3, pp. 137–167. New York: Academic Press.

Ho P, Slavazza D, Chang D, Bassi K, Chang K (1990): In: *Peptides: Chemistry, Structure and Biology*, Proceedings of the 11th American Peptide Symposium, Rivier JE, Marshall GR, eds., pp. 993-995. Leiden: Escom.

Hruby VJ (1982): *Life Sci* 31:189–199.

Hruby VJ: In: *Peptides: Chemistry, Structure and Biology*, Proceedings of the 13th American Peptide Symposium, Hodges RS, Smith JA, eds. Leiden: Escom (in press).

Hruby VJ, Al-Obeidi F, Kazmierski W (1990a): *Biochem J* 268:249–262.

Hruby VJ, Al-Obeidi F, Sanderson DG, Smith DD (1990b): In *Innovation and Perspectives in Solid Phase Synthesis: Peptides, Polypeptides and Oligonucleotides*, Epton R, ed., pp. 197–203. Birmingham, UK: S.P.C.C.

Inukai N, Nakano K, Murakami M (1968): *Bull Chem Soc Jpn* 41:182–186.

Isied SS, Kuehn CG, Lyon JM, Merrifield RB (1982): *J Am Chem Soc* 104:2632–2634.

Kates SA, Solé NA, Johnson CR, Hudson D, Barany G, Albericio F (1993a): *Tetrahedron Lett* 34:1549–1552.

Kates SA, Daniels SB, Albericio F (1993b): *Anal Biochem* 212:303–310.

Kessler H (1982): *Angew Chem Int Ed Engl* 21:512–523.

König W, Geiger R (1981): In: *Perspectives in Peptide Chemistry*, Eberle A, Geiger R, Wieland T, eds., pp. 31–44. Basel: Karger.

Kopple KD (1972): *J Pharm Sci* 61:1345–1356.

Lebl M, Hruby VJ (1984): *Tetrahedron Lett* 25:2067–2068.

Lyttle MH, Hudson D (1992): In: *Peptides: Chemistry and Biology*, Proceedings of the 12th American Peptide Symposium, Smith JA, Rivier JE, eds., pp. 583-584. Leiden: Escom.

Mazur S, Jayalekshmy P (1979): *J Am Chem Soc* 101:677–683.

McMurray JS (1991): *Tetrahedron Lett* 32:7679–7682.

Meldal M (1992): *Tetrahedron Lett* 33:3077–3080.

Mitchell AR, Merrifield RB (1985): In *Peptides: Structure and Function*, Proceedings of the 9th American Peptide Symposium, Deber CM, Hruby VJ, Kopple KD, eds., pp. 289–292. Rockford, Illinois: Pierce Chemical.

Mott AW, Slomczynska U, Barany G (1986): In: *Forum Peptides Le Cap d'Agde 1984*, Castro B, Martinez J, eds., pp. 321–324. Nancy, France: Les Impressions Dohr.

Munson MC, Barany G (1993): *J Am Chem Soc* 115:10203–10216.

Munson MC, Lebl M, Slaninová J, Barany G (1993): *Pept Res* 6:155–159.

Munson MC, García-Echeverría C, Albericio F, Barany G (1992): *J Org Chem* 57:3013–3018.

Mutter M, Tuchscherer GG, Miller C, Altmann K-H, Carey RI, Wyss DF, Labhardt AM, Rivier JE (1992): *J Am Chem Soc* 114:1463–1470.

Neugebauer W, Willick G (1993): In: *Peptides 1992*, Proceedings of the 22d European Peptide Symposium, Schneider CH, Eberle AN, eds., pp. 395-396. Leiden: Escom.

Nishino N, Xu M, Mihara H, Fujimoto T, Ueno Y, Kumagai H (1992a): *Tetrahedron Lett* 33:1479–1482.

Nishino N, Xu M, Mihara H, Fujimoto T, Ohba M, Ueno Y, Kumagai H (1992b): *J Chem Soc Chem Commun*:180–181.

Ösapay G, Taylor JW (1990): *J Am Chem Soc* 112:6046–6051.

Ösapay G, Profit A, Taylor JW (1990): *Tetrahedron Lett* 31:6121–6124.

Ösapay G, Bouvier M, Taylor JW (1991): In: *Techniques in Protein Chemistry*, Villafranca JJ, ed., pp. 221-321. San Diego: Academic Press.

Ovchinnikov YA, Ivanov VT (1982): In: *The Proteins*, Neurath H, Hill RL, eds., pp. 307–642. New York: Academic Press.

Photaki I (1976): In: *Topics in Sulfur Chemistry*, Senning A, ed., Vol. 1, pp. 111–183. Stuttgart: Georg Thieme.

Plaué S (1990): *Int J Pept Protein Res* 35:510–517.

Ploux O, Chassaing G, Marquet A (1987): *Int J Pept Protein Res* 29:162–169.

Ponsati B, Giralt E, Andreu D (1990): *Tetrahedron* 46:8255–8266.

Rizo J, Gierasch LM (1992): *Annu Rev Biochem* 61:387–418.

Rothe M, Sander A, Fischer W, Mastle W, Nelson B (1977): In: *Peptides*, Proceedings of the 5th American Peptide Symposium, Goodman M, Meienhofer J, eds., pp. 506-509. New York: John Wiley.

Rovero P, Quartara L, Fabbri G (1991): *Tetrahedron Lett* 32:2639–2642.

Royo M, García-Echeverría C, Giralt E, Eritja R, Albericio F (1992): *Tetrahedron Lett* 33:2391–2394.

Schiller PW, Nguyen TM-D, Lemieux C (1988): *Tetrahedron* 44:733–743.

Schiller PW, Nguyen TM-D, Miller J (1985): *Int J Pept Protein Res* 25:171–177.

Schiller PW, Nguyen TM-D, Maziak LA, Wilkes BC, Lemieux C (1987): *J Med Chem* 30:2094–2099.

Schiller PW, Weltrowska G, Nguyen TM-D, Lemieux C, Chung NN, Marsden BJ, Wilkes BC (1991): *J Med Chem* 34:3125–3132.

Schmidt U (1986): *Pure Appl Chem* 58:295–301.

Schwyzer R, Gorup B (1958): *Helv Chim Acta* 41:2199–2205.

Seidel C, Klein C, Empl B, Bayer H, Lin M, Batz H-G (1990): In: *Peptides 1990*, Proceedings of the 21st European Peptide Symposium, Giralt E, Andreu D, eds., pp. 236-237. Leiden: Escom.

Small PW, Sherrington DC (1989): *J Chem Soc Chem Commun*:1589–1590.

Smith DD, Slaninova J, Hruby VJ (1992): *J Med Chem* 35:1558–1563.

Solé NA, Kates SA, Albericio F, Barany G: In: *Peptides: Chemistry, Structure and Biology*, Proceedings of the 13th American Peptide Symposium, Hodges RS, Smith JA, eds. Leiden: Escom (in press).

Spinella MJ, Malik AB, Everitt J, Andersen TT (1991): *Proc Natl Acad Sci USA* 88:7443–7446.

Tonelli AE (1986): In: *Cyclic Polymers*, Semlyen JA, ed., pp. 261-284. London: Elsevier.

Tromelin A, Fulachier M-H, Mourier G, Ménez A (1992): *Tetrahedron Lett* 33:5197–5200.

Trzeciak A, Bannwarth W (1992): *Tetrahedron Lett* 33:4557–4560.

Xu M, Nishino N, Mihara H, Fujimoto T, Izumiya N (1992): *Chem Lett*:191–194.

Yajima H, Fujii N, Funakoshi S, Watanabe T, Murayama E, Otaka A (1988): *Tetrahedron* 44:805–819.

Zalipsky S, Albericio F, Barany G (1985): In: *Peptides: Structure and Function*, Proceedings of the 9th American Peptide Symposium, Deber CM, Hruby VJ, Kopple KD, eds., pp. 257-260. Rockford, Illinois: Pierce Chemical.

5

ENZYMATIC SEMISYNTHESIS OF GROWTH HORMONE-RELEASING FACTOR AND POTENT ANALOGS

Jacob Bongers, Arthur M. Felix, and Edgar P. Heimer

Introduction

The potential value of enzymes in peptide synthesis is derived from the highly selective nature of these catalysts. Proteolytic enzymes can catalyze regioselective acylations, thereby eliminating the need for side-chain-protecting groups in favorable cases. The rigid stereoselectivity of the proteases ensures optically pure products, even from racemic starting materials. These properties make biocatalysis especially attractive for convergent synthetic strategies employing segment condensations in which racemization is often a concern with conventional stoichiometric coupling reagents. In addition, enzymatic segment condensations can be performed for segments without the side-chain-protecting groups that often create solubility problems and require additional stages of deprotection.

In this chapter, we review recent methods developed for the C-terminal amidation of unprotected peptides via an α-amidating enzyme-catalyzed oxidative mechanism and, alternatively, using various protease-catalyzed acyl-transfer routes. We also describe a protease-catalyzed segment condensation used to incorporate unnatural amino acids into the N terminus of a

Peptides: Design, Synthesis, and Biological Activity
Channa Basava and G. M. Anantharamaiah, Editors
©1994 *Birkhäuser Boston*

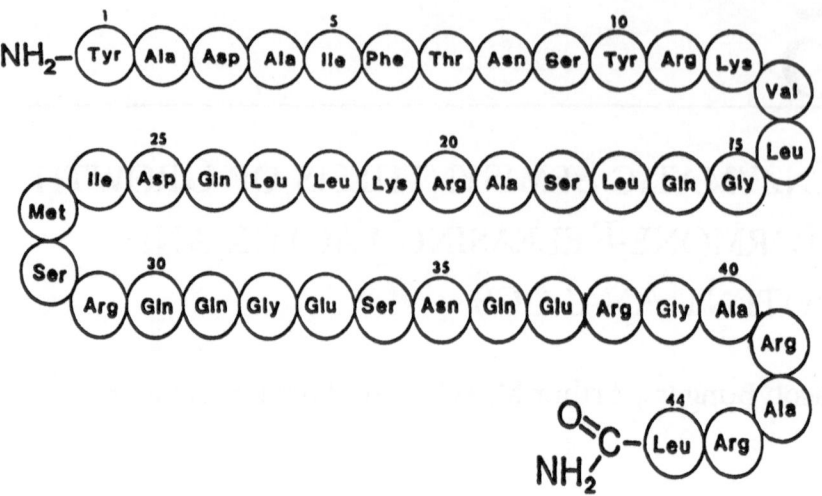

Figure 5-1. Human growth hormone-releasing factor.

peptide hormone analog. These methods were developed for the synthesis of human growth hormone-releasing factor (GRF) and analogs with the goal of using unprotected precursors that could be generated by recombinant DNA synthesis. However, the procedures that are reported may be applied generically to other peptide systems. The parent GRF hormone, GRF(1–44)-NH$_2$ (Figure 5–1), is produced in the hypothalamus and stimulates the secretion of growth hormone by the pituitary gland (Frohman and Jansson, 1986; Guillemin et al., 1982; Rivier et al., 1982). GRF(1–44)-NH$_2$ and the equipotent fragment, GRF(1–29)-NH$_2$ (Ling et al., 1984), are used in clinical studies for the treatment of growth disorders in children (Vance et al., 1990).

The parent hormone and analogs may also have applications for the enhancement of growth performance in domestic livestock (Dubreuil et al., 1990; Petitclerc et al., 1987; Pommier et al., 1990). We have described a GRF analog, [desNH$_2$Tyr[1],D-Ala[2],Ala[15]]-GRF(1–29)-NH$_2$ (Heimer et al., 1989), with an intrinsic potency four- to fivefold higher than the parent hormone in vitro (Heimer et al., 1989) and an extended in vivo half-life (Campbell et al., 1992a). The superpotency of this analog in vitro is attributed to the replacement of the native Gly[15] residue by Ala that enhances the α-helicity and increases its amphiphilic character (Felix et al., 1987; Fry et al., 1992; Madison et al., 1989), which is important to receptor binding (Campbell et al., 1992b). Replacement of the native Tyr[1]-Ala[2] by desNH$_2$Tyr[1]-D-Ala[2] results in increased metabolic stability by conferring resistance to proteolysis by dipeptidyl aminopeptidase IV (Bongers et al., 1992a; Frohman et al., 1986, 1989).

Protease-Catalyzed Peptide Synthesis

There is a growing interest in the proteases as efficient and selective catalysts in peptide synthesis (Chaiken et al., 1982; Fruton, 1982; Jakubke, 1987; Jakubke et al., 1985; Nakanishi and Matsuno, 1988; Wong and Wang, 1991). The use of nuclease and ligase enzymes for manipulating DNA has been instrumental in the development of recombinant DNA technology. Unfortunately for the peptide chemist, there are no enzymes equivalent to the DNA ligases that can be isolated from the complex multimeric ribosome for the in vitro splicing of peptides and proteins. In the absence of a natural "peptidyl ligase," one is left primarily with the proteolytic enzymes for the catalysis of selective acyl transfers. Because the natural role of proteases is to catalyze the hydrolysis of peptide bonds, then in theory they must also catalyze the reverse reaction, peptide bond synthesis. Enzymes have evolved to function only within a rather narrow physiological range of conditions, however, and thus the main difficulty in adapting proteases for use as ligases is the need to find conditions to favor peptide synthesis over hydrolysis without constricting the kinetic pathway provided by the enzyme in the process, that is, without severely degrading the activity of the enzyme. The two existing approaches to this problem are the thermodynamic and kinetic methods of protease-catalyzed peptide synthesis.

Thermodynamically controlled or "reverse proteolysis" syntheses employ conditions that shift the aminolysis/hydrolysis equilibrium toward aminolysis (eq 1):

$$RCO_2^- + {}^+H_3NR' \xrightleftharpoons{K_{syn}} RCONHR' + H_2O \qquad (1)$$

The foregoing aminolysis/hydrolysis equilibrium can be catalyzed by a protease with equal efficiency in either direction, as demanded by the principle of microscopic reversibility. In aqueous solution, the largest component of the thermodynamic barrier to synthesis is ionization of the acyl and amino components to the unreactive carboxylate and ammonium ions (eq 2):

$$RCO_2^- + {}^+H_3NR' \xrightleftharpoons{K_{ion}} RCO_2H + H_2NR' \xrightleftharpoons{K_{am}} RCONHR' + H_2O \quad (2)$$

The extent of synthesis, then, is given by the product of the competing ionization and aminolysis equilibria, that is, $K_{syn} = K_{ion}K_{am} = (Ka_2/Ka_1)K_{syn}$ where Ka_1 and Ka_2 are the acid-ionization constants for RCO_2H and $^+H_3NR'$, respectively. In aqueous solution near neutral pH, K_{syn} is only about 0.5 ($\Delta G \sim 0.4$ kcal mol^{-1}) for the most favorable reactants, that is, polypeptides or N- or C-protected amino acids (pKa$_1 \sim 4$, pKa$_2 \sim 8$) (Fruton, 1982). The equilibrium yield is minuscule ($\Delta G \sim 5$ kcal mol^{-1}) for small unblocked oligopeptide and amino acid reactants (pKa$_1$ $\sim$ 2.0–2.5; pKa$_2$ $\sim$ 9.0–9.5).

The equilibrium yield of a thermodynamically controlled coupling can be raised manyfold by employing less polar nonaqueous co-solvents (Homandberg et al., 1978) to suppress ionization of the α-CO$_2$H group of the acyl component, that is, lower the value of Ka$_1$. However, enzymes are often deactivated or inhibited to some degree by co-solvents. Other tactics for maximizing equilibrium yields include the use of a large molar excess of one of the reactants or continuous removal of the product by precipitation, extraction, or specific complexation.

Kinetically controlled syntheses (eq 3) (Schellenberger and Jakubke, 1991) employ a C-terminal ester (RCO$_2$X) that serves as an acyl donor and reacts with the enzyme (EH) yielding a highly electrophilic acyl–enzyme complex (RCOE). This complex undergoes displacement by an added nucleophile (H$_2$NR') to give a transient "burst" of the desired peptide product (RCONHR'). A competing hydrolysis converts this complex to the undesired acid (RCO$_2$H).

$$RCO_2X + EH \rightleftharpoons RCO_2X \cdot EH \xrightarrow[-XOH]{} RCOE \begin{cases} \xrightarrow{+H_2O} RCO_2H + EH \\ \xrightarrow{+H_2NR'} RCONHR' + EH \end{cases} \quad (3)$$

As the supply of ester substrate is depleted, the new peptide bond will be degraded by the protease causing the concentration of RCONHR' to reach a maximum and then slowly decay to the final equilibrium concentration determined by K$_{syn}$. For preparative purposes, the protease is deactivated at the point of maximum product accumulation. The yield in a kinetically controlled coupling, then, is not determined by K$_{syn}$ but rather by the relative initial rates of aminolysis and hydrolysis. One generally seeks to manipulate the initial reactants and conditions so as to maximize the ratio of aminolysis versus hydrolysis and thereby minimize the loss of ester starting material to hydrolysis.

Enzymatic C-Terminal Amidations of GRF and Analogs

α-Amidating Enzyme

An amidated C terminus is often required by peptide hormones and other bioactive peptides for full receptor binding affinity or to prevent proteolytic degradation by carboxypeptidases. Unfortunately, C-terminal amides cannot be produced by existing recombinant methods because the bacterial expression hosts lack the proper α-amidating enzyme (α-AE) (Bradbury et al., 1982). This posttranslational modification is accomplished by an α-AE-catalyzed O_2 oxidation of the C-terminal glycine of a Gly-extended precursor to produce an α-hydroxyglycyl intermediate that subsequently decomposes to form the peptide amide and glyoxylate (Eipper et al., 1992) (eq 4):

$$RCONHCH_2CO_2^- \xrightarrow[+ \frac{1}{2}O_2]{[\alpha\text{-AE}]} RCONHCH(OH)CO_2^- \xrightarrow[-OCHCO_2^-]{} RCONH_2 \qquad (4)$$

The α-AE requires ascorbate as a cofactor in addition to molecular oxygen.

We have reported in vitro C-terminal amidations of synthetic Gly-extended GRF peptides by a purified recombinant α-AE (Bongers et al., 1992b, 1992e). The substrates, GRF(1–44)-Gly-OH, GRF(1–29)-Gly-OH, and [Ala^{15}]-GRF(1–29)-Gly-OH (prepared by solid-phase synthesis) were enzymatically converted to the respective products, GRF(1–44)-NH$_2$, GRF(1–29)-NH$_2$, and [Ala^{15}]-GRF(1–29)-NH$_2$. Conversion to the amides by α-AE catalysis was nearly quantitative, and practical yields of about 75% were obtained after preparative HPLC purification of the reaction mixtures. All the products gave satisfactory chemical analyses and were bioequivalent in vitro (growth hormone-releasing activities and receptor-binding affinities).

We also observed by HPLC the transient accumulation of an α-hydroxyglycyl peptide intermediate in the synthesis of the potent analog [Ala^{15}]-GRF(1–29)-NH$_2$, and isolated and characterized this product (Bongers et al., 1992b, 1992e). Using this purified α-hydroxyglycyl intermediate we found that this recombinant α-AE was bifunctional, catalyzing both the oxidation and decomposition steps of the amidation process.

The advantage of the α-AE for preparing peptide amides, aside from the high yields, is that a suitable recombinant Gly-extended precursor can be prepared for virtually any desired target peptide. It is thus a general method and a natural complement to recombinant DNA methods. Because this enzyme is not yet commercially available in bulk quantities, it is useful to look at alternate routes to C-terminal amides via acyl transfers utilizing more readily available proteases (Bongers et al., 1991, 1992c, 1992d; Breddam et al., 1991; Morihara, 1991; Sakina et al., 1988).

Trypsin-Catalyzed Direct Amidation

Protease-catalyzed C-terminal amidation was at first carried out by direct amidation using ammonia as the nucleophile. Porcine trypsin was used to activate the Arg^{29}-OH residue in [Ala^{15}]-GRF(1–29)-OH, and amidation was carried out in 1.4 M NH$_3$/NH$_4$OAc buffer (pH 8.3) containing 95% (vol/

vol) 1,4-butanediol co-solvent to form [Ala^{15}]-GRF(1-29)-NH$_2$ (Bongers et al., 1991). A stable equilibrium between the acid and amide (eq 5) was established with K$_{syn}$ ~ 0.33:

$$[Ala^{15}]\text{-GRF(1-29)-OH} + NH_3 \xrightleftharpoons[\text{[trypsin]}]{K_{syn}} [Ala^{15}]\text{-GRF(1-29)-NH}_2 + H_2O \qquad (5)$$

Attempts to drive this equilibrium further toward ammonolysis by raising the pH or by adding more NH$_3$/NH$_4$OAc resulted in deactivation of trypsin. In addition to the rather low equilibrium yield (25%) of amide in this semisynthesis, trypsin catalysis was quite sluggish, and thus large amounts of trypsin were needed to amidate a given amount of substrate in a reasonable length of time. The low trypsin activity is partly the result using a high content of co-solvent, which is a shortcoming suffered by many thermodynamically controlled enzymatic syntheses. In addition, ammonia is probably an exceedingly poor nucleophile for the trypsin-activated complex.

An interesting aspect of the foregoing direct amidation was that competing proteolytic degradations of the internal tryptic cleavage sites at Lys^{21}, Arg^{20}, Lys^{12}, and Arg^{11} were suppressed by using a 1,4-butanediol co-solvent at 85% or greater (vol/vol) and pH of 8 or lower. The only side product detected during the reaction under these conditions was a minor amount (3%) of [Ala^{15}]-GRF(1-29)-O(CH$_2$)$_4$OH from the trypsin-catalyzed acylation of the 1,4-butanediol co-solvent. This ester side product was isolated and identified by mass spectrometry.

Trypsin-Catalyzed Coupling of Leucine Amide to a C-Terminal Acid

We recently used trypsin to couple Leu-NH$_2$ to the Arg^{43}-OH residue of the precursor GRF(1-43)-OH to produce GRF(1-44)-NH$_2$ (Bongers et al., 1992c) (eq 6):

$$\text{GRF(1-43)-OH} + \text{Leu-NH}_2 \xrightleftharpoons[\text{[trypsin]}]{} \text{GRF(1-44)-NH}_2 + H_2O \qquad (6)$$

Yields of 60%–70% were obtained at 22°C using a large molar excess of Leu-NH$_2$ (1 M) in either 75% (vol/vol) N,N'-dimethylacetamide (DMAC) or 95% (vol/vol) 1,4-butanediol. Catalysis was severalfold more efficient in the DMAC system. The semisynthetic GRF(1-44)-NH$_2$ was purified and shown to be chemically and biologically equivalent to a chemically synthesized standard.

The yield of GRF(1-44)-NH$_2$ was limited by competing transpeptidations at Arg^{41} and Arg^{38} that gave [Leu^{42}]-GRF(1-42)-NH$_2$ and [Leu^{39}]-GRF(1-39)-NH$_2$ side products. As in the case of the trypsin-catalyzed direct amidation, we were able to suppress degradation of the remaining internal sites at Lys[21], Arg[20], Lys[12], and Arg[11] in this synthesis by the use of co-solvents. The overall catalytic activity of trypsin (synthetic and proteolytic) decreased gradually with an increasing percentage of DMAC and then fell precipitously to undetectable levels at more than 76% DMAC. This abrupt loss of activity was reversed by merely adding water to bring DMAC to 76% or less.

The synthesis obeyed Michaelis–Menten kinetics, that is, a hyperbolic dependence of the rate of synthesis on the concentration of GRF(1–43)-OH substrate, albeit with a relatively high K_m (10.8 mM). The reaction also showed saturation with respect to the Leu-NH$_2$ nucleophile with the maximum rate of synthesis occurring for [Leu-NH$_2$]=1.0 M or more. We demonstrated that GRF(1–44)-NH$_2$ could be produced at an initial rate of 450 mg h^{-1} (mg trypsin)$^{-1}$ for an initial GRF(1–43)-OH concentration of 130 mg ml^{-1} (23 mM) in 1.0 M Leu-NH$_2$ (75% DMAC, pH 8.2, 22°C).

Carboxypeptidase Y-Catalyzed Transpeptidation

Breddam and co-workers (1991) have developed a semisynthesis of GRF(1–29)-NH$_2$ from the precursor [Ala[29]]-GRF(1–29)-OH via carboxypeptidase Y-(CPD-Y-) catalyzed exchange of the Ala[29]-OH residue for Arg-NH$_2$ (eq 7):

$$[Ala^{29}]\text{–}GRF(1\text{–}29)\text{–}OH + Arg\text{–}NH_2 \underset{[CPD\text{-}Y]}{\rightleftharpoons} GRF(1\text{–}29)\text{–}NH_2 + Ala\text{–}OH \qquad (7)$$

CPD-Y, an exoprotease from brewer's yeast, is well suited for this type of semisynthetic modification because it will not degrade internal peptide bonds as has been described for endoproteases such as trypsin. Ala[29]-OH was chosen as a favorable leaving group for this transpeptidation on the basis of model studies with the substrates Bzl-Met-Ser-X-OH (X = Ala, Leu, Arg). It was demonstrated (Breddam et al., 1991) that [Ala[29]]-GRF(1–29)-OH (2 mM) could be converted to GRF(1–29)-NH$_2$ (87% in 150 min) by CPD-Y catalysis in aqueous 1.5 M H-Arg-NH$_2$ (pH 8).

Two-Stage Enzymatic Semisynthesis of a Superpotent GRF Analog

We have combined this CPD-Y transpeptidation with a V8 protease-catalyzed segment condensation to create a two-stage semisynthetic route (Bongers et al., 1992d) to the superpotent analog, [desNH$_2$Tyr[1],D-Ala[2],Ala[15]]-GRF(1–29)-NH$_2$, from a precursor potentially accessible by recombinant DNA synthesis, [Ala[15,29]]-GRF(4–29)-OH (eq 8):

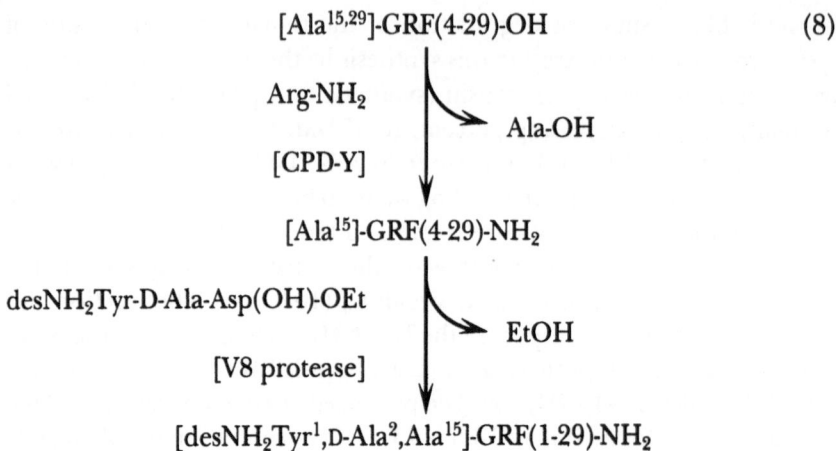

$[\text{Ala}^{15,29}]$-GRF(4-29)-OH   (8)

Arg-NH$_2$ → Ala-OH

[CPD-Y]

$[\text{Ala}^{15}]$-GRF(4-29)-NH$_2$

desNH$_2$Tyr-D-Ala-Asp(OH)-OEt   → EtOH

[V8 protease]

$[\text{desNH}_2\text{Tyr}^1,\text{D-Ala}^2,\text{Ala}^{15}]$-GRF(1-29)-NH$_2$

In the first stage, the precursor, $[\text{Ala}^{15,29}]$-GRF(4–29)-OH, was converted to the amidated segment, $[\text{Ala}^{15}]$-GRF(4-29)-NH$_2$, by the method of Breddam et al. (1991), that is, carboxypeptidase Y-catalyzed transpeptidation in 1.0 M Arg-NH$_2$. This CPD-Y-catalyzed step was limited to conversions of 75%–80% (62% isolated yield after HPLC purification) because of competing hydrolysis to form the side product $[\text{Ala}^{15}]$-GRF(4–28)-OH. The final product, $[\text{desNH}_2\text{Tyr}^1,\text{D-Ala}^2,\text{Ala}^{15}]$-GRF(1-29)-NH$_2$, was then prepared by V8 protease-catalyzed, kinetically controlled acylation of $[\text{Ala}^{15}]$-GRF(4-29)-NH$_2$ using desNH$_2$Tyr-D-Ala-Asp(OH)-OEt in 20% (vol/vol) DMSO (pH 8.2, 37°C) (Bongers et al., 1992d). The V8 protease (protease from the V8 strain of *Staphylococcus aureus*, endoprotease Glu-C) is a serine endoprotease specific for cleavage at Glu-X and, to a lesser extent, Asp-X bonds (Drapeau et al., 1972; Houmard and Drapeau, 1972; Sørenson et al., 1991). Conversion of $[\text{Ala}^{15}]$-GRF(4–29)-NH$_2$ to $[\text{desNH}_2\text{Tyr}^1,\text{D-Ala}^2,\text{Ala}^{15}]$-GRF(1-29)-NH$_2$, using a fivefold molar excess of the acyl component, desNH$_2$Tyr-D-Ala-Asp(OH)-OEt, was limited to 55%–60% (49% isolated yield) by a competing proteolysis at Asp^{25}-Ile^{26} that generated several side products. The hydrolysis product, desNH$_2$Tyr-D-Ala-Asp(OH)-OH, was also generated as well as a very minor amount of desNH$_2$Tyr-D-Ala-Asp-NHC(CH$_2$OH)$_3$ from V8 protease-catalyzed acylation of the Tris buffer. The semisynthetic analog was purified, fully characterized, and determined to possess the full biological activity of the chemically prepared standard.

We subsequently found that this V8 protease-catalyzed segment condensation is accelerated about 100 fold by use of the α-4-nitrobenzyl ester, desNH$_2$Tyr-D-Ala-Asp(OH)-ONb, in place of the original α-ethyl ester (Bongers et al., 1992d). In addition to requiring much less enzyme, use of desNH$_2$Tyr-D-Ala-Asp(OH)-ONb resulted in 90% conversion of $[\text{Ala}^{15}]$-GRF(4–29)-NH$_2$ to the final product (15% DMF, pH 8.1, 37°C) with no detectable loss of product to the slow proteolysis at Asp^{25}-Ile^{26}.

Maximizing enzyme specificity for the ester-leaving group of the acyl component in order to prevent proteolytic side reactions was originally suggested by the model studies of Schellenberger et al. (1991). This principle has implications for protease-catalyzed condensations of minimally protected polypeptide segments containing multiple competing proteolytic cleavage sites. The foregoing semisynthesis is a practical illustration of this principle. The V8-catalyzed coupling demonstrates that endoprotease-catalyzed segment condensations can be performed for polypeptides that contain multiple competing proteolytic cleavage sites by accelerating synthesis relative to proteolysis by use of an appropriate ester-leaving group for the acyl component.

These studies demonstrate that an intermediate-length peptide containing unnatural amino acids at the N terminus and an amide at the C terminus can be prepared efficiently and in good yield and purity by enzymatic semisynthesis. The use of enzymatic methods, combined with chemical or recombinant DNA technology, presents a usable alternative for the large-scale production of intermediate-length peptides.

REFERENCES

Bongers J, Lambros T, Ahmad M, Heimer EP (1992a): *Biochim Biophys Acta* 1122:147–153.

Bongers J, Heimer EP, Campbell RM, Felix AM, Merkler DJ(1992b): In: *Proceedings of the 12th American Peptide Symposium*, Rivier JE, Smith JA, eds., pp. 458–459. Leiden: ESCOM.

Bongers J, Offord RE, Felix AM, Campbell RM, Heimer EP (1992c): *Int J Pept Protein Res* 40:268–273.

Bongers J, Lambros T, Liu W, Ahmad M, Campbell RM, Felix AM, Heimer EP (1992d): *J Med Chem* 35:3934–3941.

Bongers J, Felix AM, Campbell RM, Lee Y, Merkler DJ, Heimer EP (1992e): *Pept Res* 5:183–189.

Bongers J, Offord RE, Felix AM, Lambros T, Liu W, Ahmad M, Campbell RM, Heimer EP (1991): *Biomed Biochim Acta* 50:S157–S162.

Bradbury AF, Finnie MDA, Smyth DG (1982): *Nature (London)* 298:686–688.

Breddam K, Widmer F, Meldal M (1991): *Int J Pept Protein Res* 37:153–160.

Campbell RM, Lee Y, Mowles TF, McIntyre KW, Ahmad M, Felix AM, Heimer EP (1992a): *Peptides* 13:787–793.

Campbell RM, Lee Y, Mowles TF, Rivier J, Heimer EP, Felix AM, Mowles TF (1992b): *Peptides* 12:569–574.

Chaiken IM, Komoriya A, Ohno M, Widmer F (1982): *Appl Biochem Biotechnol* 7:385–399.

Drapeau GR, Boily Y, Houmard J (1972): *J Biol Chem* 247:6720–6726.

Dubreuil P, Petitclerc D, Pelletier G, Gaudreau P, Farmer C, Mowles TF, Brazeau P (1990): *J Anim Sci* 68:1254–1268.

Eipper BA, Stoffers DA, Mains RE (1992): *Annu Rev Neurosci* 15:57–85.

Felix AM, Heimer EP, Mowles TF, Eiseinbeis H, Leung T, Lambros TJ, Ahmad M,

Wang C-T, Brazeau P (1987): In: *Proceedings of the 19th European Peptide Symposium*, Theodoropoulos D, ed., pp. 481–484. Berlin: de Gruyter.

Frohman LA, Jansson J-O (1986): *Endocr Rev* 7:223–253.

Frohman LA, Downs TR, Heimer EP, Felix AM (1989): *J Clin Invest* 83:1533–1540.

Frohman LA. Downs TR, Williams TC, Heimer EP, Pan Y-CE, Felix AM (1986): *J Clin Invest* 78:906–913.

Fruton JS (1982): *Adv Enzymol Relat Areas Mol Biol* 53:239–306.

Fry D, Madison VS, Greely D, Felix AM, Heimer EP, Frohman L, Campbell RM, Mowles TF, Toome V, Wegrzynski BB (1992): *Biopolymers* 32:649–666.

Guillemin R, Brazeau P, Böhlen P, Esch F, Ling N, Wehrenberg WB (1982): *Science* 218:585–587.

Heimer EP, Ahmad M, Lambros T, McGarty T, Wang C-T, Mowles TF, Maines S, Felix AM (1989): In: *Synthetic Peptides: Approaches to Biological Problems*, Symposia on Molecular and Cellular Biology, New Series, Vol. 86, Tam J, Kaiser ET, eds., pp. 309–319. New York: Liss.

Homandberg GA, Mattis JA, Laskowski M, Jr. (1978): *Biochemistry* 17:5220–5227.

Houmard J, Drapeau GR (1972): *Proc Natl Acad Sci USA* 69:3506–3509.

Jakubke H-D (1987): In: *The Peptides*, Vol. 9, Udenfriend S, Meienhofer J, eds, pp. 103–165. San Diego: Academic Press.

Jakubke H-D, Kuhl P, Konnecke A (1985): *Angew Chem Int Ed Engl* 24:85–93.

Kullmann W (1985): *Enzymatic Peptide Synthesis*. Boca Raton: CRC Press.

Ling N, Baird A, Wehrenberg WB, Ueno N, Munegumi T, Brazeau P (1984): *Biochem Biophys Res Commun* 123:854–861.

Madison V, Berkovitch-Yellin Z, Fry D, Greely D, Toome V (1989): In: *Synthetic Peptides: Approaches to Biological Problems*, UCLA Symposia on Molecular and Cellular Biology, New Series, Vol. 86, Tam J, Kaiser ET, eds., pp. 109–123. New York: Liss.

Morihara K (1991): *Biomed Biochim Acta* 50:S15–S18.

Nakanishi K, Matsuno R (1988): *Adv Biotechnol Processes* 10:173–202.

Petitclerc D, Pelletier G, Lapierre H, Gaudreau P, Couture P, Dubreuil P, Morisset J, Brazeau P (1987): *J Anim Sci* 65:996–1005.

Pommier SA, Dubreuil P, Pelletier G, Gaudreau P, Farmer C, Mowles TF, Brazeau P (1990): *J Anim Sci* 68:1291–1298.

Rivier J, Spiess J, Thorner M, Vale W (1982): *Nature (London)* 300:276–278.

Sakina K, Keiko K, Morihara K, Yajima H (1988): *Chem & Pharm Bull (Tokyo)* 36:4345–4354.

Schellenberger V, Jakubke H-D (1991): *Angew Chem Int Ed Engl* 30:1437–1449.

Schellenberger V, Gorner A, Konnecke A, Jakubke H-D (1991): *Pept Res* 4:265–269.

Sorensen SB, Sorensen TL, Breddam K (1991): *FEBS Lett* 294:195–197.

Vance ML (1990): *Clin Chem* 36:415–420.

Wong C-T, Wang K-T (1991): *Experientia (Basel)* 47:1123–1129.

6

RECENT DEVELOPMENTS IN THE SYNTHESIS OF GLYCOPEPTIDES

Horst Kunz

Introduction

Glycoproteins are important carriers of biological selectivity, in particular, in recognition processes on membranes. Their linkage regions are characterized by *N*- or *O*-glycosidic bonds between the carbohydrate parts and the peptide backbone. Because glycosidic bonds are sensitive to reaction conditions frequently applied in peptide chemistry, attention must be paid to mild protecting group techniques throughout the synthesis of glycopeptides. The Fmoc group, which is removed with the weak base morpholine, and the allylic protecting groups were demonstrated to be particularly useful tools in the chemical synthesis of glycopeptides. The allylic protection, which is cleaved off under neutral conditions by palladium(0)-catalyzed allyl transfer reactions, was extended to a new anchoring principle in solid-phase synthesis. In addition, enzymatic reactions were revealed to be efficient in glycopeptide chemistry.

Carbohydrates of Glycoproteins: Tools in Biological Selectivity

During the past decades it has been recognized that the carbohydrate parts of natural glycoconjugates, glycoproteins and glycolipids, exhibit key func-

Peptides: Design, Synthesis, and Biological Activity
Channa Basava and G. M. Anantharamaiah, Editors
©1994 *Birkhäuser Boston*

tions in biological selection processes; in particular, on membranes. The organized distribution of complex proteins within the multicellular organisms obviously deserves a third level of selectivity in addition to the first level, which is the translation of information by DNA, and the second level, consisting of the selective reactivity of proteins and peptides, for example, as enzymes. On this third level, carbohydrates of glycoproteins constitute recognition signals in immunodifferentiations, in the binding and passage of serum components, for example, enzymes, hormones, or carrier proteins, through membranes, in the docking of viruses or bacteria to cells and in intercell communication (Brandley et al., 1986). When one considers these roles of the carbohydrates of glycoproteins as labels in biological selection processes, the increasing interest in glycopeptides, which are partial structures of natural glycoproteins, becomes evident.

Linkage Regions of Mammalian Glycoproteins

In spite of the great variety of glycoproteins, only a few types of linkage regions between the peptide and carbohydrate parts occur in nature. Most frequently found are *N*-glycoproteins, which typically contain the *N*-glycosidic bond between the side-chain amide of an asparagine and *N*-acetyl glucosamine 1. The *O*-glycoproteins constitute the second important type of these conjugates. In mammals, they occur in the two major forms: Proteoglycans are characterized by the β-*O*-xylosyl serine linkage 2, while the mucin-type proteins contain the typical α-*O*-glycosidic linkage between *N*-acetylgalactosamine and serine or threonine 3 (Montreuil, 1982) (Scheme 6–1).

It should be noted that the carbohydrate side chains are coupled to the peptide backbone by glycosidic bonds in all natural glycoproteins. As these glycosidic structures are more or less sensitive to acids and, in addition, the *O*-glycosyl serine and threonine linkages (2 and 3) are also decomposed easily by a base-catalyzed β-elimination of the entire carbohydrate, special

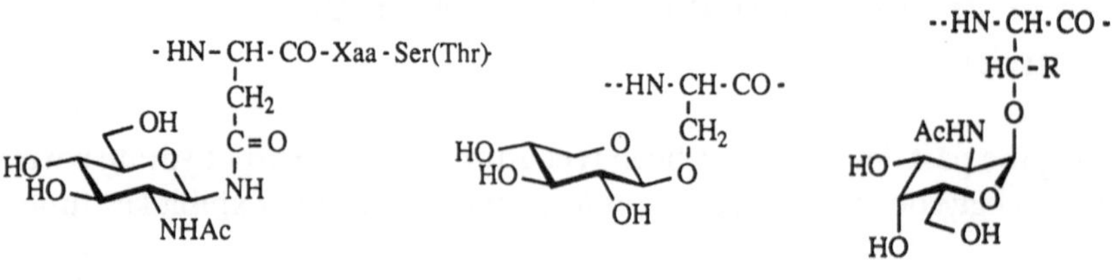

Scheme 6–1.

emphasis has to be given to mild reaction conditions in all steps throughout the glycopeptide synthesis (Kunz, 1987). The construction of the oligosaccharides (Paulsen, 1982; Schmidt, 1986) and their glycosidic coupling to the amino acid derivatives (Kunz, 1987, 1992) are additional preconditions for the successful synthesis of glycopeptides.

The Fmoc Group in Glycopeptide Synthesis

The (9-fluorenyl) methoxycarbonyl Fmoc group (Carpino et al., 1970) is frequently applied in peptide chemistry. Its removal is usually carried out with piperidine. An efficient and general application of the Fmoc group in glycopeptide synthesis (Lacombe et al., 1983; Schultheiss-Reimann et al., 1983) became possible when it was demonstrated that the weak base morpholine, which is sufficient for the selective removal of the Fmoc group, does not affect the sensitive O-glycosyl serine and threonine linkages (Schultheiss-Reimann et al., 1983). Under these conditions, the N-deblocking of the glycosyl serine and threonine derivatives 4 with the tumor-associated Tn antigen side chain was achieved quantitatively. The O-glycosidic bonds of the products 5, prone to easy base-catalyzed β-elimination, remain untouched (Scheme 6-2).

After this problem had been solved, further chain extension could be carried out without difficulties (Kunz et al., 1986, 1990; Paulsen et al., 1987). This chemistry has been successfully adopted in the solid-phase synthesis of glycopeptides (Lüning et al., 1989; Peters et al., 1989).

The Allyloxycarbonyl Group

Although the allyloxycarbonyl (Aloc) group has been known for more than 30 years (Stevens and Watanabe, 1950), it was not considered useful for peptide synthesis because of the unselective or rough deblocking conditions (hydrogenation or treatment with strong acids). We found, however,

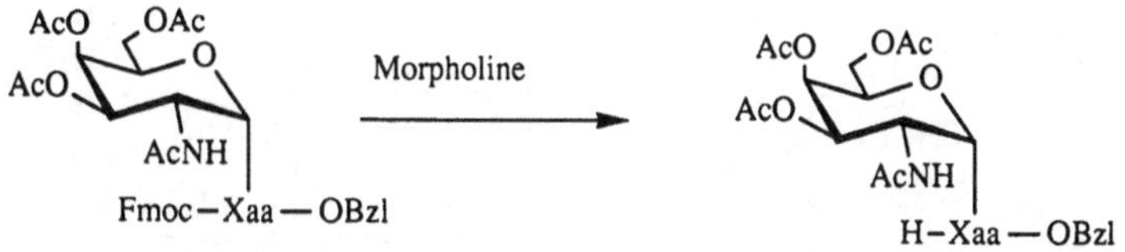

4a: Xaa = Ser 86%,
4b: Xaa = Thr 85%

5a: Xaa = Ser
5b: Xaa = Thr   yield: quant.

Scheme 6-2.

that the use of the allyloxycarbonyl group together with a novel cleavage method, that is, the palladium(0)-catalyzed allyl transfer to weakly basic or neutral nucleophiles (Kunz et al., 1984a), is very efficient in the synthesis of peptides and glycopeptides. In this sense, the Aloc group was removed from the complex fucosyl chitobiose asparagine conjugate 6 (Scheme 6–3) with complete selectivity (Kunz et al., 1988a). The numerous other blocking groups as well as the N- and O-glycosidic bonds remained absolutely unaffected.

Chain extension of the product 7 furnished the trisaccharide tripeptide 8 almost quantitatively (see Scheme 6–3). Because the Aloc group was acid stable, the *tert*-butyl ester of 8 was selectively removable to yield the carboxy-deblocked glycopeptide 9 (Kunz et al., 1988a). It is important to note that the acid stability of the O-glycosidic bonds strongly depends on the protecting group pattern within the carbohydrate portion. Although a glycopeptide analogous to 8 with O-benzyl ether-type protection in the fucose unit suffered complete cleavage of the fucoside bond on treatment with trifluoroacetic acid, the fucoside linkage of the O-acetyl-protected compounds 8 and 9 are stable under identical conditions. This result reveals an important effect of indirect protection. Protonation occurs first at the carbonyl oxygens of the O- and N-acetyl groups. Thus, a Coulomb repulsion is generated that prevents proton attack at the otherwise sensitive O-glycosidic bonds.

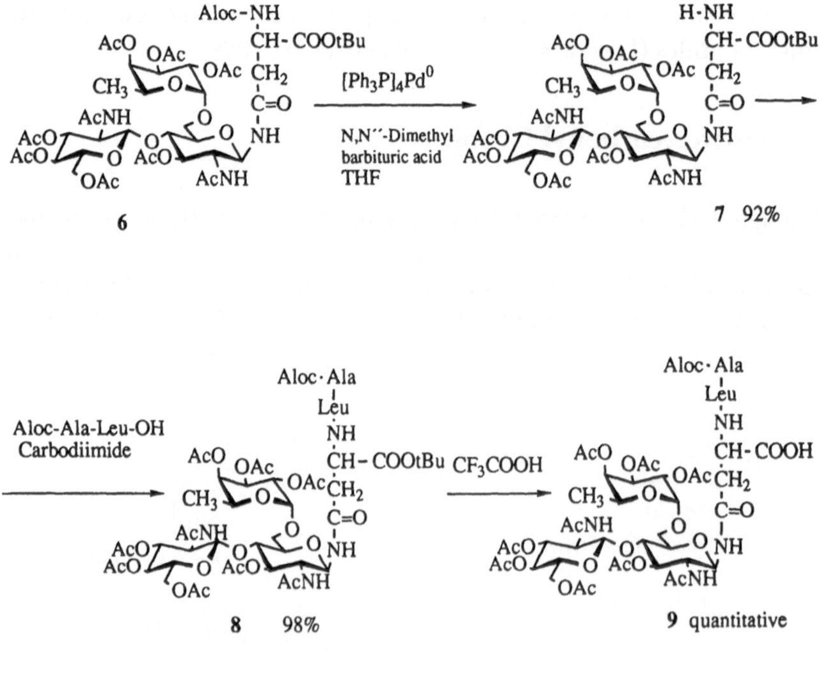

Scheme 6–3.

The Allyl Ester as the Carboxy Protection

Even before the Aloc group, we applied the allyl ester as the C-terminal protection in the synthesis of peptides and glycopeptides (Kunz et al., 1984b). Its removal by palladium(0)-catalyzed allyl transfer, usually to morpholine (Kunz et al., 1984b) or *N*-methyl aniline (Ciommer et al., 1991), provides very efficient and mild deblocking of the carboxy function. Furthermore, the allyl ester can advantageously be combined with the Fmoc group. Both these protections can selectively be removed even from sensitive *O*-glyco-peptides, for example, **10** (Scheme 6–4). The Fmoc group was cleaved off by using morpholine to give **11**, thus leaving the allyl ester and the O-glycosyl threonine bond intact. To cleave the allyl ester, the Pd(0)-catalyzed reaction to obtain **12** was carried out by application of *N*-methyl aniline as the allyl trapping agent, which is too weakly basic to affect the Fmoc group (Ciommer et al., 1991) (see Scheme 6–4).

The selectively deblocked components **11** and **12** were condensed to furnish the complex glycopeptide **13** with the tumor-associated T-antigen disaccharide side chain (Ciommer et al., 1991). Appropriate application of this technique allows the successful synthesis of *N*- and *O*-glycopeptides with more extended peptide sequences.

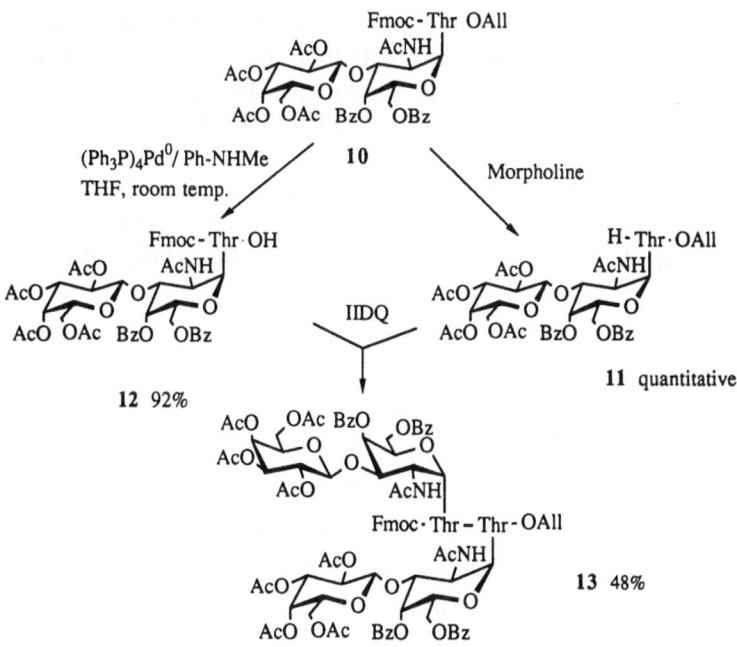

Scheme 6–4.

The Allylic Anchoring Principle in Solid-Phase Synthesis

The favorable properties of the allylic protecting groups were transferred to the solid-phase synthesis by the development of a new allylic anchoring principle **14** (Kunz et al., 1987, 1988b). Applying the Pd(0)-catalyzed cleavage, the synthesized peptides and glycopeptides can be detached from the polymeric support under practically neutral conditions (Scheme 6–5). The prevailing detachment conditions can be suitably adjusted by an appropriate choice of the allyl-trapping nucleophile. Weak bases, such as morpholine or *N*-methyl aniline, as well as neutral or weakly acidic compounds, for example, *N,N'*-dimethyl barbituric acid, can be selected for this purpose.

A particularly useful version of the allylic anchoring principle consists in the polymeric esters of the 4-hydroxycrotonyl-aminomethyl structure (HYCRAM™; HYCRAM is a trademark of Orpegen Company, Heidelberg, Germany). The improved HYCRAM anchor with an β-alanine as the standard amino acid inserted between the aminomethyl polymer and the hydroxycrotonyl moiety was used for the construction of the polymer-linked peptide T **15** (Scheme 6–6) carrying two *O*-glycosidic and one *N*-glycosidic side chains (Kunz et al., 1992). In this synthesis, the Fmoc group, removable with morpholine, served as the temporary amino protection. Using the Pd(0)-catalyzed allyl transfer reaction carried out in DMSO containing solvents and with *N*-methyl aniline as the allyl acceptor, the complex glyco-octapeptide was released from the polymeric support without affecting the *tert*-butyl-type side-chain protection or the *N*- and *O*-glycosidic bonds.

After purification by preparative HPLC, the triglycosyl peptide T **16** (see Scheme 6–6) was isolated in a yield of 40% (0.5 g) (Kunz et al., 1992). Peptide T is a partial sequence of gp 120 of the HIV-1 virus, which was found to inhibit the binding of the virus to the CD4 receptor of T4 cells (Brenneman et al., 1988). The efficiency of the allylic anchoring method has been demonstrated in a number of glycopeptide syntheses and in the large-scale synthesis of pharmaceutical peptides (Birr et al., 1992).

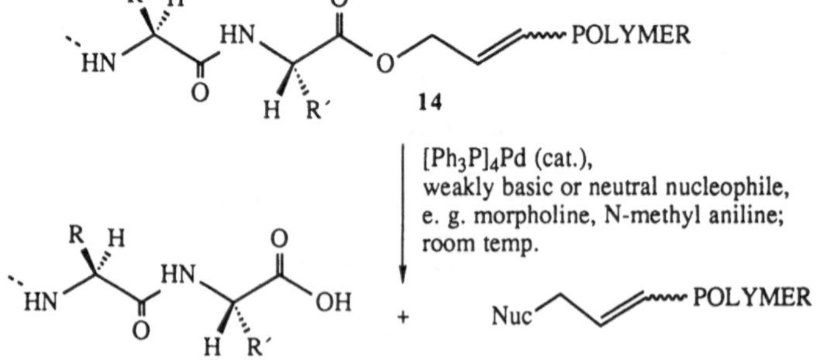

Scheme 6–5.

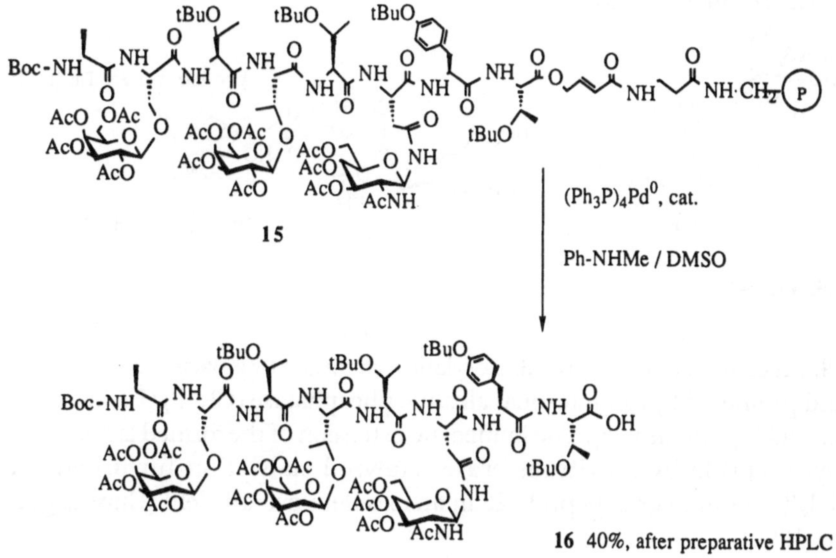
15
(Ph3P)4Pd0, cat.
Ph-NHMe / DMSO
16 40%, after preparative HPLC

Scheme 6–6.

Enzymatic Methods in Glycopeptide Synthesis

Because enzymes operate selectively and under mild conditions, they are considered interesting tools in the glycopeptide chemistry. The selective hydrolysis of the glycopeptide *n*-heptyl ester **17**, catalyzed by lipase (Braun et al., 1992), illustrates the interesting aspects of this technology (Scheme 6–7). The enzyme exclusively cleaves the heptyl ester from the sterically demanding substrate. The other blocking groups and the O-glycosidic linkages of the product **18** remained untouched.

Of particular use are chain extensions in the saccharide part of glycopeptides by applying glycosyltransferases (Paulson et al., 1989). The efficiency of this methodology has been demonstrated on the *N*-glycopeptide

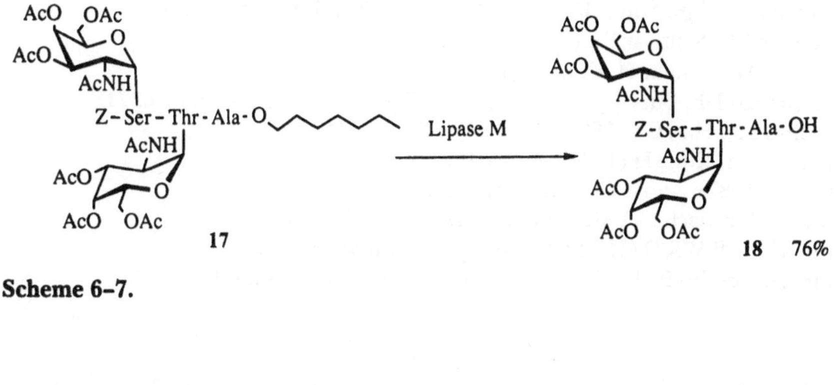
Z-Ser-Thr-Ala-O
Lipase M
Z-Ser-Thr-Ala-OH
17
18 76%

Scheme 6–7.

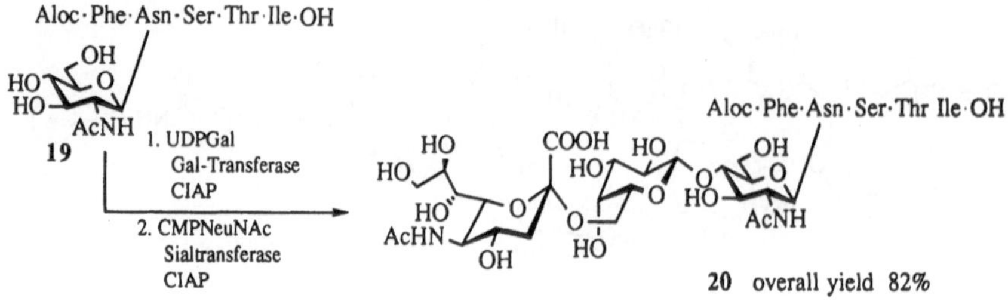

Scheme 6–8.

19, which was subjected to galactosylation catalyzed by galactosyltransferases and promoted by calf intestinal alkaline phosphatase (CIAP) (Unverzagt et al., 1990) (Scheme 6–8). The immediate extension of the formed lactosamine glycopeptide by sialyltransferase-catalyzed sialylation furnished the sialyllactosamin glycopeptide **20** in an excellent overall yield (Unverzagt et al., 1990).

Conclusion and Outlook

The preparative methods developed during the past decade now make available glycopeptides that are partial structures of biologically interesting glycoproteins. Using the modified Fmoc procedure and the allyl protecting groups in combination with *tert*-butyl- and benzyl-type protection, glycopeptides with simple saccharide parts are now accessible almost routinely either in solution or on solid phase. Glycopeptides with more complex side chains, for example, fucosyl-containing compounds, require more advanced technologies. However, chemical methods and enzymatic techniques that are now available allow the efficient construction even of such complex glycoconjugates.

REFERENCES

Birr C, Becker G, Nyuyen-Trong RM, Kunz H, Kosch W (1992): In: *Peptides: Chemistry and Biology*, Smith JA, Rivier JE, eds., p. 674. Leiden: ESCOM.

Brandley BK, Schnaar RL (1986): *J Leukocyte Biol* 40:97.

Braun P, Waldmann H, Kunz H (1992): *Synlett* 1992:39.

Brenneman DE, Buzy JM, Ruff MR, Pert CB (1988): *Drug Dev Res* 15:371.

Carpino LA, Han GY (1970): *J Am Chem Soc* 92:5748.

Ciommer M, Kunz H (1991): *Synlett* 1991:593.

Kunz H (1987): *Angew Chem Int Ed Engl* 26:294.

Kunz H, Birnbach S (1986): *Angew Chem Int Ed Engl* 25:360.

Kunz H, Brill WK-D (1992): *Trends Glycosci Glycotechnol* 4:61.

Kunz H, Dombo B (1987): Ger. Par. Appl. P 3720269.3, June 19, 1987.

Kunz H, Dombo B (1988b): *Angew Chem Int Ed Engl* 27:711.

Kunz H, Kosch WM, März J (1992): In: *Peptides: Chemistry and Biology*, Smith JA, Rivier JE, eds., p. 502. Leiden: ESCOM.

Kunz H, Unverzagt C (1984a): *Angew Chem Int Ed Engl* 23:436.

Kunz H, Unverzagt C (1988a): *Angew Chem Int Ed Engl* 27:1697.

Kunz H, Waldmann H (1984b): *Angew Chem Int Ed Engl* 23:71.

Kunz H, Birnbach S, Wernig P (1990): *Carbohydr Res* 202:207.

Lacombe JM, Pavia AA (1983): *J Org Chem* 48:2557.

Lüning B, Norberg T, Tejbrant T (1989): *Glycoconjugate J* 6:5.

Montreuil J (1982): In: *Comprehensive Biochemistry*, Vol. 19, B II, Neuberger A, van Deenen LLM, eds., p. 1. Amsterdam: Elsevier.

Paulsen H (1982): *Angew Chem Int Ed Engl* 21:155.

Paulsen H, Schultz M (1987): *Carbohydr Res* 159:37.

Paulson JC, Colley KC (1989): *J Biol Chem* 264:17615.

Peters S, Bielefeldt T, Meldal M, Bock K, Paulsen H (1992): *J Chem Soc Perkin Trans I* 1992:1163.

Schmidt RR (1986): *Angew Chem Int Ed Engl* 25:212.

Schultheiss-Reimann P, Kunz H (1983): *Angew Chem Int Ed Engl* 22:62.

Stevens CM, Watanabe R (1950): *J Am Chem Soc* 72:725.

Unverzagt C, Kunz H, Paulson JC (1990): *J Am Chem Soc* 112:9308.

II

PEPTIDE DESIGN
AND APPLICATIONS

7

SYNTHESIS, CHARACTERIZATIONS, AND MEDICAL APPLICATIONS OF BIOELASTIC MATERIALS

D. Channe Gowda, Timothy M. Parker, R. Dean Harris, and Dan W. Urry

Introduction

Bioelastic materials are elastomeric polypeptides composed of repeating sequences. They are a relatively new class of polymers that may also be called elastic protein-based polymers, having their origins in repeating sequences found in the mammalian elastic protein, elastin. The most striking and longest sequence between cross-links in pig and cow is the polypentapeptide–(PPP), poly(VPGVG) or $(Val^1-Pro^2-Gly^3-Val^4-Gly^5)_n$, where n is 11 (Sandberg et al., 1985; Yeh et al., 1987). Another repeat first found in porcine elastin is a polytetrapeptide–(PTP), poly(VPGG) or $(Val^1-Pro^2-Gly^3-Gly^4)_n$, but this repeat has not been found to occur with n greater than 2 without substitution (Sandberg et al., 1981). The next most common recurring sequence in mammalian elastin is a polyhexapeptide–(PHP), poly(APGVGV) or $(Ala^1-Pro^2-Gly^3-Val^4-Gly^5-Val^6)_n$ where, with but a couple of isomorphous hydrophobic residue replacements such as Val by Ile or Leu, n is 8 in man (Indik et al., 1987). The monomers, oligomers, and high polymers of these repeats have been synthesized and conformationally characterized (Urry and Long, 1976). The high polymers of these repeating sequences have been cross-linked into sheets, rods, and tubes, and the PPP and PTP have been found to be elastomeric with the former being capable

Peptides: Design, Synthesis, and Biological Activity
Channa Basava and G. M. Anantharamaiah, Editors
©1994 *Birkhäuser Boston*

of an elastic modulus similar to that of the natural elastic fiber (Urry et al., 1976, 1981, 1982).

The parent elastic protein-based polymer, poly(VPGVG), can be minimally modified within the allowable conformational constraints of the β-spiral structure, (1) to exhibit a range of elastic moduli (Urry, 1990), (2) to have variable rates of degradation (Urry et al., 1992a), (3) to have the potential for various modes of drug delivery (Urry, 1991), (4) to perform free energy transduction involving the intensive variables of temperature, pressure, chemical potential, mechanical force, and electrochemical potential (Urry, 1992), (5) to be prepared with functional enzyme sites, for example, for lyslyl oxidase (Kagan et al., 1980), prolyl hydroxylase (Urry et al., 1979), protein kinases, and phosphatases (Pattanaik et al., 1991), and (6) to be prepared with cell attachment sequences (Nicol et al., 1992) that impart the properties of cell attachment, spreading, and growth to confluence to a matrix that otherwise does not exhibit cell attachment properties.

The parent elastic protein-based polymer, poly(VPGVG), and its γ-irradiation cross-linked elastomeric matrix, designated as X^{20}-poly(VPGVG), exhibit remarkable biocompatibility (Urry et al., 1991), and the matrix is a particularly useful form for a number of medical applications. Because of its potential as a biomaterial to be desired in large quantity, a number of approaches to the synthesis of the polypentapeptide of elastin have been undertaken. The primary problems with chemical syntheses have been purity and obtaining very high molecular weights. Further, because all the amino acid residues indicated as residue X into polymers with the general formula poly[f_v(GVGVP),f_x(GXGVP)] where $f_v + f_x = 1$ have been introduced, the problems of adequate side-chain-blocking groups and deblocking procedures have been sufficiently solved to obtain essentially impurity-free, protein-based polymers retained by 50-kDa cutoff membranes. This was necessary, for example, for the development of the hydrophobicity scale (Urry et al., 1992b). The ability to introduce all the amino acid residues into these high molecular weight polymers, has been a satisfying development that has taken several years of effort to achieve. Because there are excellent reviews available on many aspects of physical characterizations (Urry, 1992, 1993) and medical applications (Urry et al., 1993) of these bioelastic materials, this review focuses mainly on the synthetic efforts but also includes some recent aspects of physical characterizations and medical applications.

Syntheses

Polypentapeptide Syntheses

A number of approaches to the synthesis of the polypentapeptide of elastin have been undertaken. Pentamer purity before polymerization is a critical factor in obtaining high molecular weight polymers in good yields, because impurities can result in termination of the polymerization process and even small amounts of racemization can alter the physical properties. The strategies and approaches utilized by this laboratory are described in the following discussion; the approaches are presented much as they evolved within this laboratory.

Synthesis of the sequential polypeptides of the repeating pentamer can be achieved by polymerizing any one of the following pentamer permutations:

A. Val-Pro-Gly-Val-Gly (VPGVG)
B. Pro-Gly-Val-Gly-Val (PGVGV)
C. Gly-Val-Gly-Val-Pro (GVGVP)
D. Val-Gly-Val-Pro-Gly (VGVPG)
E. Gly-Val-Pro-Gly-Val (GVPGV)

Sequences B and E are of lesser interest as they have a bulky, optically active amino acid at their C termini that could result in low yields and racemic products. Sequences A and D are of interest because they have the least sterically hindering and optically inactive Gly in the C-terminal position. Sequence C is also promising as it has the least hindered Gly amino acid at the N terminus and a Pro at the C terminus, which will not result in racemization on activation and coupling of the carboxyl group.

In the early studies, permutation A was chosen (Urry et al., 1974a) because it best contains the repeating conformational unit that involves a hydrogen bond between Val^1 C–O and the Val^4 N-H. The approach used in the synthesis of this pentamer consists of a strategy of separately synthesizing the Val-Pro dimer and the Gly-Val-Gly trimer, then coupling these to give the pentamer. This is referred to as a 2 + 3 coupling strategy. The t-butyloxycarbonyl (Boc) group was used for α-amino protection, and its removal was achieved with HCl/dioxane. The coupling reactions were carried out with dicyclohexylcarbodiimide (DCC) (Sheehan and Hess, 1955). The PPP preparation (Urry et al., 1974b) was carried out by converting the pentamer to the pentachlorophenyl ester (OPcp) (Kupryszewski, 1961) or p-nitrophenyl ester (ONp) (Bodanszky and Du Vigneaud, 1959), removing the protecting Boc group, and polymerizing the peptide active ester in dimethylformamide (DMF). The result was a PPP with $n \sim 18$ (Urry et al., 1975).

In the second approach, a 3 + 2 coupling strategy was used (Prasad et al., 1985); the tripeptide Val-Pro-Gly and the dipeptide Val-Gly were synthesized separately and coupled to obtain the pentamer. The Boc group was used for α-amino protection, and coupling was achieved by means of the mixed anhydride (MA) (Vaughan and Osato, 1952), the 1-ethyl-3-(3-dimethylamino)propyl carbodiimide (EDCI) (Sheehan et al., 1965), or the active ester method (Sakakibara and Inukai, 1964). The pentapeptide ben-

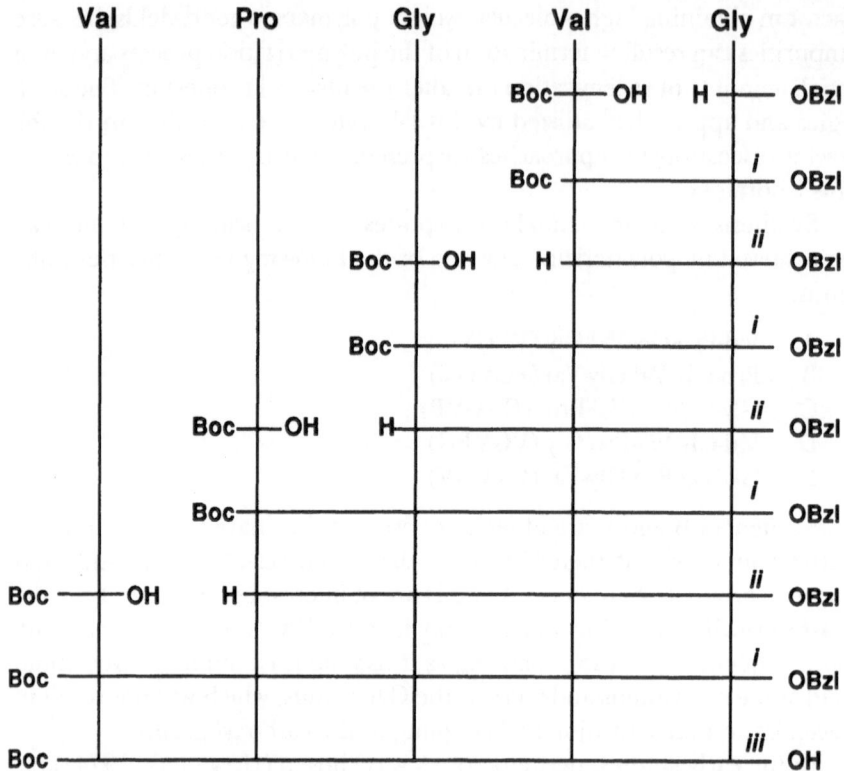

I. **isobutylchloroformate**
ii. **HCl/dioxane**
iii. **H₂/Pd-C**

Scheme 7–1. Schematic representation of the synthesis of Boc-Val-Pro-Gly-Val-Gly-OH.

zyl ester was hydrogenated to free acid, converted to ONp, deblocked with trifluoroacetic acid (TFA), and polymerized for 14 days in dimethylsulfoxide (DMSO) in the presence of triethylamine. The reaction was terminated by the addition of H-Val-OCH₃·HCl to give a C-terminal methyl ester. This approach gave a PPP in which $n = 40$ by end-group analysis.

For large-scale preparation of the pentamer, a simple and inexpensive method is desired. For that purpose, MA coupling at each stage of the synthesis is a useful approach (Scheme 7–1). In this approach, the synthesis proceeded smoothly to the tetrapeptide stage. The reaction of Boc-Val with PGVG-OBzl by the MA method gave a mixture of the desired product and N-isobutyloxycarbonyl-PGVG-OBzl in about a 60:40 ratio. This difficulty with MA coupling was overcome by adding 1-hydroxybenzotriazole (HOBt)

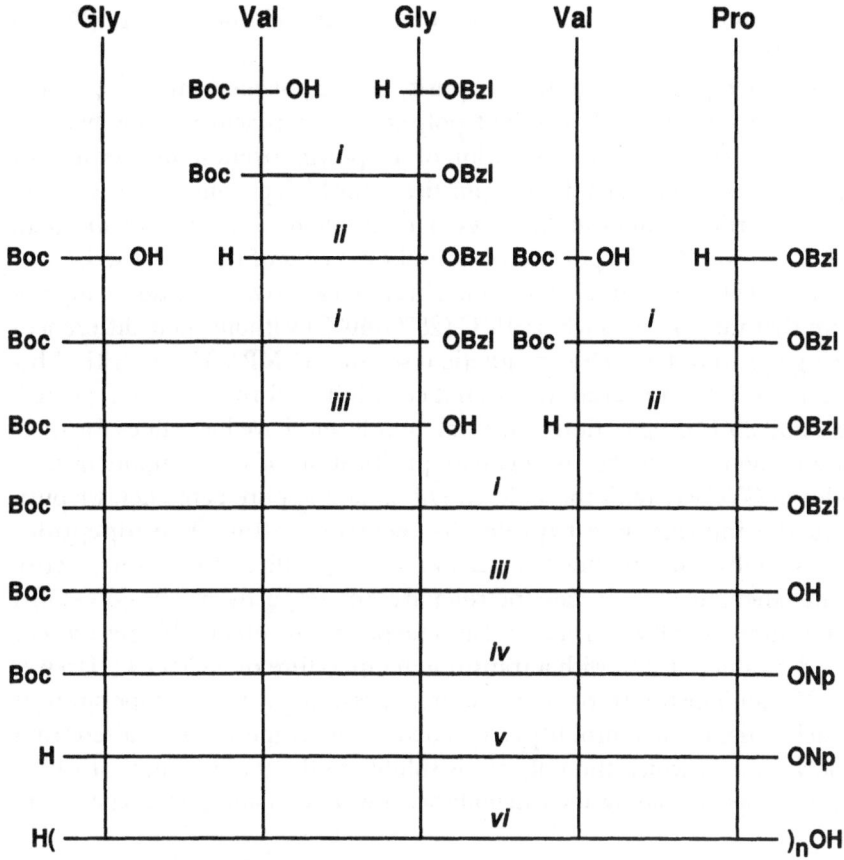

i. isobutylchloroformate
ii. HCl/dioxane
iii. H₂/Pd-C(10%)
iv. bis(p-nitrophenyl)carbonate
v. trifluoroacetic acid
vi. dimethylsulfoxide/N-methylmorpholine

Scheme 7–2. Schematic representation of the synthesis of poly(GVGVP).

to the reaction mixture before the addition of PGVG-OBzl. The result was a very good yield of the desired product (Prasad et al., 1985).

The synthesis of permutation C, GVGVP, is considered next; this repeat was polymerized by Bell et al. (1975) using OPcp activation of the carboxyl. Bell et al. reported a high polymer yield of 44% with $n = 22$. In preparing this pentamer, we used a 3 + 2 approach (Scheme 7–2). The pentamer buildup strategy was to synthesize the dipeptide VP and the tripeptide GVG and to couple the two fragments to give Boc-GVGVP-OBzl. The problem of by-product formation was encountered here also when Boc-Val-OH was coupled to H-Pro-OBzl but was overcome by the addition of HOBt (Prasad et al., 1985).

As noted previously, pentamer purity before polymerization is essential to obtain high molecular weight polymers in satisfactory yields because impurities can result in termination of the polymerization process and be-cause inclusion of even minor impurities in the high polymer alters its physi-cal properties in undesirable ways. The problems of purity are stringent because two different polymerizations, both being of molecular weight re-tained by 50-kDa cutoff dialysis membranes, can have transition tempera-ture that vary by as much as 15°C (25°C–40°C) without their differences being apparent by nuclear magnetic resonance (NMR). This is critical be-cause the 40°C preparation does not cross-link to form elastomeric matri-ces, and 30°C preparations cross-link poorly and have low values for their elastic moduli. The key is adequate purification of the component pep-tides of GVGVP. With this objective of obtaining pure pentamer, we puri-fied the intermediate peptides by recrystallization. The dipeptides Boc-VP-OBzl and the Boc-VG-OBzl were recrystallized from ether/petro-leum ether and ethyl acetate/petroleum ether, respectively; Boc-GVG-OBzl was also recrystallized from ethyl acetate:petroleum ether. This gives a very good product of PPP with a transition temperature of 25.5°±1°C (Urry et al., 1992c). The transition temperature, T_t, is defined as the temperature at which half-maximal turbidity is obtained as the temperature is raised from a low value at which the polymer is soluble to the temperatures at which hydrophobicity folding and assembly occur with reversible phase separation.

Methods of Polymerizations

A screening effort was undertaken to determine the activation and poly-merization conditions that would give the highest yields of high molecular weight PPP: these studies are summarized in Table 7–1. The yields are given in terms of the quantity of polymer retained in 3,500-M_r cutoff tubing after extensive dialysis against water. A number of syntheses have been carried out using p-nitrophenyl esters (ONp), o-nitrophenyl esters (ONo), m-nitrophenyl esters (ONm), pentachlorophenyl ester (OPcp), and trichlorophenyl ester (OTcp), with and without HOBt (Bodanszky, 1955; Bodanszky et al., 1972; Yamamoto and Hayakawa, 1982). Using the GVGVP permutation, both ONp and ONo activation gave high yields, but in the latter case the molecular weight remained in the 15,000 range. Moreover, the desired very high molecular weight was obtained with ONp. Further dialysis using 50,000-M_r cut-off dialysis tubing indicated a 79% yield, from the pentamer, of a polymer of more than 50,000 daltons. Best estimates of n are of the order of 200. When the VPGVG permutation was used with ONp, the value of T_t was higher. Because the GVGVP permutation gave

Table 7-1. Comparison of Different Solution Polymerizations
to Obtain High Polymers of the PPP of Elastin

Number	Method of Synthesis Polymerization	Yield (%) after 3500-M_r Cutoff Dialysis
1	H-VPGVG-ONp	70–80 (several attempts)
2	H-VPGVG-ONp/0.2 equiv HOBt	78
3	H-VPGVG-ONp/1.0 equiv HOBt	59
4	H-VPGVG-ONo	93
5	H-VPGVG-ONm	74
6	H-VPGVG-OPcp	40
7	H-GVGVP-OTcp	52
8	H-GVGVP-ONp	94
9	H-GVGVP-ONo	91
10	H-GVGVP-OH/EDCI	11
11	H-GVGVP-OH/EDCI/HOBt	85
12	H-GVGVP-OH/EDCI/HOSu	82
13	H-GVGVP-OH/DIC/HOSu	77

high yield of very high molecular weight, for the purpose of synthesis the pentamer GVGVP is used; it is abbreviated as poly(GVGVP). For the secondary structural reason of a hydrogen bond between Val[1] CO and the Val[4] NH, the polypeptide is most commonly referred to as poly(VPGVG) in our discussion.

EDCI, DCC, and N,N-diisopropylcarbodiimide (DIC) were also used as polymerizing agents in the presence of HOBt or N-hydroxysuccinimide (HOSu). It was found that EDCI in the presence of HOBt gave equally good polymers comparable to the ONp approach (Nicol et al., 1992; Urry et al., 1991). This method is useful when the longer chain peptides do not form active esters easily. The method was demonstrated during the polymerization of elastin sequences and tricosapeptides (manuscript in preparation).

Syntheses of Poly[f_v(GVGVP),f_x(GXGVP)] Where X Is Any Naturally Occurring Amino Acid Residue

After having checked the feasibility of preparing the PPP on a large scale in a pure, simple, and inexpensive way, the next effort was to introduce the naturally occurring amino acids that were necessary, for example, to develop the T_t-based hydrophobicity scale (Table 7–2; Figure 7–1). Importantly, the molecular conformation of poly(VPGVG) allows for chemical substitution, when done in a manner that does not disrupt conformation or elasticity. The Pro[2] and Gly[3] residues are essential for retaining the type II β-turn; in general, these positions cannot be changed. Improper placing of even a CH$_2$ moiety can change properties in undesirable ways. Substitution of an L-Ala residue for Gly[5] results in a granular precipitate on raising

Table 7-2. Hydrophobicity Scale for Proteins Based on Inverse Temperature Transitions

Residue X		T_t, linearly extrapolated to $f_x = 1$	Correlation Coefficient
Lys(NMeN, reduced)[a]		-130°C	1.000
Trp	(W)	-90°C	0.993
Tyr	(Y)	-55° C	0.999
Phe	(F)	-30° C	0.999
His (pH 8)	(H^o)	-10°C	1.000
Pro	(P)	(-8°C)	calculated
Leu	(L)	5°C	0.999
Ile	(I)	10°C	0.999
Met	(M)	20°C	0.996
Val	(V)	24°C	reference
Glu(COOCH$_3$)	(E^m)	25°C	1.000
Glu(COOH)	(E^o)	30°C	1.000
Cys	(C)	30°C	1.000
His (pH 4)	(H^+)	30°C	1.000
Lys(NH$_2$)	(K^o)	35°C	0.936
Asp(COOH)	(D^o)	45°C	0.994
Ala	(A)	45°C	0.997
HyP		50°C	0.998
Asn	(N)	50°C	0.997
Ser	(S)	50°C	0.997
Thr	(T)	50°C	0.999
Gly	(G)	55°C	0.000
Arg	(R)	60°C	1.000
Gln	(Q)	60°C	0.999
Lys(NH$_3^+$)	(K^+)	120°C	0.999
Tyr(ϕ - O^-)	(Y^-)	120°C	0.996
Lys(NMeN, oxidized)[a]		120°C	1.000
Asp(COO$^-$)	(D^-)	170°C	0.999
Glu(COO$^-$)	(E^-)	250°C	1.000
Ser(PO$_4^=$)		1000°C	1.000

[a] NMeN is for N-methyl nicotinamide pendant on a lysyl side chain, i.e., N-methyl incotinate attached by amide linkage to the ϵ- NH$_2$ of Lys, and the reduced state is N-methyl-1, 6-dihydronicotinamide.

the temperature and destroys elasticity (Urry, 1983). Therefore, this position cannot be altered. An interaction that is important in the hydrophobic folding process occurs between the Val^1 γ-CH$_3$ and the Pro^2 δ-CH$_2$ (Chang et al., 1989; Urry et al., 1977, 1989). Fidelity of substitution is achieved at position 1 with β-branched amino acids (Urry et al., 1986a). For example, an Ala residue in position 1 results in a polymer that undergoes an irreversible thermally induced aggregation (Rapaka et al., 1978). On the other hand, an Ile residue in position 1 results in an elastic matrix with excellent properties (Urry et al., 1986b). It is particularly fortunate that position 4 is available for all possible residue substitutions with the general formula poly[f$_v$(VPGVG),f$_x$(VPGXG)] where f$_v$ and f$_x$ are mole fractions with f$_v$ + f$_x$ = 1 and X is the guest residue. Using the 20 naturally occurring amino acids,

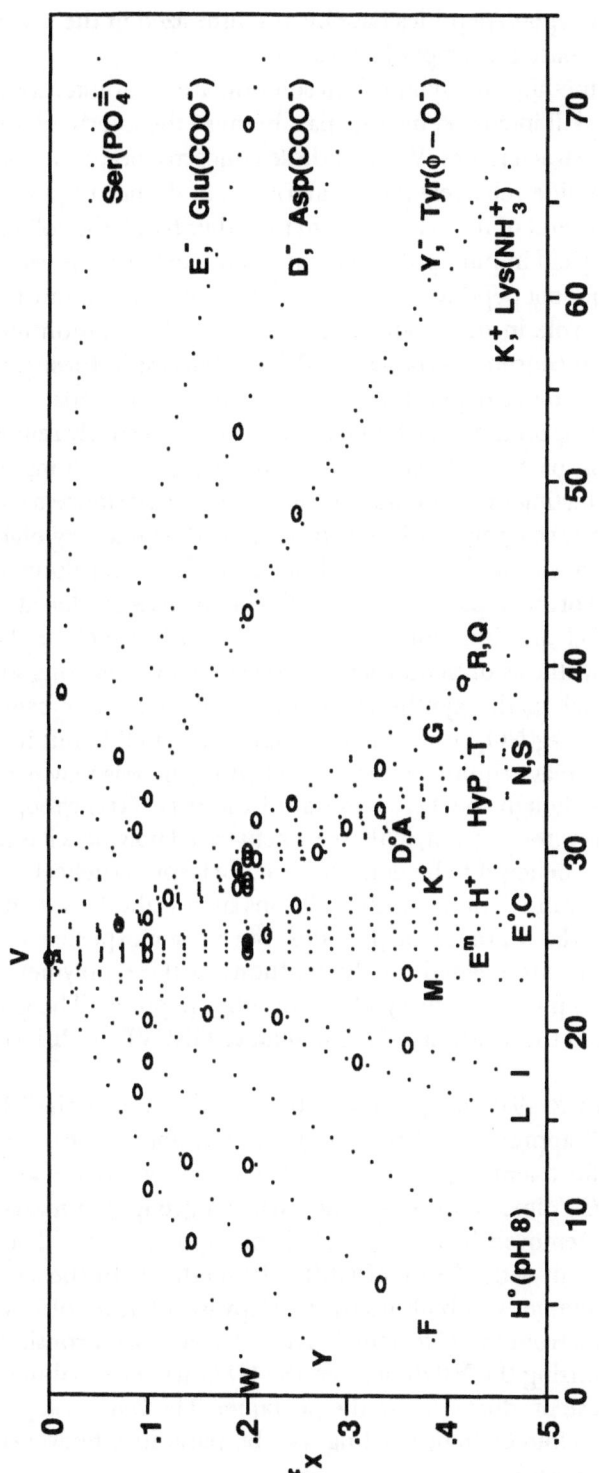

Figure 7–1. Temperature of inverse temperature transition, T_t for poly[f_v(VPGVG),f_X(VPGXG)].

more than 200 polypentapeptides have been synthesized in the process of developing the T_t-based hydrophobicity scale.

The classical methods for synthesis in solution are labor intensive, time consuming, and skill intensive, in large part because the intermediates differ in solubility characteristics. With all these concerns, however, the solution methods provide relatively pure materials that do not require much purification at the end of the synthesis. On the other hand, the solid-phase syntheses always yield impure products that require extensive purification even at the component peptide stage. As we mentioned earlier, purity plays a very important role in these polymers; therefore, the solution method has routinely been chosen to synthesize GXGVP. Success in these protein-based polymer syntheses depends not so much on the methods of activation and coupling as on the availability of an array of selectively removable protecting groups, particularly side-chain-protecting groups. Complete removal of the protecting groups employed is of great importance to obtain a desired protein-based polymer in satisfactory yield with a very high molecular weight and with a high degree of purity; if this is not done, an inseparable mixture of incompletely deprotected side chains is produced within a given polymer chain. Situations have often arisen in which applicable methods in the synthesis of peptides to remove certain protecting groups cannot be applied to the synthesis of these polymers. For example, hydrogenolysis of $Arg(NO_2)$ is normally complete within 2 h, but in these polymers removal may require a week or the hydrogenolysis may never go to completion. Although the TFA removal of the trityl (Trt) group from peptides proceeds within 30 min, in these protein-based polymers it is nearly impossible. This is believed to be derived from the β-spiral (helical nature) of these polymers. Mild deprotecting conditions such as the TFA treatment are preferred for the synthesis of peptides, but in our experience more rigorous conditions are needed for the synthesis of these polymers than those which are employed in the synthesis of other peptides. The general approaches used in the synthesis of the pentamer GXGVP are briefly discussed next.

The pentamer GXGVP was synthesized by a stepwise approach (Scheme 7-3) or the 3 + 2 approach (Scheme 7-4). In both approaches, the Boc group was used for α-amino protection, as has been mentioned, and was removed with HCl/dioxane or TFA. The carboxyl group was masked by benzyl ester and removed by hydrogenolysis or saponification. The coupling was carried out with MA or EDCI/HOBt methods. In the stepwise approach, the pentamer was built up by the stepwise addition of Boc-protected amino acids from the C terminal. The 3 + 2 approach consists of a strategy of synthesizing the VP dimer and the GXG trimer separately and then coupling these products to give the pentamer. The Boc pentapeptide acid was converted into ONp by reacting with bis-paranitrophenyl carbonate (Bis-PNPC) in pyridine.

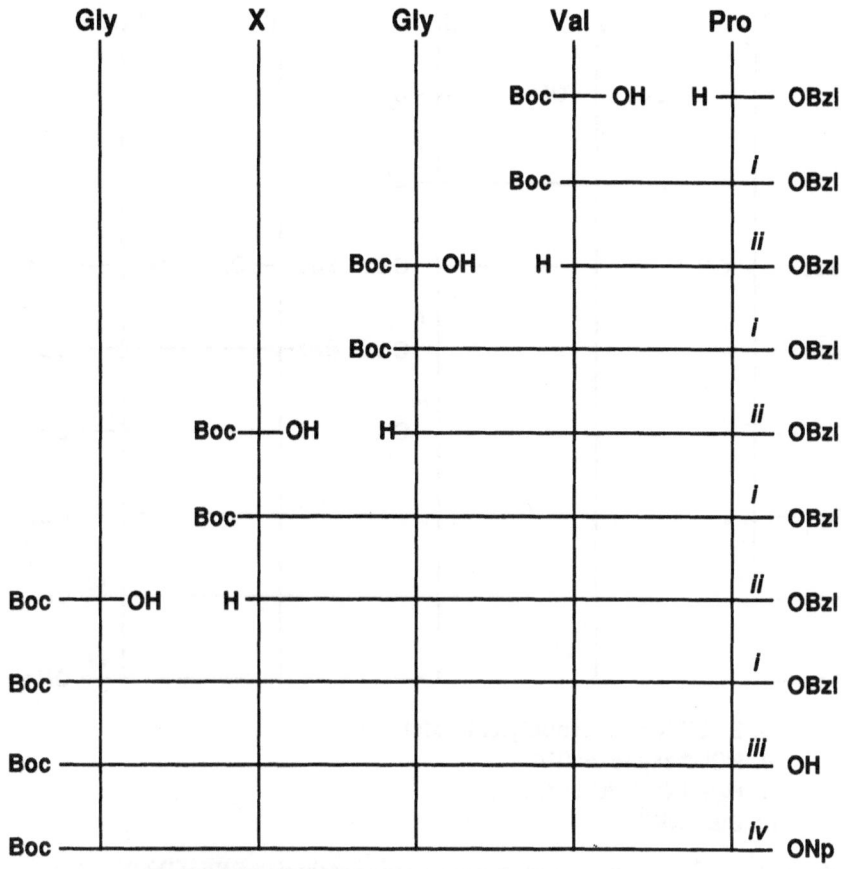

Scheme 7–3. Schematic representation of stepwise synthesis of Boc-GXGVP-ONp.

The Boc-GXGVP-ONp was mixed with Boc-GVGVP-ONp in the required ratios and deblocked together with TFA. A 1 M solution of the TFA salt in DMSO was polymerized for 14 days using 1.6 equiv of N-methylmorpholine (NMM) as base. The polymer was dissolved or suspended in water, dialyzed using 3500-M_r cutoff dialysis tubing, and lyophilized. The side-chain-protecting groups were removed by low or high HF procedures. This product was base treated with 1 N NaOH, dialyzed using 50-kDa cutoff dialysis tubing, and lyophilized to obtain poly[f_v(GVGVP),f_x(GXGVP)]. The different side-chain-protecting groups used for trifunctional amino acids and the problems faced during their cleavage are discussed next.

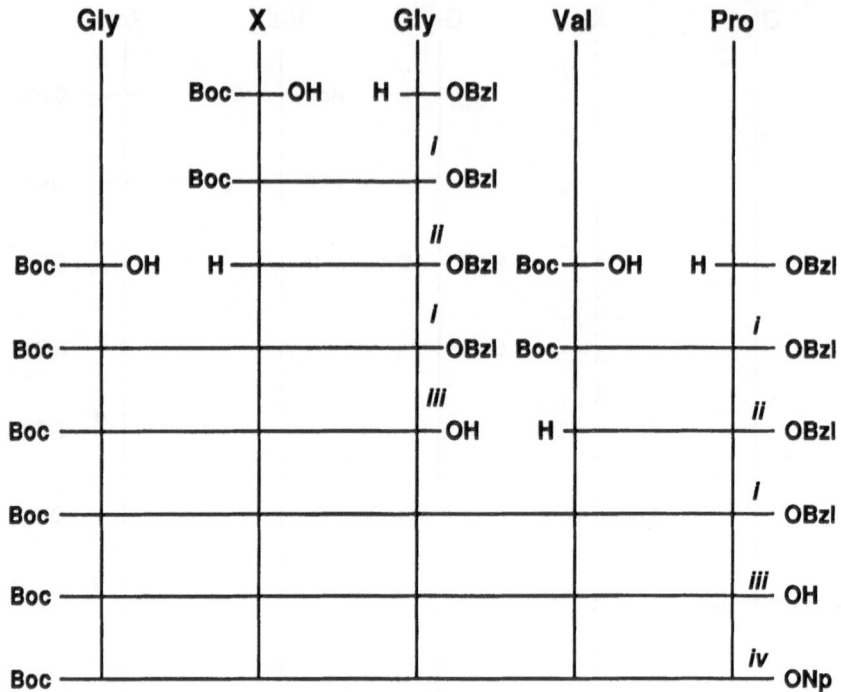

I. **EDCI/HOBt or isobutylchloroformate**
II. **HCl/dioxane or TFA**
III. **H₂/Pd-C (10%) or NaOH**
Iv. **Bis-PNPC**

Scheme 7–4. Schematic representation of the synthesis of Boc-GXGVP-ONp by (3 + 2) fragment coupling method.

Aspartic Acid and Glutamic Acid

The most common side reaction of the Asp residue is cyclization to form succinimide and the subsequent reopening of the ring to yield undesirable β-aspartyl peptides (Bodansky et al., 1978; Nicolis et al., 1989; Tam et al., 1988). Like Asp, Glu can also undergo cyclization leading to the subsequent formation of γ-Glu peptides, but this is not as serious as with Asp. The result of this side reaction is the formation of undesired products such as the free α-carboxyl, resulting in a lower pKa. In the early synthesis (Zhang et al., 1989), the side-chain function of Glu was protected by methyl ester and deblocked by base treatment with NaOH. Surprisingly, the correct pKa of Glu, 4.4, was obtained. The synthesis was subsequently repeated following the same procedure but the same result without the side reaction could not be obtained. Then, the synthesis was carried out with benzyl, t-butyl protection, and again the pKa was low. Finally, a study was conducted by synthesizing Glu containing a 25-mer on solid phase with methyl (OCH_3), benzyl (OBzl), and cyclohexyl (OCHx) protection. Only with the preparation using the cyclohexyl ester-protecting group (Urry et al., 1992d) was the pKa routinely obtained as in the earlier synthesis. The synthesis with cyclohexyl protection was repeated in solution phase and the correct pKa was obtained. The same side-chain protection yielded the best result when it was also applied to Asp. This protecting group was also used in the synthesis of elastin sequence W4 (a 52-amino-acid polymer with only one Glu) and with tricosapeptides synthesized to enhance hydrophobicity-induced pKa shifts (Urry et al., 1992e).

Arginine and Lysine

The guanidino side chain function of Arg is a strong nucleophile and is easily acylated during coupling if it is not protected. In our earlier studies, the NO_2 group was chosen to protect the guanidino function of Arg. The synthesis proceeded smoothly to the pentapeptide stage, and the pentamer was polymerized to obtain the polymers. Unfortunately, this group posed problems as it could not be removed by any of the known deblocking procedures such as hydrogenation (Copeland and Oroszlan, 1988) or transfer hydrogenation (Anantharamaiah and Sivanandaiah, 1977). In the second approach, the most widely used tosyl (Tos) group (Mazur, 1968) was used and the pentamer was built up by the 3 + 2 approach. The pentamer ONp was mixed with Boc-GVGVP-ONp, deblocked, polymerized, dialyzed, and lyophilized. The tosyl group was carefully deblocked with high HF in the presence of p-cresol at 0°C. The result was a very good yield of the desired product.

Protection of the ε-amino group of lysine is mandatory because it is a good nucleophile. In the coupling reactions it competes with the α-amino group for the acylating agent. Because the Boc group is used for temporary α-amino protection, the benzlyloxycarbonyl (Z) group can be used for the semipermanent blocking of the ε-amino group (Bergmann et al., 1935; Erickson and Merrifield, 1973a). The pentamer was built by the 3 + 2 coupling strategy, and the C-terminal OBzl was removed by saponification. After polymerization, the attempt to remove the Z group by hydrogenation remained incomplete, even after several days. In the second approach, the more acid-resistant 2-chlorobenzyloxycarbonyl (2-ClZ) group (Erickson and Merrifield, 1973b) was used and was removed by low HF treatment at 0°C for 2 h. Maintenance of the temperature at 0°C during the HF treatment is very important; the yield of polymer of greater than 50 kDa is very low at elevated temperatures because of damage to the peptide backbone. When compared to the histidine deblocking, however, the temperature problem with lysine is trivial.

Histidine

Histidine is one of the most problematic amino acids in peptide synthesis; this is also true in the synthesis of these protein-based polymers. The two main problems associated with the use of histidine are acylation of unprotected histidine and racemization. In these syntheses, however, the main problem is the removal of the side-chain-protecting groups while retaining the high molecular weight polymer. Initially, the most commonly used tosyl group (Fuji and Sakakibara, 1974) was employed to protect the imidazole function of histidine but the synthesis of pentamer was not fruitful. In the second approach, the benzyl group (du Vigneaud and Behrens, 1937) was used without success. In the third approach, another popular method utilizing the benzyloxymethyl (Bom) protecting group (Brown and Jones, 1981; Brown et al., 1982) was used. The pentamer was synthesized by the stepwise approach and polymerized. According to the literature, the Bom group can be deprotected by using either HF or hydrogenation (Brown and Jones, 1981; Brown et al., 1982). In both deprotecting methods, the polymer chain was broken resulting in low molecular weights (<50 kDa) and the limited yield of polymers had low histidine content. The deblocking was repeated with different scavengers such as anisole, thioanisole, p-cresol, or imidazole with different concentrations of HF without fruitful results.

In another approach, Dnp was used and the polymer was synthesized (Losse and Krychowski, 1971). The deprotection of this group was tried using all reported deblocking procedures, but the blocking group could not be removed using the known methods. Finally, the acid-sensitive trityl group (Sieber and Riniker, 1987) was used and the histidine was introduced as Fmoc-His(Trt)-OH. The last amino acid, Gly, was introduced as Ddz-Gly-OH to obtain the pentamer. The pentamer ONp was deblocked with 2% TFA and mixed with TFA · GVGVP-ONp, polymerized, dialyzed, and lyophilized. The polymer was treated with 100% TFA and checked with ^{13}C NMR, which indicated the presence of the trityl group. Finally, 72 h of hydrogenation was required for complete removal of the trityl group, but the yield of the polymer was very low. This amino acid is still in need of a very good side-chain-protecting group, like the OCHx for Asp or Glu, to obtain better results.

Serine, Threonine, and Tyrosine

The side chain of Ser contains a primary hydroxyl group while a secondary hydroxyl group is present in Thr. The alcoholic hydroxyl groups are sufficiently nucleophilic to compete with the amino group in coupling reactions, especially if highly reactive acylating agents are used. In such cases, protection of the Ser side chain is often desirable, and protection of the

Thr hydroxyl function is less necessary. In the presence of base, the hydroxyl group of Tyr is more reactive than that of Ser; therefore, the protection of Tyr is necessary. The risk of O-acylation can be avoided in all three amino acids by the protection of the hydroxyl group.

Synthesis of the Ser-, Thr-, and Tyr-containing pentamers proceeded using benzyl (Bzl) protection (Mizoguchi et al., 1968; Sugano and Miyoshi, 1976). However, removal of this group by hydrogenation, even after several days, was incomplete. Subsequently, this problem was solved by deprotection with HF. The improved synthesis of Tyr-containing polymers was carried out by a combination of 2,6-dichloro-benzyl (2,6-Cl$_2$-Bzl) protection and HF deprotection (Erickson and Merrifield, 1973b; Tam et al., 1983) in the presence of dimethyl sulfide and p-cresol scavengers. This gave very good results for the Tyr-containing polymers (Luan et al., 1992).

Asparagine and Glutamine

The side-chain carboxamides in both Asn and Gln residues are primary amides, which are more accessible to hydrolytic action than are the secondary amides of the peptide bonds. The synthesis of the pentamers containing these amino acids was carried out by the 3 + 2 approach without side-chain protection. The coupling reactions were carried out with EDCI/HOBt, and deprotection of Boc was effected by 100% TFA. After polymerization, the reaction was terminated by the addition of H-Val-OCH$_3$ to avoid the base treatment used to remove the terminal ONps. With these modifications, a very good yield of the desired product was obtained.

Tryptophan

The well-known sensitivity of indole to acids and oxidation leads to the production of complex mixtures, which are usually colored (pink to dark red) and consist of components that were not studied in detail. Such general decomposition will occur in deprotection steps, for example, with HBr in acetic acid or HBr in TFA (Boissonnas et al., 1958; Theodoropoulos and Fruton, 1962) and to a lesser extent even in neat TFA. In the latter medium, working at 0°C and in an inert atmosphere, Yajima et al. (1970) reduced the decomposition considerably. Scavengers that can trap cations, mostly thiols and thioethers, can prevent alkylation as well as the general oxidative decomposition. In the synthesis of these protein-based polymers, the Trp-containing pentamer utilized neat TFA deblocking in the presence of 1,2-ethanedithiol scavenger by the stepwise approach. The result was satisfactory and was confirmed by values of T$_t$, DSC, and ^{13}C NMR, and ^{1}H NMR (Luan et al., 1992).

Methionine and Cysteine

The presence of Met is the source of two different kinds of problems in peptide synthesis. Met can interfere with the removal of protecting groups from the side chain of other residues, and side reactions can occur that are directly related to the side chain of the Met residue. The undesired reactions that affect the thioether group are oxidation, alkylation, and decomposition by reduction with sodium in liquid ammonia. In the removal of protecting groups, catalytic hydrogenation is problematic because of the poisoning effect of the sulfur atom in the form of a sulfide. By carrying out all operations involving Met in an inert atmosphere, for example, under nitrogen or argon, oxidation can be reasonably prevented. More serious damage can take place in Met side chains by *S*-alkylation than by oxidation. Acidolytic removal of the Boc group, *t*-butyl esters, and ethers will cause *S*-*t*-butylation (Siber et al., 1970). The pentamer synthesis was carried out by the stepwise approach using resorcinol as the scavenger during deblocking, after addition of the Met residue. The C-terminal benzyl ester was removed by catalytic transfer hydrogenation using ammonium formate and 10% palladium on carbon. The pentamer ONp was purified on a silica gel column and mixed with Boc-GVGVP-ONp, deblocked, polymerized, dialyzed, and lyophilized.

The pronounced reactivity of the thiol group of Cys renders its protection mandatory. In the first approach, *t*-butyl protection was used to build up the pentamer. Deprotection by known procedures posed problems. In the second approach, the methylbenzyl group was used, but its removal using HF in the presence of *p*-cresol and thiocresol was not satisfactory. Like His, this amino acid is also in need of a better side-chain-protecting group to obtain the best results.

Other Amino Acids

The pentamers containing Gly, Ala, Leu, Val, Ile, or Phe require no special preparative methods. These pentamers were synthesized either by the 3 + 2 or the stepwise approach without any difficulties.

Syntheses of Polytetrapeptides with the General Formula Poly[f_v(VPGG),f_x(XPGG)]

A series of polytetrapeptides have been considered in relationship to cell attachment and the prevention of adhesions applications. These have the general structural formula poly[f_v(VPGG),f_x(XPGG)] where f_v and f_x are mole fractions with $f_v + f_v = 1$ and X is any naturally occurring amino acid or a chemical modification thereof. The synthesis of tetrapeptide, XPGG, can be achieved using the permutation GGXP because this permutation gave a very high molecular weight polymer when determined by the value of T_t. In the first approach (Luan et al., 1991; Urry et al., 1986b), Boc-GG-OBzl was prepared using EDCI/HOBt for coupling and was hydrogenated to give the acid. Boc-XP-OBzl was synthesized by the mixed anhydride method in the presence of HOBt, deblocked, and coupled with Boc-GG-OH using EDCI/HOBt to give Boc-GGXP-OBzl. After hydrogenating to the acid, it was converted to ONp by reacting with bis-PNPC. After removing the Boc group, the active ester was polymerized, dialyzed against water using a 50,000-M_r cutoff dialysis tubing, and lyophilized.

In the second approach (Nicol et al., 1993), the tetrapeptide was prepared by stepwise addition of Boc amino acids from the C terminus. Boc-XP-OBzl was synthesized by the mixed anhydride method in the presence of HOBt, deblocked, and coupled with Boc-Gly-OH using EDCI/HOBt to obtain Boc-GXP-OBzl. This was again deblocked and coupled with Boc-Gly-OH using EDCI/HOBt and the resulting tetrapeptide, after hydrogenating to the acid, was converted to ONp. The Boc group was removed, and the tetramer was polymerized, dialyzed, and lyophilized to obtain the polytetrapeptide. This approach gave a very good yield as compared to the first approach.

Synthesis of the Kinase Site, Arg-Gly-Tyr-Ser-Leu-Gly

In an effort to test how phosphorylation could shift the temperature of an inverse temperature transition (Pattanaik et al., 1991), a kinase site was introduced. Specifically, the cyclic AMP-dependent protein kinase site, (Arg-Gly-Tyr-Ser-Leu-Gly), that is, RGYSLG, of chicken egg lysozyme was synthesized on solid phase and copolymerized with IPGVG to give poly[30(IPGVG), (RGYSLG)]. The synthesis of RGYSLG by solid phase follows.

The hexapeptide was synthesized by the solid-phase technique (Merrifield, 1964) starting from the Boc-Gly-OCH$_2$-C$_6$H$_4$ resin. The Boc group was used for temporary amino protection, and its removal was effected by 40% TFA in methylene chloride. DCC/HOBt was used as the coupling reagent. The side-chain functions of Arg, Ser, and Tyr were protected by tosyl, benzyl, and 2,6-dichlorobenzyl derivatives, respectively. After completion of the sequence, the protected peptide was cleaved from the resin by transesterification with 2-dimethylaminoethanol (Barton et al., 1973) and purified over silica gel. The protected hexapeptide was mixed with Boc-IPGVG-OH at the appropriate ratio, treated with TFA to remove the Boc group, polymerized using EDCI/HOBt in the presence of NMM as base, dialyzed using 3500-M_r cutoff dialysis tubing, and lyophilized. The protecting groups of the hexapeptide were then deblocked by a low–high HF deprotection procedure (Tam et al., 1983), dialyzed, and lyophilized.

Syntheses of the Cell Attachment Sequences Gly-Arg-Gly-Asp-Ser-Pro, Arg-Glu-Asp-Val-Phe-Pro-Gly, Arg-Glu-Asp-Val-Tyr-Pro-Gly, Arg-Glu-Asp-Val-Pro, and Gly-Arg-Glu-Asp-Val-Pro

Unmodified X^{20}-poly(GVGVP) provides very poor support for cell attachment when tested in the absence of serum. Cell adhesion properties of X^{20}-poly(GVGVP) can be achieved by the covalent incorporation of RGDS, the primary cell attachment sequence of fibronectin. In this direction, RGDS was synthesized as GRGDSP, the actual sequence within fibronectin, and polymerized with GVGVP at different ratios (Nicol et al., 1992). Similarly, REDV, another amino acid sequence within fibronectin, was shown to mediate melanoma cell adhesion. When as GREDVY this sequence is attached to glycophase glass, it is reported to be specific for human endothelial cell spreading. It was synthesized as REDVFPG, REDVYPG, REDVP, and GREDVP, each of which was polymerized with GVGVP at a ratio of 20:1 (Nicol et al., in press). The syntheses of these sequences are briefly discussed next.

The synthesis of Boc-Gly-Arg(Tos)-Gly-Asp(OCHx)-Ser(Bzl)-Pro-ONp was carried out by classical solution methods following a 3 + 3 approach (Scheme 7–5). In this synthesis, Boc chemistry was used with EDCI/HOBt as the coupling method. The side-chain functions of Arg, Asp, and Ser were protected by tosyl, cyclohexyl, and benzyl groups, respectively. The C-terminus carboxyl group was protected by phenacyl ester, and its removal was achieved by Zn:90% acetic acid. The Boc hexapeptide ONp was prepared by reacting the acid with bis-*p*-nitrophenylcarbonate. This was mixed with Boc-GVGVP-ONp at different ratios, deblocked, polymerized, dialyzed, and lyophilized. The side-chain-protecting groups were deblocked with a low–high HF procedure to obtain poly[n(GVGVP),(GRGDSP)]. In another approach, Boc chemistry was combined with Ddz protection for some amino acids and the side-chain function of aspartic acid was protected by *t*-butyl ester and C-terminal carboxyl by benzyl ester (Nicol et al., 1992). The product is good in both approaches, with lower yield in the latter approach.

The syntheses of the two heptapeptides, Boc-Arg(Tos)-Glu(OCHx)-Asp(OCHx)-Val-Phe-Pro-Gly-OH and Boc-Arg(Tos)-Glu(OCHx)-Asp(OCHx)-Val-Tyr(2,6-Cl$_2$-Bzl)-Pro-Gly-OH, were carried out by the solid-phase technique starting from the Boc-Gly-OCH$_2$-C$_6$H$_4$ resin and following the same procedure as explained for the synthesis of the kinase site. The hexapeptide Boc-Gly-Arg(Tos)-Glu(OCHx)-Asp(OCHx)-Val-Pro-OH and the pentapeptide Boc-Arg(Tos)-Glu(OCHx)-Asp(OCHx)-Val-Pro-OH were synthesized by the solution-phase method. The materials and methods are the same as those described in the synthesis of the pentamer GXGVP, each of which was converted to ONp by reacting with bis-*p*-nitrophenyl carbonate and mixed with Boc-GVGVP-ONp at a ratio of 20:1, deblocked, polymer-

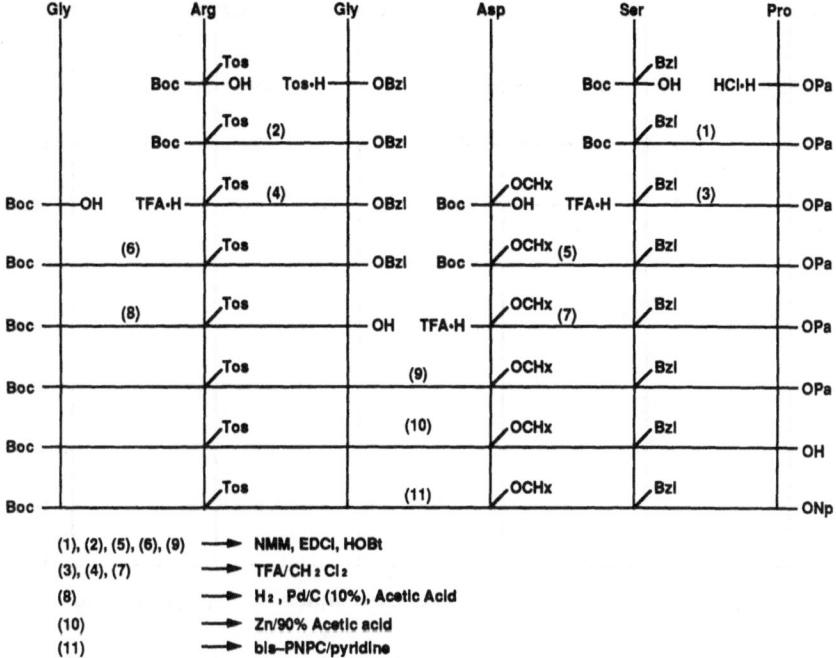

Scheme 7-5. Schematic representation of the synthesis of Boc-GR(Tos)GD(OCHx) S(Bzl)P-ONp.

ized, dialyzed, and lyophilized. The protecting groups are cleaved with HF, dialyzed using 50-kDa cutoff dialysis tubing, and lyophilized.

Syntheses of Polytricosapeptides

In an effort to enhance hydrophobicity-induced pKa shifts (Urry et al., 1992e), a series of polytricosapeptides with the general formula poly(GXGFP GVGVP GVGFP GFGFP GVGVP GVGFP), poly(GXGFP GVGVP GVGVP GVGVP GFGFP GFGFP), and poly(GXGVP GFGFP GFGVP GVGVP GFGFP GVGVP) have been synthesized where X = Glu, Asp, Lys, or His. These tricosapeptides were synthesized by the [(5 + 5 + 5) + (5 + 5 + 5)] fragment coupling strategy in solution phase (Scheme 7–6). The pentamers required for this purpose are synthesized with appropriate side-chain protection as previously described. In the syntheses, the Boc group was used for Nᵃ protection, and its removal was effected by TFA. All coupling reactions and polymerizations were carried out by the EDCI/HOBt method, and the final deprotection was effected by HF. More details of syntheses and product verification are presented elsewhere.

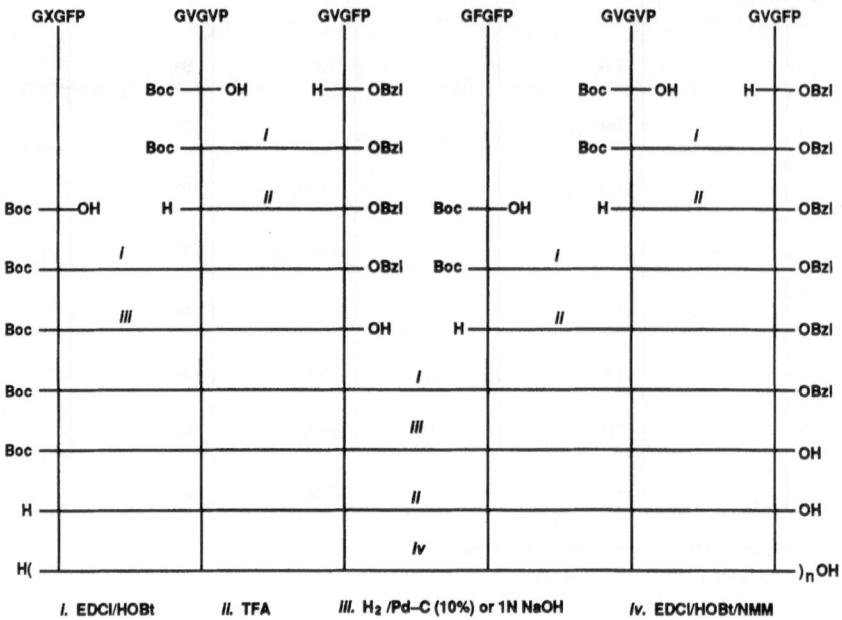

Scheme 7-6. Schematic representation of the synthesis of Polytricosapeptides.

Other Protein-Based Polymer Syntheses

In addition to the foregoing syntheses, a number of other polymers such as poly(GVGIP), poly[f_v(GVGVP), f_x(GVGFP)], poly[f_v(GVGIP), f_x(GXGIP)] where X = Glu, Asp, or Lys, poly(GVGVAP), poly(AGVPGLGVG), poly(AGVPGFGVG), and a number of other sequences from elastin have also been synthesized with substitution at position 1. In an effort to gain a measure of control over the rate of nonenzymatic degradation of bioelastic materials, several polypentapeptides containing glycolic acid have also been synthesized (Urry et al., in press). In addressing the effect on T_t of changing the oxidation/reduction, N-methylnicotinamide was attached by carboxamide linkage to the Lys residue in poly[0.73(GVGVP),0.27(GKGVP)] (Urry et al., 1992f). The syntheses of these protein-based polymers constitute only a fraction of the more than 1000 such syntheses carried out in this laboratory during the past quarter of a century.

Verification of Syntheses

In addition to the standard peptide chemistry procedures, the syntheses are routinely verified by temperature profiles of aggregation (and pH dependence thereof when composition indicates), which are an informative

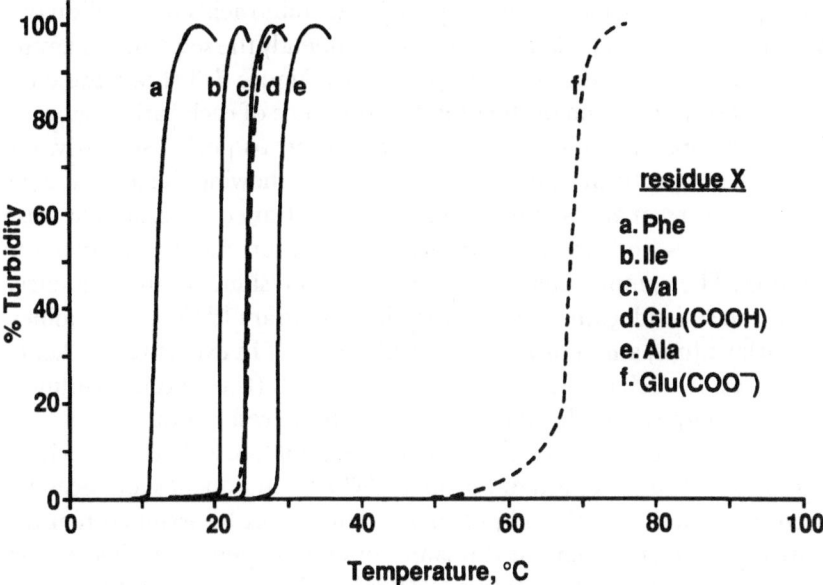

Figure 7-2. Temperature profiles for turbidity formation, TP$_t$s for poly[0.8(VPGVG), 0.2(VPGXG)], i.e., $f_X = 0.2$.

initial screening method. The syntheses are also routinely verified by amino acid analysis, by one-dimensional proton and ^{13}C NMR, and, when warranted, by two-dimensional NMR, circular dichroism, optical rotatory dispersion, and quantitative acid–base titrations.

The PPP and the analogs considered are all soluble in water when a sufficiently low temperature can be reached without freezing. When the temperature is raised toward the physiological range, these polymers associate by means of hydrophobic intermolecular interactions to form cloudy suspensions: on standing, the aggregates settle. In the case of PPP, what forms on the bottom of the vial is a dense viscoelastic phase called a coacervate. The coacervate phase is approximately 50% peptide and 50% water. The process of coacervation for PPP and most of its analogs is reversible; that is, when the temperature is lowered, the coacervate slowly redissolves. The temperature profiles of turbidity formation, TPτs, of sequences that form viscoelastic phases are characterized primarily by profiles that steepen as the concentration is increased whereas sequences that irreversibly form aggregates are characterized by a translation of the profile to a lower temperature on increasing the concentration. Simple curves are obtained for pure syntheses in both cases. Inhomogeneous sequences and impurities are often detected by complex profiles. The temperature profiles for turbidity formation for the high concentration limits of the PPP and a series of analogs are given in Figure 7-2.

It is possible to demonstrate the purity and amino acid composition of a polypeptide and even to demonstrate independently the sequence of amino acids using ^{13}C and proton NMR approaches; Figure 7–3 shows the complete ^{13}C NMR spectrum of the PPP. The presence of each carbon atom of the PPP is apparent as is the absence of extraneous peaks. Similarly, the proton NMR spectrum of the PPP (Figure 7–4), showing the assignments of all proton resonances and the absence of extraneous peaks that arise from impurities, verifies the amino acid composition and the purity of the syntheses. The complexities arise from identical residues in the sequences (e.g., of the 30 residues in polytricosapeptides, there are 12 glycines, 6 valines, 5 phenylalanines, and 6 prolines), which can result in extensive overlap of resonances. In such cases, multidimensional NMR (two- and three-dimensional) techniques have been employed to achieve resolution.

Amino acid analyses provide another important tool with which to check the purity and composition of polymers. When component sequences are mixed in a reaction flask and polymerized, it cannot be assumed that the purified product polymer has the same component peptide ratios as were placed in the reaction flask. While NMR is helpful, more accurate analyses of ratios are often required, such as when a cell attachment sequence is included in a 20:1 ratio. For such cases an HPLC amino acid system that can determine picomolar quantities of amino acids is utilized. The amino acid analysis of poly[20(GVGVP),(GRGDSP)] is shown in Figure 7–5.

Preparation of Cross-linked Matrices

A simple, effective means of obtaining a cross-linked matrix is by γ-irradiation cross-linking using a ^{60}Co source. Those compositions that form viscoelastic phases can be cast into various shapes, including tubes and sheets. First, PPP is dissolved in water in a 250 mg/ml concentration. The solution is then placed in a mold and centrifuged with the temperature maintained at 10°C below the transition for 1 h. It is then is centrifuged for an additional 4 h while maintaining the temperature 10°C above the transition. Next, the coacervate phase is checked for uniformity. If it does not contain any irregularities such as bubbles, it is γ-irradiated with a 20-Mrad dose of ^{60}Co to achieve the cross-links that result in an insoluble matrix. The molds are then opened in a laminar flow hood using sterile conditions and placed in a tube containing sterile water. Similarly, the analogs of PPP can be prepared for cross-linking by maintaining the temperature 10°C below and then 10°C above the transition during centrifugation.

Interestingly, PPP withstands γ-irradiation without detectable residue destruction. To date, the sites involved in the cross-linking have not been determined and are at such low levels as not to be apparent in the amino acid analysis data. As shown in Figure 7–6, composition of the HPLC chro-

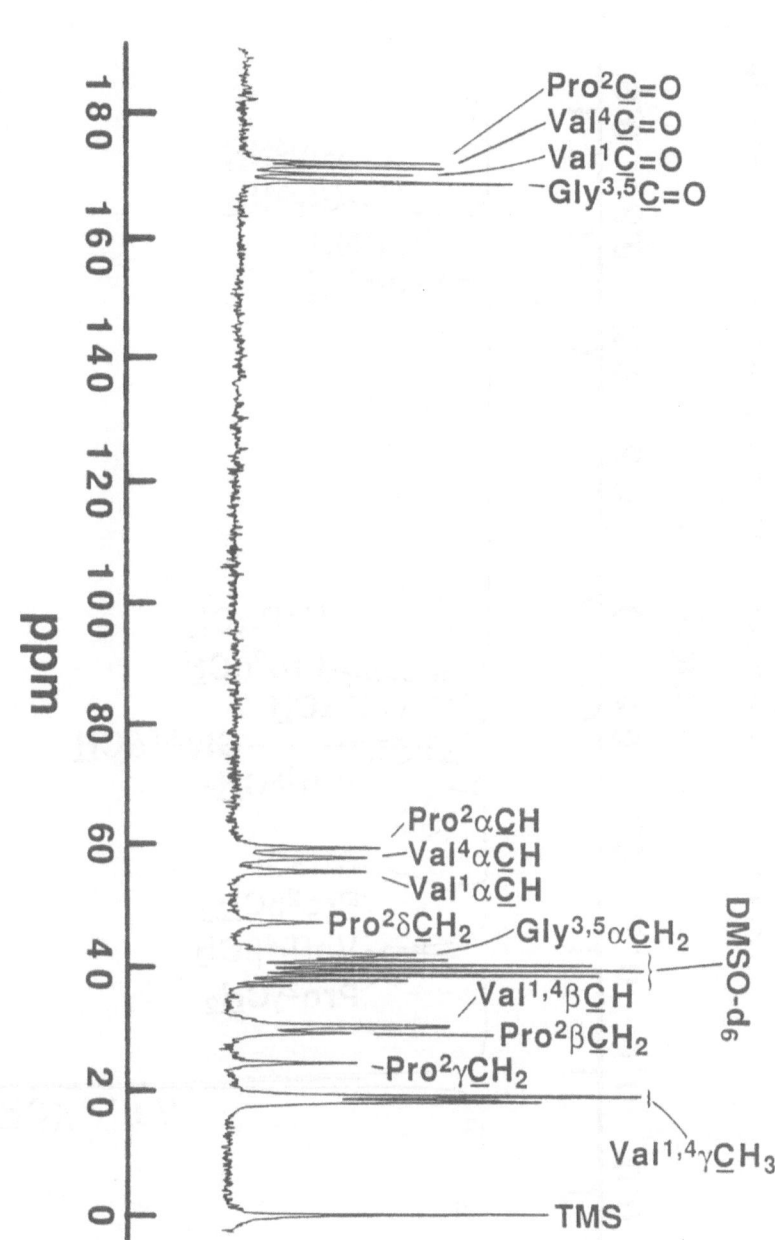

Figure 7-3. ^{13}C NMR spectra of PPP at 25 MHz in DMSO.

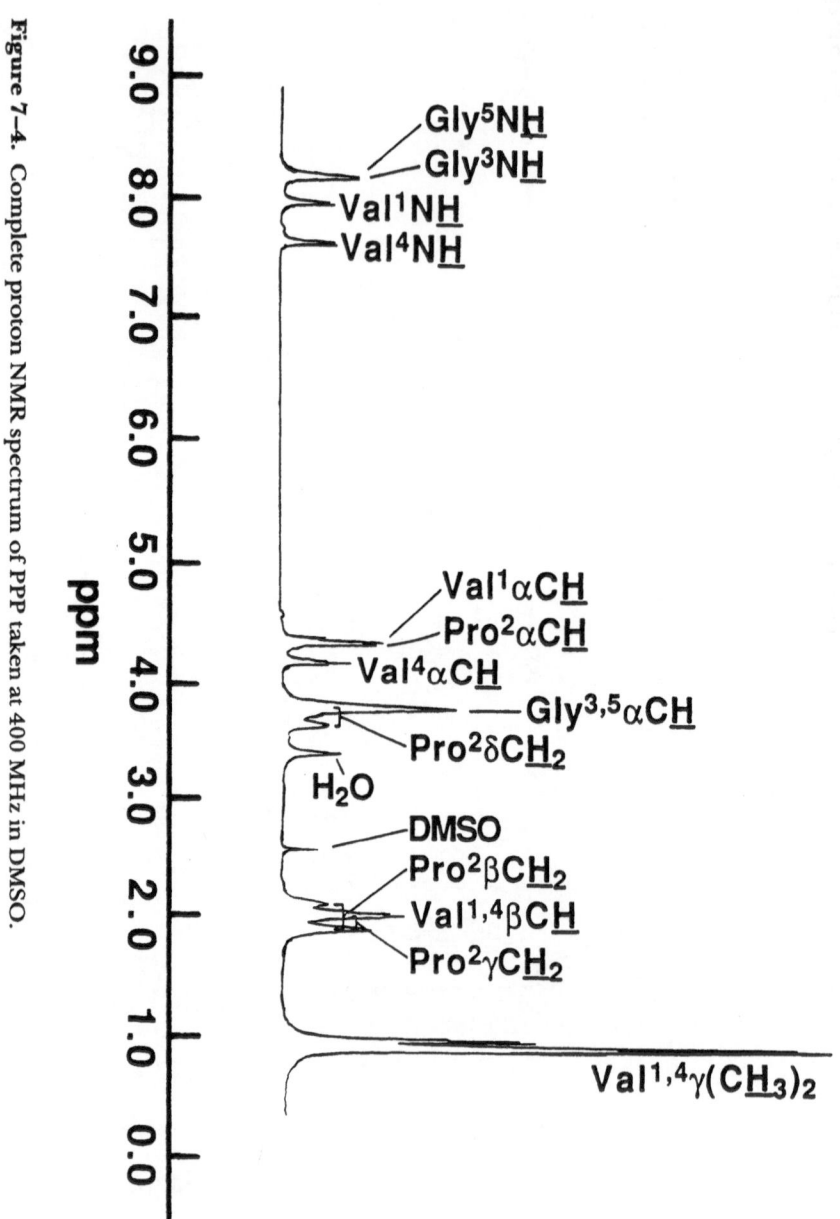

Figure 7–4. Complete proton NMR spectrum of PPP taken at 400 MHz in DMSO.

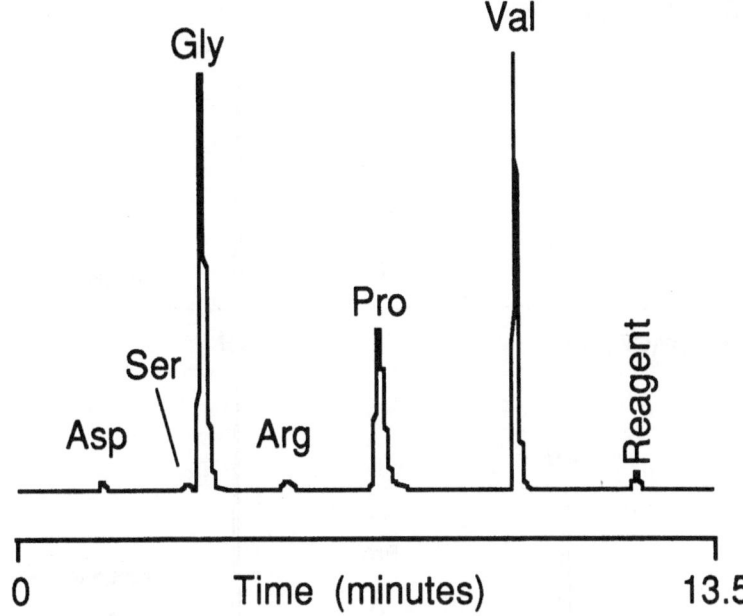

Figure 7–5. HPLC chromatogram of acid-hydrolyzed poly[20(GVGVP),(GRGDSP)].

matograms for hydrolysates of both poly(GVGVP) and X^{20}-poly(GVGVP) demonstrate no detectable effect of the 20-Mrad γ-irradiation (Urry et al., 1992c). Further, all 20 natural amino acids and the redox couple *N*-methylnicotinamide withstand γ-irradiation with little detectable residue destruction (manuscript in preparation). In addition to γ-irradiation cross-linking, electron beam irradiation cross-linking appears promising.

General Physical Characterizations

The general physical characterizations may be grouped as (a) mechanical studies, (b) ultrastructural studies, (c) conformational studies, (d) dynamics studies, (e) acid–base titrations, and (f) thermodynamic studies such as differential scanning calorimetry. These physical properties of synthetic biomaterials have been extensively reviewed (Urry, 1992, 1993). A brief discussion of mechanical studies and acid–base titrations follows.

Mechanical Studies

The mechanical studies for characterization of elasticity are most commonly stress/strain curves for determination of elastic modulus and

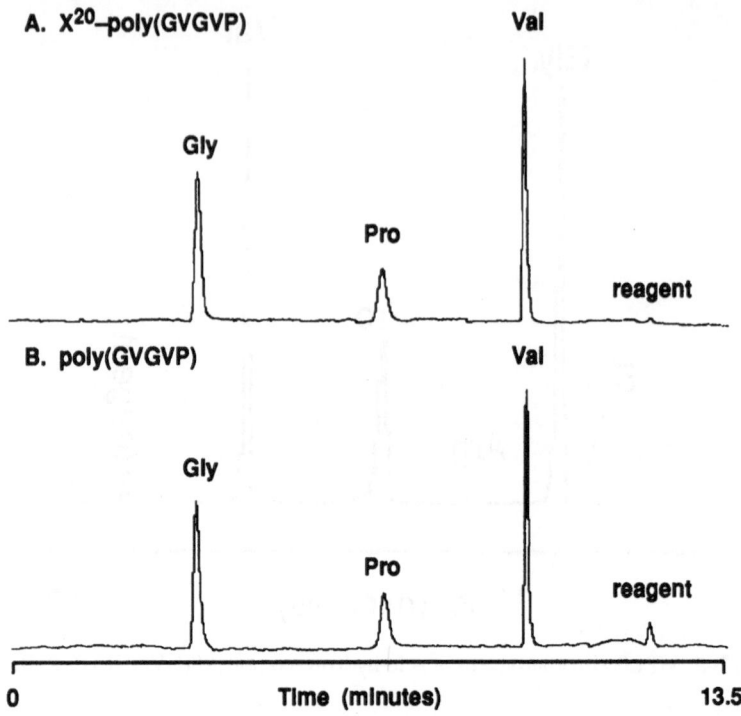

Figure 7-6. HPLC chromatograms of acid-hydrolyzed poly[VPGVG) before and after 20-Mrad γ-irradiation.

thermoelasticity studies for assessing the entropic contribution to elasto-meric force. The elastic (Young's) modulus for X^{20}-poly(GVGVP) is about 1×10^6 dynes/cm² with little or no hysteresis, and extensions of as much as 200% have been observed. The elastic modulus resulting from γ-irradia-tion has been found to be proportional to the square of the γ-irradiation dose, that is, a doubling of the dose quadruples the elastic modulus. De-pending on the composition, the elastic modulus for a 20-Mrad dose can vary from 10^5 to 10^9 dynes/cm². It is very important to mention that the impure polymer always gives a weak elastomeric band with low elastic modu-lus. Thermoelasticity studies involve stretching a band of elastomer to a fixed length and then monitoring force (f) as the temperature (T) is varied. A dramatic increase in force is observed as the temperature is raised through the transition. Above the transition, however, a plot of $\ln(f/T)$ versus T gives a near-zero slope such that the ratio of internal energy component of force (f_e) to total elastomeric force; that is, f_e/f, is of the order of $1/10$. On the basis of these results and their associated classical arguments, X^{20}-poly(GVGVP) is a dominantly entropic elastomer, as is natural elastin. The remarkable durability exhibited by natural elastin, apparently capable of billions of stretch/relaxation cycles in the aortic arch, is also a potential for these synthetic elastomers.

Acid–Base Titrations

Acid–base titrations are used to determine the pKa of ionizable side chains and have also been used to demonstrate stretch-induced increases in pKa for the synthetic elastomers. By these titrations, the number of ionizable amino acids can also be determined quantitatively. It is very important to note here that small changes in the polymers (presence of impurities, incomplete deblocking of side-chain-protecting groups and cyclic imide formation) can produce significantly different pKa values. For example, the base treatment deprotection of the OCHx group from Asp polymers gives low pKa values whereas HF deprotection gives the correct pKa. Similarly, the use of methyl ester to protect the γ-carboxyl group of Glu produces a polymer with pKa as low as 3.5. With OCHx protection and deprotection with HF, however, the polymer produces a correct pKa value of 4.4. Further, it has been shown that proper design at nanometric dimensions can dramatically change the pKa of an amino acid side chain. For example, the pKa of a Glu residue has been shifted, by design and synthesis, from 4.3 to 8.1.

Medical Applications

Given the properties of the bioelastic materials just noted, it is possible to design and synthesize elastomeric polypeptides capable of exhibiting additional properties and functions with both medical and nonmedical applications. For medical applications, it is first necessary to demonstrate adequate biocompatability for each protein-based polymer composition.

Biocompatibility of a Bioelastic Material

Because of the dynamic and dominantly hydrophobic structure of poly(GVGVP), it had been anticipated that it and its γ-irradiation cross-linked matrix would be biocompatible. Following the American Society for Testing Materials (ASTM) recommendations for a set of biological tests required to establish biocompatibility for materials in contact with tissues, tissue fluids, and blood, 11 tests were performed on poly(GVGVP) and the elastic matrix, X^{20}-poly(GVGVP) (Urry et al., 1991). With the results following in parentheses, these were "(1) the Ames mutagenicity test (non-mutagenic), (2) cytotoxicity-agarose overlay (non-toxic), (3) acute systemic toxicity (non-toxic), (4) intracutaneous toxicity (non-toxic), (5) muscle implantation (favorable), (6) acute intraperitoneal toxicity (non-toxic), (7) systemic antigenicity (non-antigenic), (8) dermal sensitization [the Magnusson and Kligman maximization method] (non-sensitizing), (9) pyrogenicity (non-pyrogenic), (10) Lee-White clotting study (normal clotting time), and (11) in vitro hemolysis test (non-hemolytic)." The result is a remarkable biocompatibility.

In addition, biocompatibility tests are under way on a member of the polytetrapeptide series, namely poly(GGAP) and X^{20}-poly(GGAP). To date, the series of tests—the Ames mutagenicity test, cytotoxicity-agarose overlay, systemic toxicity, Kligman sensitization, and hemolysis—indicate good biocompatibility.

Medical Applications

The medical applications of these bioelastic materials have been extensively reviewed (Urry et al., 1993). A few of these are discussed here.

We have shown in cell adhesion studies that X^{-20}poly(GVGVP) is a poor substrate for cell adhesion (Nicol et al., 1992). As no fibrous capsule forms around it when implanted, the matrix and other states of the material have potential for use in the prevention of postsurgical adhesions. Specific studies under way include a contaminated peritoneal model using the rat (Hoban et al., in press), a strabismus surgery model using the rabbit eye (Elsas et al., 1992), and, in a study just beginning, a total artificial heart model as a bridge to transplantation, using the calf.

The synthetic incorporation of RGDS, the cell attachment site of fibronectin, as GRGDSP into the matrix results in a material with cell attachment properties equivalent to those of fibronectin-coated tissue culture plastic (Nicol et al., 1992). Thus, the biocompatibility and appropriate mechanical properties of these bioelastic materials, combined with the capacity for incorporation of bioactive peptide sequences, indicate their potential for development as matrices for tissue reconstruction.

Further, these materials can be designed to swell or to contract in a manner to effect drug delivery by use of any of a number of intensive variables, that is, to perform free energy transduction as a means of achieving drug delivery. This is made especially attractive because, in addition to being able to swell or to contract, they can be designed to contain chemical clocks that would control the rate of degradation as desired (Urry et al., in press).

In addition to the medical applications just mentioned that are under development, these biomaterials can also be considered in a number of nonmedical applications such as biomimetics, molecular machines, transducers (sensors and actuators), superabsorbents, biodegradable plastics, and delivery systems for herbicides, pesticides, growth factors, and fertilizers.

Acknowledgments

This work was supported in part by contracts DAAL03-92-C-0005 (to R.D.H.) from the U.S. Department of the Army, the U.S. Army Research Office, and N00014-89-J-1970 (to D.W.U.) from the U.S. Department of the Navy, Office of Naval Research. The authors wish to acknowledge the many members of the Laboratory of Molecular Biophysics, past and present, who have contributed so extensively to the work reviewed here.

REFERENCES

Anantharamaiah GM, Sivanandaiah KM (1977): *J Chem Soc Perkin Trans* I:490–491.
Barton MA, Lemieux RU, Savoie JY (1973): *J Am Chem Soc* 95:4501–4506.
Bell JR, Boohan RC, Jones JH, Moore RM (1975): *Int J Pept Protein Res* 7:229–234.
Bergmann M, Zervas L, Ross WF (1935): *J Biol Chem* 111:245–260.
Bodanszky M (1955): *Nature (London)* 175:685.
Bodanszky M, duVigneaud V (1959): *J Am Chem Soc* 81:5688–5691.
Bodanszky M, Tolle JC, Deshmane SS, Bodanszyk A (1978): *Int J Pept Protein Res* 12:57–68.
Bodanszky M, Bath RJ, Chang A, Fink ML, Funk KW, Greenwald SM, Klausner YS (1972): In: *Chemistry and Biology of Peptides*, Meinhofer J, ed., p. 203. Ann Arbor, Michigan: Ann Arbor Scientific.
Boissonnas RA, Guttmann ST, Huguenin RL, Jaquenoud P-A, Sandrin ED (1958): *Helv Chim Acta* 41:1867–1882.
Brown T, Jones JH (1981): *J Chem Soc Chem Commun* 648–649.
Brown T, Jones JH, Richards JD (1982): *J Chem Soc Perkin Trans* I:1553–1561.
Chang DK, Venkatachalam CM, Prasad KU, Urry DW (1989): *J Biomol Struct & Dyn* 6:851–858.
Copeland T, Oroszlan S (1988): *Gen Anal Technol* 5:109–115.
du Vigneaud V, Behrens OK (1937): *J Biol Chem* 117:27–36.
Elsas FJ, Gowda DC, Urry DW (1992): *Pediatr Ophthalmol Strabismus* 29:284–286.
Erickson BW, Merrifield RB (1973a): *J Am Chem Soc* 95:3757–3763.
Erickson BW, Merrifield RB (1973b): *J Am Chem Soc* 95:3750–3756.
Fuji T, Sakakibara S (1974): *Bull Chem Soc Jpn* 47:3146–3151.
Hoban LD, Pierce M, Quance J, Hayward I, McKee A, Gowda DC, Urry DW, Williams T: *J Surg Res* (in press).
Indik Z, Yeh H, Ornstein-Goldstein N, Sheppard P, Anderson N, Rosenbloom J, Peltonen L, Rosenbloom J (1987): *Proc Natl Acad Sci USA* 84:5680–5684.
Kagan HM, Tseng L, Trackman PC, Okamoto K, Rapaka RS, Urry DW (1980): *J Biol Chem* 255:3656–3659.
Kupryszewski G (1961): *Res Chem* 35:595.
Losse G, Krychowski J (1971): *Tetrahedron Lett* 4121–4128.
Luan C-H, Parker TM, Gowda DC, Urry DW (1992): *Biopolymers* 32:1251–1261.
Luan C-H, Parker TM, Prasad KU, Urry DU (1991): *Biopolymers* 31:465–475.
Mazur RH (1968): *Experientia (Basel)* 24:661.
Merrifield RB (1964): *Biochemistry* 3:1385–1390.
Mizoguchi T, Levin G, Woolley DW, Stewart JM (1968): *J Org Chem* 33:903–904.

Nicol A, Gowda DC, Urry DW (1992): *J Biomed Mater Res* 26:393–413.

Nicol A, Gowda DC, Parker TM, Urry DW (1993): *J Biomed Mater Res* 27:801–810.

Nicol A, Gowda DC, Parker TM, Urry DW (1993): In: *Biotechnology of Bioactive Polymers*, Gebelein CG, Carraher CE, Jr., eds. New York: Plenum.

Nicolis E, Pedroso E, Giralt E (1989): *Tetrahedron Lett* 30:497–506.

Pattanaik A, Gowda DC, Urry DW (1991): *Biochem Biophys Res Commun* 178:539–545.

Prasad KU, Iqbal MA, Urry DW (1985): *Int J Pept Protein Res* 25:408–413.

Rapaka RS, Okamoto K, Urry DW (1978): *Int J Pept Protein Res* 12:81–92.

Sakakibara S, Inukai N (1964): *Bull Chem Soc Jpn* 37:1231–1232.

Sandberg LB, Soskel NT, Leslie JG (1981): *N Engl J Med* 304:566–579.

Sandberg LB, Leslie JG, Leach CT, Torres VL, Smith AR, Smith DW (1985): *Pathol Biol* 33:266–274.

Sheehan JC, Hess GP (1955): *J Am Chem Soc* 77:1067–1068.

Sheehan JC, Preston J, Cruickshank PA (1965): *J Am Chem Soc* 87:2492–2493.

Sieber P, Riniker B (1987): *Tetrahedron Lett* 28:6031–6034.

Sieber P, Riniker B, Brugger M, Kamber B, Ritten W (1970): *Helv Chim Acta* 53:2135–2150.

Sugano H, Miyoshi M (1976): *J Org Chem* 41:2352–2353.

Tam JP, Heath WF, Merrifield RB (1983): *J Am Chem Soc* 105:6442–6455.

Tam JP, Riemen MW, Merrifield RB (1988): *Pept Res* 1:6–18.

Theodoropoulos D, Fruton JS (1962): *Biochemistry* 1:933–937.

Urry DW (1983): *Ultrastruct Pathol* 4:227–251.

Urry DW (1990): *Mater Res Soc Symp Proc* 174:243–250.

Urry DW (1991): In: *Cosmetic and Pharmaceutical Applications of Polymers*, Gebelein CG, Cheng TC, Yang VC, eds., pp. 181–192. New York: Plenum.

Urry DW (1992): *Prog Biophys Mol Biol* 57:23–57.

Urry DW (1993): *Angew Chem Int Ed Engl* 32:819–841.

Urry DW, Long MM (1976): *CRC Crit Rev Biochem* 4:1–45.

Urry DW, Harris RD, Long MM (1981): *Biomater Med Devices Artif Organs* 9:181–194.

Urry DW, Harris RD, Long MM (1982): *J Biomed Mater Res* 16:11–16.

Urry DW, Cunningham WD, Ohnishi T (1974a): *Biochemistry* 13:609–616.

Urry DW, Long MM, Cox BA, Ohnishi T, Mitchell LW, Jacobs M (1974b): *Biochim Biophys Acta* 371:597–602.

Urry DW, Gowda DC, Harris CM, Harris RD: In: *Polymeric Drugs and Drug Delivery Systems*, Ottenbrite RM, ed. Washington, DC: American Chemistry Society (in press, 1994).

Urry DW, Khaled MA, Rapaka RS, Okamoto K (1977): *Biochem Biophys Res Commun* 79:700–706.

Urry DW, Long MM, Harris RD, Prasad KU (1986a): *Biopolymers* 25:1939–1953.

Urry DW, Harris RD, Long MM, Prasad KU (1986b): *Int J Pept Protein Res* 28:649–660.

Urry DW, Mitchell LW, Ohnishi T, Long MM (1975): *J Mol Biol* 96:101–117.

Urry DW, Parker TM, Reid MC, Gowda DC (1991): *J Bioact Compat Polym* 6:263–282.

Urry DW, Okamoto K, Harris RD, Hendrix CF, Long MM (1976): *Biochemistry* 15:4083–4089.

Urry DW, Sugano H, Prasad KU, Long MM, Bhatnagar RS (1979): *Biochem Biophys Res Commun* 90:194–198.

Urry DW, Gowda DC, Harris C, Harris RD, Cox BA (1992a): *J Am Chem Soc (Polymer Preprints)* 33(2):84–85.

Urry DW, Gowda DC, Parker TM, Luan C-H, Reid MC, Harris CM, Pattanaik A,

Harris RD (1992b): *Biopolymers* 32:1243–1250.

Urry DW, Parker TM, Nicol A, Pattanaik A, Minehan DS, Gowda DC, Morrow C, Pherson DT (1992c): *J Am Chem Soc* 66:399–402.

Urry DW, Peng SQ, Parker TM (1992d): *Biopolymers* 32:373–379.

Urry DW, Gowda DC, Peng SQ, Parker TM, Harris RD (1992e): *J Am Chem Soc* 114:8716–8717.

Urry DW, Hayes LC, Gowda DC, Harris CM, Harris RD (1992f): *Biochem Biophys Res Comm* 188:611–617.

Urry DW, Chang DK, Krishna R, Huang DH, Trapane TL, Prasad KU (1989): *Biopolymers* 28:819–833.

Urry DW, Nicol A, Gowda DC, Hoban LD, McKee A, Williams T, Olsen DB, Cox BA (1993): In: *Biotechnological Polymers: Medical, Pharmaceutical and Industrial Applications, A Conferences in Print*, Gebelein CG, ed. pp 82–103. Atlanta, Georgia: Technomic Publishing.

Vaughan JR, Jr., Osato RL (1952): *J Am Chem Soc (Div Polym Mater* 74:676–678.

Yajima H, Kawatani H, Watanabe H (1970): *Chem & Pharm Bull (Tokyo)* 18:1279–1283.

Yamamoto H, Hayakawa T (1982): *Biopolymers* 21:1137–1047.

Yeh H, Ornstein-Goldstein N, Indik Z, Sheppard P, Anderson N, Rosenbloom Rosenbloom JC, Cicila GC, Yoon K, Rosenbloom J (1987): *Collagen Relat Res* 7:235–249.

Zhang H, Prasad KU, Urry DW (1989): *J Protein Chem* 8:173–182.

8

SYNTHETIC PEPTIDES IN THE STUDY OF VIRAL FUSION, INFLAMMATION, AND ATHEROSCLEROSIS

Ewan M. Tytler, Jere P. Segrest, and G. M. Anantharamaiah

Introduction

The principal area of research in this laboratory, the study of the structure and function of plasma lipoproteins, is stimulated by the fact that coronary artery disease (CAD) is the number one cause of death in the United States. CAD is caused by the deposition of cholesterol in the arteries, resulting in atherosclerosis or "hardening of the arteries." A complete discussion of the pathology of atherosclerosis is not within the scope of this chapter, but the following summary may prove useful.

Atherosclerosis is a cascade of events leading to occlusion of arteries in which many factors are involved. The exact sequence of events is not clear. Cholesterol is transported through the body by plasma lipoproteins. It is known that high levels of plasma low density lipoprotein (LDL) correlate positively with CAD while high levels of high density lipoprotein (HDL) correlate negatively with CAD (Maciejko et al., 1983). These lipoproteins have also been called "bad" and "good" cholesterol, respectively. HDL reduces cholesterol buildup and protects arteries from hardening or narrowing from cholesterol deposition. Individual risk of developing CAD includes strong inheritable genetic factors, but this risk can be modified by diet and exercise. Many inherited lipid disorders can cause atherosclerosis and CAD.

Peptides: Design, Synthesis, and Biological Activity
Channa Basava and G. M. Anantharamaiah, Editors
©1994 *Birkhäuser Boston*

In general, these disorders elevate plasma cholesterol levels, especially LDL cholesterol levels. Atherosclerosis is accelerated by a diet high in cholesterol and saturated fat, which raises plasma cholesterol levels. Individuals with high circulating LDL cholesterol are especially at risk for CAD.

There is an inverse relationship between plasma HDL levels and the incidence of atherosclerosis (Maciejko et al., 1983). HDL acts on cell membranes to "soak up" excess cholesterol. The active component of HDL is a apolipoprotein A-I (apo A-I), which activates the plasma enzyme lecithin cholesterol acyl transferase (LCAT). LCAT esterifies cholesterol (Soutar et al., 1975), the cholesterol ester is sequestered in the core of HDL particles and ultimately unloaded into the liver (Mahley et al., 1984).

Much research on the structure and function of apo A-I has been simulated by its potential role in the prevention of atherosclerosis. Apo A-I has several other biological activities in addition to its role in reverse cholesterol transport. Experiments from our and other laboratories have demonstrated that apo A-I can interact with membranes and perhaps assist in cell membrane repair mechanisms. The specialized structural motif of apo A-I that is thought to be responsible for the membrane interaction, called the *amphipathic helix* (Segrest et al., 1974), is described in detail later. In this chapter, we describe various facets of the amphipathic helix, and, through the design of synthetic peptides that mimic the biological activities of apo A-I, we dissect the effects of these structures on cells.

The presence of the structures in apo A-I that can interact with membranes gave an important clue that this protein can also act on other cells in the body such as neutrophils, which are involved in inflammatory disorders including arthritis. Inflammation is caused by the activation of the neutrophils (Weissman, 1977). Experiments have shown that apo A-I suppresses neutrophil activation caused by many activators (Blackburn et al., 1991). There is epidemiologic evidence that arthritis patients possess low levels of HDL (Heldenberg et al., 1983); thus, these individuals also have higher risk of developing CAD (Maciejko et al., 1983).

Because of an alarming increase in cases of acquired immunodeficiency syndrome (AIDS), our laboratory investigated possible links between the levels of HDL and AIDS. We noticed that AIDS patients possessed low levels of HDL; however, it is not yet clear if these patients develop AIDS disease because of low levels of HDL or if the onset of the disease causes reduction in levels of HDL in these patients. In our studies, apo A-I inhibited virus-induced fusion of cultured cells infected with the AIDS virus, thus inhibiting virus multiplication (Owens et al., 1990).

All the foregoing evidence led us to conclude that HDL and apo A-I act as cell protection agents and may actually assist in cell repair. We describe here how we have used synthetic peptide analogs of apolipoproteins to understand some of the cellular basis of the onset and progression of CAD, inflammatory disorders, and viral infections.

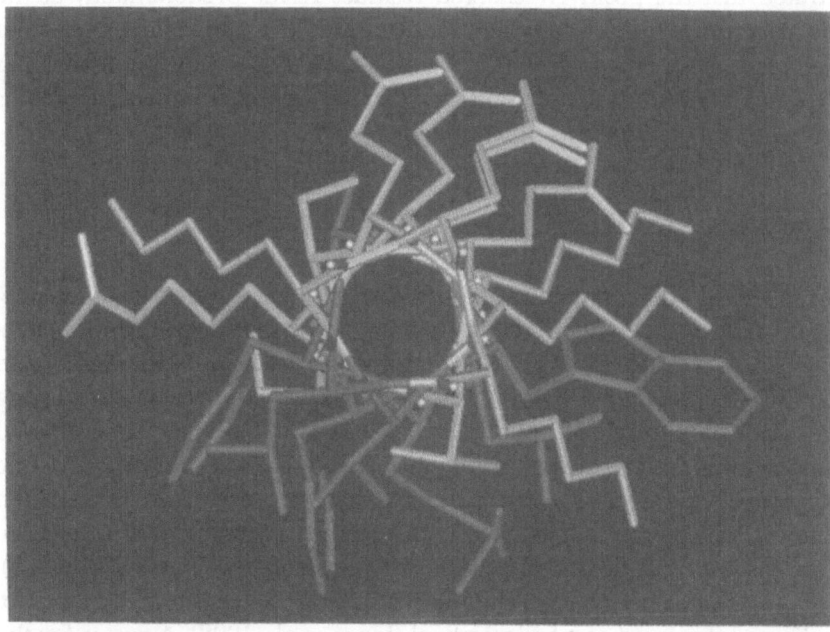

Figure 8-1. The amphipathic helix. Residues 33–53 of apolipoprotein C-I (Segrest et al., 1974) modeled as an idealized α-helix on a Silicon Graphics IRIS Indigo Elan 4000 workstation using SYBYL software (TRIPOS Associates). Helix is viewed from amino terminus with polar face oriented toward top of photograph. Hydrophobic residues are shaded.

The Amphipathic Helix

For a protein to interact with lipids, it must be able to fold into a structure that can complement the lipid structure. The first lipid-associating structure described was the transmembrane alpha (α–) helix of glycophorin (Segrest et al., 1972). A transmembrane helix allows a protein to be anchored in a lipid membrane. The helix thus allows proteins to span biological membranes and thus provides chemical communication between the inside and outside of a membrane. Segrest et al. (1974) discovered that the sequences of exchangeable apolipoproteins C-I, C-II, and C-III, when folded into an α-helical conformation, are arranged such that the hydrophobic residues are located on one side of the α-helix while the hydrophilic residues are located on the opposite side of the helix (Figure 8–1). This sided α-helix, which can associate with both the hydrophobic environment of the hydrocarbon chains of membrane phospholipids and an aqueous environment, is thus called an amphipathic (literal meaning: having passion on both sides) helix because of these properties. Initial findings also demonstrated that the positively charged residues reside predominantly at the polar–nonpolar interface while the negatively charged residues reside at the center of the polar face (Segrest et al., 1974). We now know that this type of arrangement is largely restricted to the amphipathic helical domains of the apolipoproteins just mentioned.

Amphipathic Helix Classes

Amphipathic helix structural motifs have also been found in other peptides and proteins that interact with biological membranes, including peptide hormones (Epand et al., 1977, Kaiser and Kizdy, 1984), amphibian peptide skin secretions (Bevins and Zasloff, 1990), and bee and wasp sting peptide toxins (Argiolas and Pisano, 1983, 1985). Differences were noted among amphipathic helices having different biological activities. We have developed computer programs that analyze differences between amphipathic helices and allow us to determine the common structural features of amphipathic helical domains having similar functions (Table 8-1). In one of these programs, called WHEEL, a sequence is folded into an α-helix and displayed as a helical wheel (Jones et al., 1992). A vector for the hydrophobicity of each amino acid in the sequence is calculated from its hydrophobicity, according to a hydrophobicity scale such as the Goldman, Engelman, Steitz (GES) scale (Cornette et al., 1987), and its radial location on the helix. Hydrophobic amino acids are given vectors pointing away from the center of the helix while polar residues are given vectors pointing toward the center of the circle. The sum of these vectors is the hydrophobic moment (Eisenberg et al., 1982), which is a measurement of the amphipathicity of the sequence. The most amphipathic sequences are found in the gp41 surface protein of the HIV virus (see Table 8-1) (Eisenberg

Table 8-1. Amphipathic Helix Classes and some of their Structural Properties

Amphipathic Helix Class	Present in	Mean Hydrophobic Moment/ Residue	Mean +/- Charge Ratio	Mean Angle Subtended by Polar Face
A	Apolipoproteins	0.43	1.06	≥ 180
G	4-Helix Bundles	0.13	1.1	≥ 180
H	Hormones	0.51	3.66	≤ 100
K	CaM-regulated Protein Kinases	0.38	15	≥ 180
L	Antibiotics, Venoms	0.37	4.0	≤ 100
M	Transmembrane Proteins	0.12	0.4	≤ 60
Y	Apo A-I, A-IV	0.37	0.86	≥ 180
Y*	HIV gp41	0.59	2.36	≥ 180

Abbreviations: CaM=calmodulin, HIV gp41= 41KDa surface glycoprotein expressed by the human immunodeficiency virus and Wesson, 1990) while the least amphipathic sequences are found in trans-membrane proteins (Table 8-1) (Segrest et al., 1990). In another program, COMBO analysis, sequences of different amphipathic helical domains are oriented according to their hydrophobic moments and the distribution of charged, neutral, nonpolar, and hydrophobic amino acids around the helices is determined (Jones et al., 1992).

Using these programs, naturally occurring amphipathic helices were grouped according to differences in the arrangement of the polar residues on the helix (see Table 8-1) (Segrest et al., 1990). This architecture also appeared to be correlated with the biological activity of the molecule. For example, apolipoprotein (class A) amphipathic helices (see Table 8-1) have positively charged residues at the polar–nonpolar interface and negatively charged residues at the center of the polar face. This charge distribution is thought to be responsible for the lipid affinity of apolipoprotein amphipathic helices. On the other hand, lytic (class L) amphipathic helices (see Table 8-1), which comprise bee and wasp venoms and amphibian antibiotics, have positively charged residues at the center of the polar face. The class A and the class L amphipathic helices appear to have opposite effects on membranes, and it follows that this must have something to do with the arrangement of the amino acids in the α-helix. This difference in charge distribution was hypothesized to be the reason for their opposite biological activities (Tytler et al., 1993). As is discussed next, we made synthetic peptide analogs of these different amphipathic helical motifs and tested the physicochemical and biological activities of these analogs.

Design of Amphipathic Helical Synthetic Peptide Analogs

It is often difficult to investigate the relationship between the structure and function of a biologically active protein. For instance, apo A-I is a 243-amino-acid protein capable of associating with lipid. To study the complex actions of large proteins, one approach has been to synthesize segments of the protein by solid-phase peptide synthesis and to determine the biological activity of these segments. Model peptide analogs are synthetic peptides in which the secondary structural features (the way in which the protein folds) are maintained while the primary structure (the amino acid sequence) is changed. This is a powerful tool for determining the structural basis for the biological activity of a peptide or a protein.

Several different strategies have been used to design peptides, with a view to determine which structural features of an amphipathic helix are necessary for a specific biological activity. These strategies can be assigned to two groups, one using naturally occurring peptide or protein sequences and the other using a consensus sequence for a group of peptide or protein sequences.

Using Naturally Occurring Sequences

One of the simplest approaches in peptide design is to take the sequence of a naturally occurring peptide with a known biological activity and synthesize a series of analogs with different chain lengths. These analogs are then assayed for biological activity, and typically a minimum chain length of peptide will be found that can mimic the biological activity of the natural peptide or protein under investigation. Because peptides are synthesized from carboxy to amino terminus in the solid-phase method (the opposite direction from in vivo synthesis), the peptides are usually truncated from the amino terminus. The researcher simply takes aliquots of peptide resin at different stages of the synthesis. This approach was used to show that the last three amino acids of the antibiotic magainin 2 was not necessary for antibacterial activity while deletion of the last six amino acids completely abolished its activity (Zasloff et al., 1988).

A naturally occurring sequence can also be "mutated" by making simple substitutions in the sequence, for example, replacing a leucine with an isoleucine residue. This can show whether the charge, hydrophobicity, or bulk of the side chain of an amino acid at a particular location is important for its biological activity. We are fortunate that natural selection often provides us with a series of naturally occurring "mutants" of a particular sequence, which allows us to make intelligent guesses as to what is important for a particular activity of a peptide. For example, several mastoparans have been isolated from different species of wasp. These mastoparans have subtle differences in their amino acid sequence and in their hemolytic activity (Argiolas and Pisano, 1983, 1984). The use of a naturally occurring sequence is, however, limited in the amount of information it can provide. More information can be provided by using consensus sequences.

Using a Consensus Sequence

A consensus sequence for a group of peptides or proteins with similar biological activity is usually created by lining up the amino acid sequences of the peptides and picking out the amino acids that occur in all or most of the sequences. The assumption is that the primary structure is the most important factor in determining the biological activity of the peptide. As is described later, this is not always the case. The investigator then makes an analog with this consensus sequence and compares its properties with that of the natural peptide.

Computer-Assisted Design of Model Peptides

Our approach to peptide design is based on the assumption that the secondary structure, and not the primary structure, is the most important factor in determining the biological activity of amphipathic helical peptides or proteins. We used a database of known amphipathic helical sequences with the COMBO and CONSENSUS computer analysis to determine the radial and axial distribution of charged, neutral, nonpolar, and hydrophobic amino acids (Jones et al., 1992). We then used this information to design consensus sequences that mimic the secondary structure of the amphipathic helical motif, and not necessarily its primary structure.

Having created a suitable consensus peptide sequence, the typical approach is to make simple substitutions in the sequence. Certain amino acids can be substituted for other amino acids with similar properties (e.g., replacement of an aspartic acid by a glutamic acid), and the analog can fold in the correct way and exert a biological effect similar to the natural sequence. Unless care is taken in the substitutions, this approach can lead to a lot of negative or uninterpretable results; this is especially true in polypeptides of longer chain length. Also, single amino acid deletions can be made in the sequence. Using this approach we showed that deletion of valine at position 10 in the apolipoprotein model peptide 18A abolished its ability to activate the enzyme LCAT, without changing its α-helicity (Anantharamaiah, 1986).

This approach to peptide design is comparable to site-directed mutagenesis in which the gene encoding for the protein is changed to produce a mutant protein with an altered primary structure. The use of model synthetic peptides allows a finer focus on the structure in question and avoids problems such as incorrect processing of the mutant proteins that can occur in site-directed mutagenesis. The investigator can determine whether the secondary structure of an amphipathic helix is important for biological function by synthesizing a series of model peptides with strategic changes in the primary structure and measure changes in the secondary structure by circular dichroism (CD) spectroscopy. The changes in secondary structure can then be correlated to biological activity of these analogs. It can thus be determined which residues are required for the correct folding of a peptide and which residues are essential for its biological activity.

Apolipoprotein Class Model Peptides

A series of apolipoprotein analogs were designed that are 18 amino acids in length; this has the potential to fold into five turns of an α-helix (Figure 8-2). The archetypical peptide, 18A (see Figure 8-2), interacts with multilamellar vesicles of dimyristoyl phosphatidylcholine to form peptide–lipid complexes similar to that formed by apo A-I (Anantharamaiah et al., 1985). Several variations were made including reverse-18A (designated 18R; see Figure 8-2), an analog in which the charges on the polar face were reversed (Anantharamaiah et al., 1985), and scrambled-18A (designated

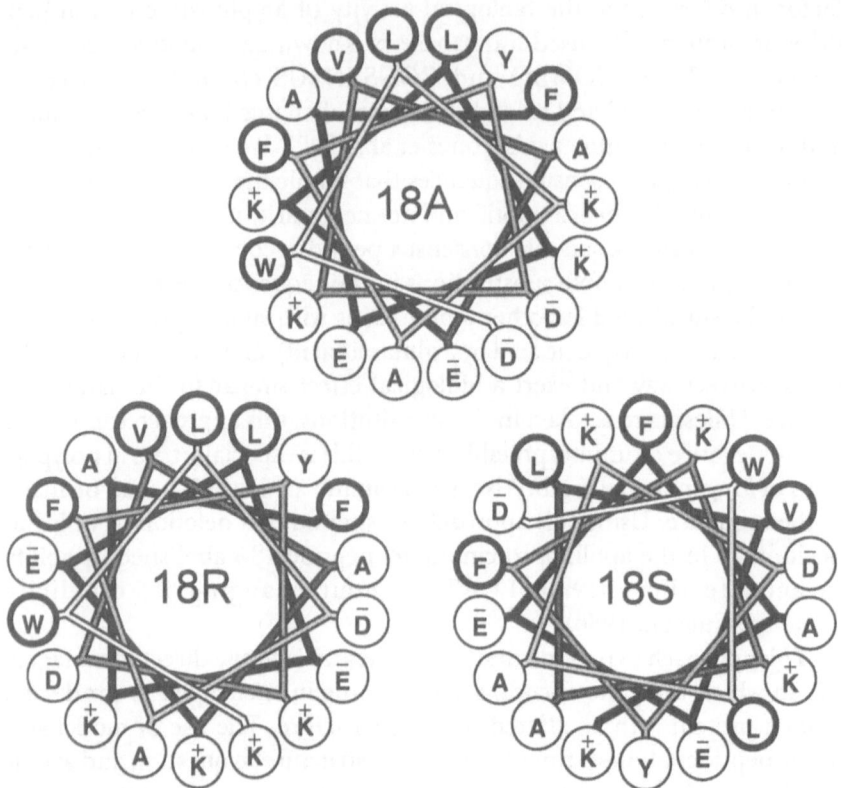

Figure 8-2. Helical wheel diagrams of apolipoprotein peptide analogs 18A, reverse-18A (18R), and scrambled-18A (18S). Single-letter amino acid code is used; hydrophobic residues are highlighted.

18S; see Figure 8-2), an analog in which the entire sequence is scrambled (Owens et al., 1990). Dimers of 18A connected by a proline (18A-Pro-18A, designated 37pA) or an alanine (18A-Ala-18A, designated 37aA) were also synthesized (Anantharamaiah et al., 1985; Owens et al., 1990) to test the cooperative effects of multiple amphipathic helical domains and the effects of an extended amphipathic helix, respectively.

The computer-assisted design approach was used to create a series of consensus peptides of apo A-I called A-I$_{con}$ (Figure 8-3). These peptides were specifically designed to mimic the properties of apo A-I. There are eight 22-mer tandem amphipathic helical repeats at the carboxy terminus of human apo A-I (Luo et al., 1986). Although the tandem repeats were recognized at both the nucleic acid and amino acid levels, there are differences in the amino acid sequences of these tandem repeats. These sequences

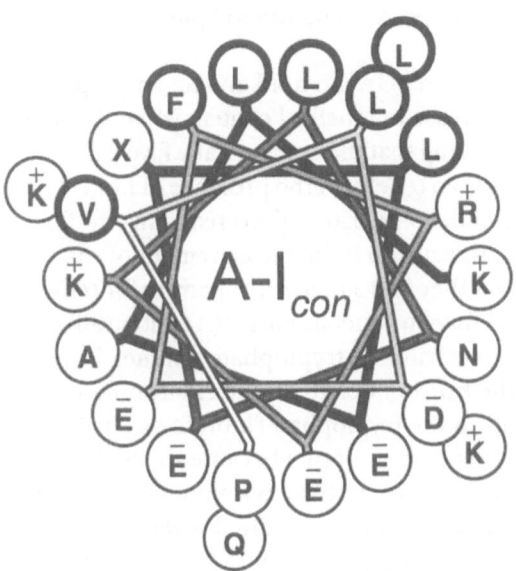

Figure 8–3. Helical wheel diagrams of 22-mer A-I$_{con}$ apolipoprotein peptide analogs. Single-letter amino acid code; hydrophobic residues are highlighted. X is glutamic acid, arginine, histidine, or alanine.

formed the database for the COMBO and CONSENSUS analyses (Jones et al., 1992) used to design a consensus sequence. Four A-I$_{con}$ consensus analogs were synthesized that were 22 amino acids in length, corresponding to the unit length of the tandem repeats (Anantharamaiah et al., 1989, 1990). These analogs differed in the residue at the 13th position on the nonpolar face of the helix that was either glutamic acid, arginine, histidine, or alanine (see Figure 8–3). These corresponded to the amino acids found at this position in the eight different amphipathic helical domains of apo A-I. We also synthesized dimers 44 amino acids long of A-I$_{con}$ (Anantharamaiah et al., 1989, 1990) to test the cooperative effects of two tandem repeats of the amphipathic helical domains of apo A-I.

Lipid Binding and Detergent Properties of Apolipoprotein Peptide Analogs

Apolipoproteins and class A synthetic peptide analogs bind to lipid. Purified apo A-I clarifies a turbid suspension of the phospholipid dimyristoyl phosphatidylcholine (DMPC). Examination of the solution using negative stain electron microscopy showed that lipoprotein particles are formed with diameters less than 100 Å. Class A synthetic peptide analogs, including 18A, also form similar particles (Anantharamaiah et al., 1985). Apo A-I and these analogs act as detergents by solubilizing lipid and forming stable micellar structures in which peptide or apo A-I is bound to lipid to form lipo-protein particles.

One of the hallmarks of interaction between lipid and an amphipathic helical peptide or protein is an increase in α-helical content when the pep-tide or protein binds to lipid, indicating that the energetically favored struc-ture of these peptides or proteins is an α-helix in the presence of lipid. This probably occurs because the potential α-helical regions rearrange to form amphipathic α-helices that can interact with lipid. Measurement of the CD spectra of the analogs showed that they had a higher propensity for α-helix formation in the presence of lipid than in aqueous buffer (Anantharamaiah et al., 1985). The fluorescence spectrum of tryptophan residues in pep-tides has been used to predict the hydrophobicity of the environment sur-rounding this amino acid. A shift in the tryptophan fluorescence maxima toward the blue end of the visible spectrum occurs because the hydropho-bic side chain of tryptophan is in a hydrophobic environment. The tryp-tophan fluorescence peak of 18A and 37pA was shifted toward the blue end of the spectrum in the presence of phospholipid (Anantharamaiah, 1986), suggesting that the tryptophan residues in these peptides were in-deed associated with lipid. None of these properties were observed in re-verse-18A. These studies indicate that the arrangement of charged amino acids on the polar face of the class A amphipathic helix is responsible for its high lipid affinity. It appears that the hydrophobic side chains of the interfacial basic residues are contributing to the hydrophobicity and amphipathicity of the class A amphipathic helix; this explains why the model peptide 18A has a higher lipid affinity than reverse-18A.

Apolipoprotein Peptide Analogs as Lecithin:Cholesterol Acyl Transferase (LCAT) Activators

It is clear from epidemiologic studies (Maciejko et al., 1983) that higher levels of HDL reduce the incidence of atherosclerosis. Apo A-I is the major activator of the plasma enzyme LCAT that esterifies cholesterol, and is involved in reversed cholesterol transport. Many apolipoproteins activate LCAT to some degree, but apo A-I is the most potent activator (Anantharamaiah et al., 1989). We initially showed that the apolipoprotein analogs 18A and 37pA both activate LCAT while reverse-18A does not (Fig-ure 8–4A) (Anantharamaiah, 1986). 37pA was much more potent than 18A. The cooperative effects of two amphipathic helices allowed 37pA to con-vert the vesicular egg lecithin substrate into discoidal complexes, which are a better substrate for LCAT (Anantharamaiah, 1986). These analogs there-fore mimic both the structure and the activity of apolipoproteins including apo A-I.

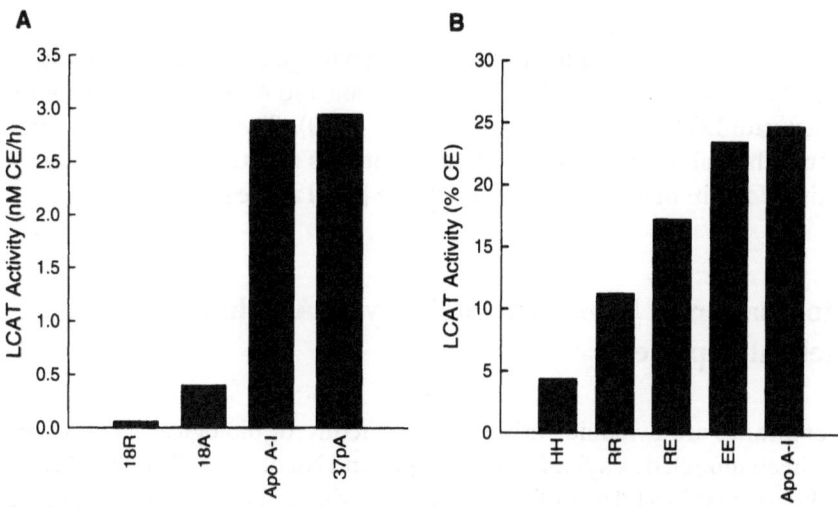

Figure 8–4. Activation of lecithin: cholesterol acyl transferase (LCAT) by apo A-I and apolipoprotein peptide analogs. LCAT activation was measured as ^{3}H-cholesterol ester (CE) formed using small unilamellar vesicles of egg lecithin as a substrate (Anantharamaiah, 1986; Anantharamaiah et al., 1990). **A.** Activation by: apo A-I, 18A, 18R, and 37pA at activator concentration of 10 μg. **B.** Activation by ([Glu[13]] A-I$_{con}$) dimer (EE), [Arg[13]] A-I$_{con}$-[Glu[13]] A-I$_{con}$(RE), ([Arg[13]] A-I$_{con}$) dimer (RR), ([His[13]] A-I$_{con}$) dimer (HH), and apo A-I at activator concentration of 25 μg.

Several laboratories have attempted to identify the major LCAT-activating domain of apo A-I. Cleavage of apo A-I by CNBr or proteolytic enzymes, procedures that produce defined fragments of apo A-I, could not locate the LCAT activation site of this apolipoprotein. As an alternative approach to determine the LCAT-activating site of apo A-I, the A-I$_{con}$ series of synthetic analogs of apo A-I was used (Anantharamaiah et al., 1989, 1990). The rationale was that the variability in the 13th residue might correlate to LCAT activation. As with the 18A series of peptides, A-I$_{con}$ dimers were more effective activators of LCAT than monomers (Anantharamaiah et al., 1989, 1990), suggesting that cooperative effects of two amphipathic helices may be involved in LCAT activation by apo A-I. We showed in two different assay systems that the 44-amino-acid A-I$_{con}$ dimer with glutamic acid at the 13th position (EE) was as effective as apo A-I in activating LCAT at low peptide concentrations (Figure 8–4B) (Anantharamaiah et al., 1989, 1990). This suggested that there was specificity within the sequence of the amphipathic helix for LCAT activation. Examination of the sequence of apo A-I showed the presence of glutamic acids at 13th position in two tandem amphipathic helical repeats in the [66–121] region of this protein. This suggested that the [66–121] region of apo A-I with glutamic acids at positions 78 and 111 is essential for LCAT activation. Supporting these conclusions were the studies of site-directed mutagenesis of apo A-I in which Glu 78, mutated to Ala, yielded a recombinant apo A-I with reduced ability to activate LCAT (Anantharamaiah et al., 1990). Physicochemical studies from other laboratories support our hypothesis that the major LCAT-activating domain of apo A-I is located in the [66–121] region of apo A-I.

Modulation of Membrane Stability by Amphipathic Helical Peptides

Membranes are dynamic entities. The structure of biological membranes has been modeled as a *fluid mosaic* (Singer and Nicolson, 1972). Membrane proteins float in a bilayer of phospholipids, where phospholipids can move laterally. There is also a degree of "flip-flop" in which lipids move from one side of the bilayer to the other. Membranes can undergo many rearrangements. Defects in the packing of phospholipids occur spontaneously in membranes and must be repaired to maintain membrane integrity. Many membrane fusion events also occur; for example, secretion involves fusion of secretory vesicles with plasma membrane. Membrane fusion requires rearrangement of the lipids within the two fusing bilayers. In this process, several intermediate *inverted* phases are thought to be formed (Cullis and de Kruijff, 1979; Ellens et al., 1989).

A fusion event can be stopped if the formation of the intermediate inverted phases is inhibited. A membrane-stabilizing agent inhibits the formation of these intermediate inverted phases by raising the temperature at which they can occur. The ability of a molecule to stabilize bilayer structure in lipids can be measured by differential scanning calorimetry (DSC). In this procedure a lipid is heated until it passes through an endothermic transition representing a change from bilayer phase to inverted hexagonal phase. This is called the bilayer-to-hexagonal-phase transition temperature (T_H) (Figure 8–5). A molecule that raises this temperature stabilizes bilayer structure, while a molecule that decreases this temperature destabilizes bilayer structure. As a rule, fusion inhibitors stabilize bilayer structure (Epand et al., 1987).

Both apo A-I and the class A analog 18A raise the T_H of phosphatidylethanolamine and thus stabilize bilayer structure (Tytler et al., 1993; Venkatachalapathi et al., 1993). Studies in our laboratory have also shown that HDL, apo A-I, and the class A synthetic peptide analogs 18A, 37aA, and 37pA inhibited albumin-induced leakage from small unilamellar vesicles, while reverse-18A did not inhibit this leakage (Liu et al., 1990). This was interpreted as resulting from apo A-I filling in the packing defects in the vesicles.

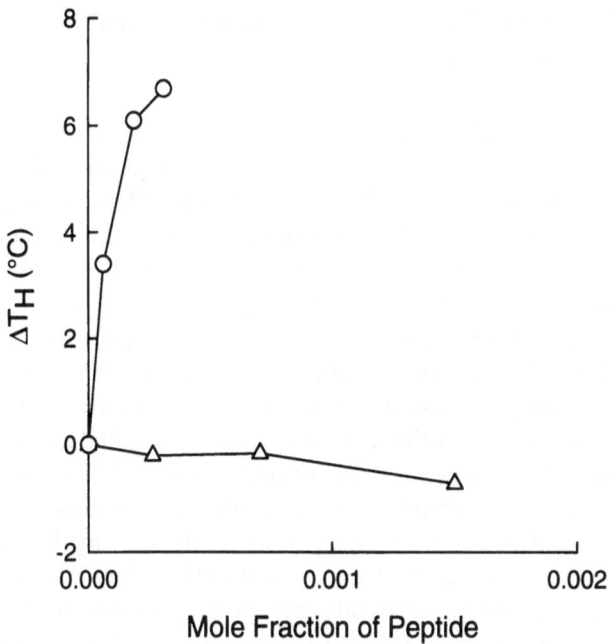

Figure 8–5. Effect of apolipoprotein A-I (*circle*) and peptide venom mastoparan (*triangle*) on bilayer to inverted hexagonal phase transition temperature (T_H) of lipid phosphatidylethanolamine measured by differential scanning calorimetry (Tytler et al., 1993; Venkatachalapathi et al., 1993).

In contrast, fusogenic agents destabilize bilayer structure. Inverted lipid intermediates are thought to be involved in membrane fusion (Ellens et al., 1989). In general, a fusogen will lower the temperature at which these inverted phases can occur. It is well known that some amphipathic peptides promote secretion (Argiolas and Pisano, 1983, 1985). The mastoparans, a group of venomous peptides isolated from wasp sting, were named for their ability to promote degranulation of mast cells and secretion of histamine (Hirai et al., 1979). Thus it appears that these class L venoms promote membrane fusion events. Mastoparan promotes secretion by several of its activities, including enzymatic cleavage of phospholipid by phospholipases, signal transduction by binding to GTPases (G proteins) (Higashijima et al., 1988; Perainin and Snyderman, 1989), and destabilizing the bilayer phase (Figure 8–5) (Tytler et al., 1993). Thus the temperature at which the inverted intermediate lipid phases involved with fusion can occur is lowered by mastoparan. Mastoparan hemolyzes red blood cells (Argiolas and Pisano, 1983) but mastoparan-dependent hemolysis can be inhibited by apo A-I (Tytler et al., 1991). These class L peptides therefore exert a biological activity on a membrane opposite to that of class A amphipathic helices.

Class A Amphipathic Helical Peptides Inhibit Neutrophil Activation

Polymorphonuclear (PMN) leukocytes or neutrophils in healthy individuals provide part of the repertoire of cells that defend the individual from infection by pathogens or other foreign organisms. These cells secrete proteases, enzymes that digest foreign organisms, and also oxygen radicals including superoxide (O_2^-), which are strong oxidizing agents. These secretions require stimulation of the cells by an activator such as immunoglobulin G (IgG). Individuals suffering from inflammatory disorders including rheumatoid arthritis have abnormally high levels of stimulated neutrophils. Instead of mounting an immune attack, the secretions from these neutrophils destroy the tissues of the individual in what is called an autoimmune response. In rheumatoid arthritis, activated neutrophils accumulate at the joints. The activated neutrophils secrete proteases that cause local inflammation. Inflammation is followed by swelling of the joints because of the formation of fluid-filled intracellular spaces called synovia. The proteases secreted by the activated neutrophils degrade the cartilage in affected joints (Janoff, 1975; Starkey et al., 1977), and thus movement of the joints is stiff and restricted. The sequence of events leading to the stimulation of neutrophils in disorders such as rheumatoid arthritis is slowly being unraveled. As autoimmune responses cannot be stopped with existing therapies, the next available step in treatment is to suppress neutrophils activated by an autoimmune response. Because individuals with high levels of apo A-I are resistant to inflammatory diseases, we have assessed the ability of apo A-I to suppress neutrophil activation (Blackburn et al., 1991).

The proteases that are released from neutrophils are stored within secretory vesicles. The secretion of proteases from activated neutrophils requires fusion of the secretory vesicles with the outer plasma membrane. It follows that inhibitors of this fusion event would suppress the secretion from activated neutrophils. Both apo A-I and the peptide analogs 37pA and [Glu^{13}] A-I$_{con}$ suppressed secretion of O_2^- and lactoferrin from neutrophils stimulated by IgG (Figure 8–6) (Blackburn et al., 1991), acting as fusion inhibitors; however, reverse-18A did not suppress secretion. [Glu^{13}] A-I$_{con}$ was a more effective inhibitor of lactoferrin release than 37pA (see Figure 8–6), which suggested that a specific type of charge distribution in the class A motif was involved in inhibition of secretion. Intact HDL did not inhibit secretion, indicating that the amphipathic helical domains of apo A-I exert the effect. About 4% of plasma apo A-I is not bound to HDL (Ishida et al., 1987); this form of apo A-I is likely to be the form that can suppress the activation of neutrophils in normal individuals. The mechanism by which neutrophil degranulation is inhibited is thought to be the ability of the class A amphipathic helix to stabilize bilayer structure in lipids by raising the bilayer to hexagonal phase transition temperature (T_H) (Tytler et al., 1993).

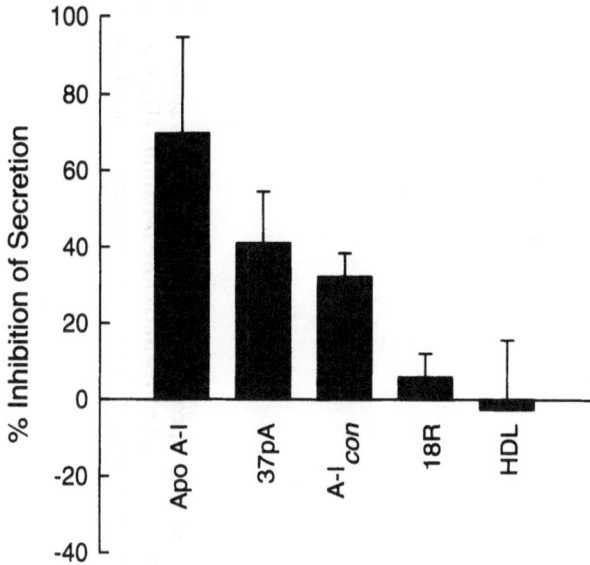

Figure 8-6. Inhibition of neutrophil degranulation by apo A-I and apolipoprotein peptide analogs. Purified neutrophils were activated by immunoglobulin IgG. Degranulation was measured as lactoferrin release using solid-phase radioimmunoassay (Blackburn et al., 1991). Inhibitor concentration was 1.5 μM.

Inhibition of Human Immunodeficiency Virus-Mediated Fusion by Amphipathic Helical Peptides

Acquired immunodeficiency syndrome (AIDS) is caused by the entry of the human immunodeficiency virus (HIV) into the infection-fighting CD4+ T-lymphocyte blood cells (Popovic et al., 1984). The presence of circulating antibodies to the HIV virus clinically defines an individual as being HIV positive. An HIV-positive person eventually loses the ability to mount an immune response and usually dies from an opportunistic infection, such as pneumonia caused by *Pneumocystis carinii*.

One approach to the treatment of HIV infection is to stop the spread of the virus within an infected individual so that the individual does not develop AIDS or the AIDS-related complex. This may ultimately lead to individuals being no longer infective and will reduce the reservoir of the virus within the population, which could lead to significant decreases in the spread of the AIDS epidemic. It has been discovered that the HIV virus promotes fusion of infected cells with uninfected cells to form giant cells called syncytia (Sodroski et al., 1986). The fusion is mediated by a segment of the gp160 surface glycoprotein called the fusion peptide (Gallaher, 1987). Figure 8-7 shows the fusion events that are thought to occur during syncy-

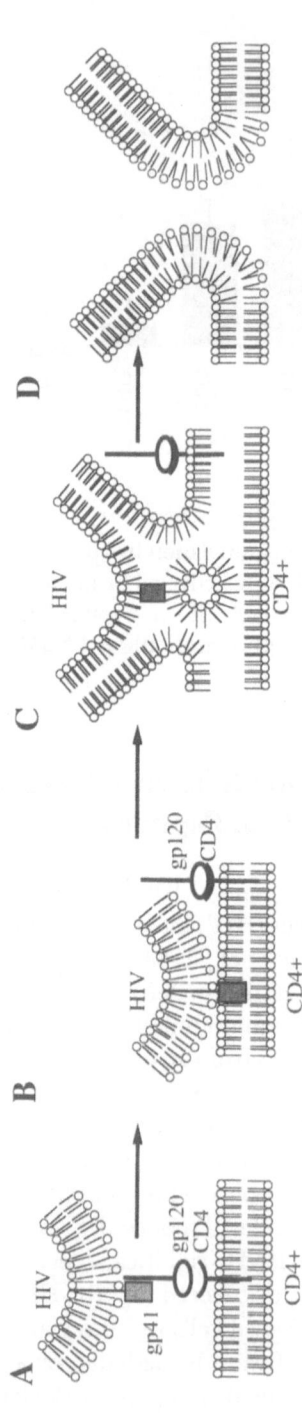

Figure 8–7. Fusion of CD4+ cells by fusion peptide of the HIV virus to form syncytium. Glycoprotein gp120 expressed on surface of HIV-infected cell interacts with CD4 receptor on surface of uninfected cell (A, bringing cell membranes into close proximity (B). Fusion domain of gp41 perturbs the membrane bilayers (B), forming putative inverted lipid intermediate (C) that results in fusion of membranes to form syncytium (D).

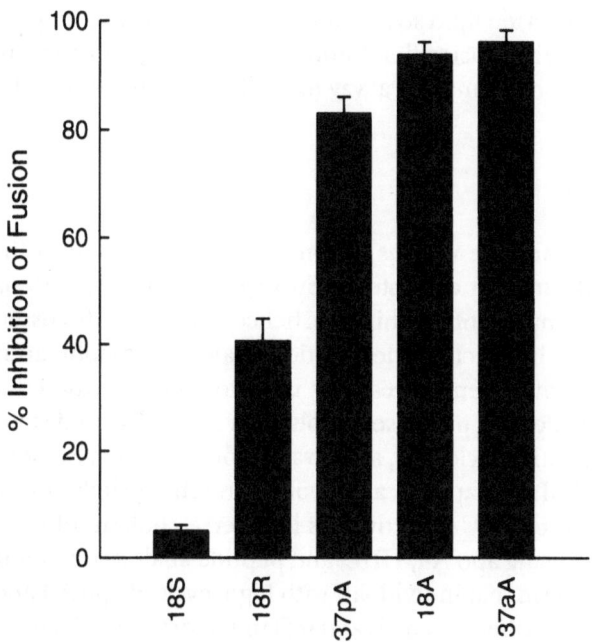

Figure 8–8. Inhibition of HIV-induced fusion by apo A-I and apolipoprotein peptide analogs. CD4+ HeLa cells were infected with recombinant *Vaccinia* virus (VVenv 1). Inhibitor concentration was 100 μ*M*.

tium formation by HIV. We have investigated the possibility of using class A model peptides as inhibitors of fusion induced by either HIV or by a recombinant *Vaccinia* virus expressing HIV gp160 (VVenv1). Apo A-I and the peptide analogs 18A, 37aA, and 37pA all inhibited HIV-dependent and VVenv1-dependent fusion of cells while reverse-18A and scrambled-18A did not (Figure 8–8) (Owens et al., 1990). We have also shown that apo A-I and the peptides 18A, 37aA, and 37pA inhibit the cell fusion mediated by the herpes simplex virus (HSV) while reverse-18A does not (Srinivas et al., 1990). We subsequently showed that A-I$_{con}$ and two synthetic fragments of apo A-I, apo A-I[1–33] and apo A-I[66–120], corresponding to residues 1–33 and 66–120, respectively, of human apo A-I, also inhibit HSV-induced fusion (Srinivas et al., 1991). Apo A-I[1–33] binds weakly to lipid and is also a weak inhibitor of syncytium formation. It thus appears that, in general, peptide analogs of apolipoproteins which can interact with lipid and that are not cytotoxic inhibit fusion mediated by envelope viruses.

   We have shown that apo A-I and these analogs stabilize lipid bilayer structure by inhibiting the formation of inverted lipid structures (Tytler et al., 1993; Venkatachalapathi et al., 1993); it is possible that the mechanism by which these peptides inhibit virus-mediated fusion is inhibition of the formation of inverted lipid structures required for fusion. Thus, the design of peptides as viral fusion inhibitors to produce greater stabilization of lipid bilayer structure may be a way to inhibit the spread of AIDS.

Conclusions

We have described the various rationales frequently used in the study of structure and function of proteins. Strategies used for the design of synthetic peptide analogs of amphipathic helices have been discussed. We have given examples in which model peptide analogs of amphipathic proteins and peptides have been successfully used to elucidate the common link between physiological processes involved in some diseased states, such as inflammation, atherosclerosis, and viral fusion. We have also demonstrated that plasma HDL and apo A-I are involved in other cellular events in addition to their role as LCAT activators in reverse cholesterol transport. Results obtained using apo A-I, HDL, and peptide analogs that mimic apo A-I support the notion that individuals with high levels of apo A-I and HDL are more resistant to atherosclerosis and inflammatory and infectious diseases. Basic research of this type has suggested a biochemical basis for the inherited susceptibility to these disorders. This understanding may allow physicians to identify individuals who are particularly at risk for these disorders and perhaps to administer prophylactic treatment with HDL-elevating agents, such as niacin, to prevent development of the disease.

Acknowledgments

This chapter includes data produced by many members of the Atherosclerosis Research Unit at the University of Alabama at Birmingham and by several of our collaborators, including Drs. Warren Blackburn, Christie Brouillette, Hong Chung, Jeff Engler, Richard Epand, David Garber, Steve Harvey, Martin Jones, Hans De Loof, Mark Mulligan, Randall Owens, Charles Schmidt, R.V and Shamala Srinivas, and Y. V. Venkatachalapathi. We are indebted to their work and their intellectual contributions. Thanks are also due to Kim Gillis, Martin Jones, Gwen Ware, and Joy Williams for their critiques of this manuscript. This research was supported by NIH grants T32 HL07632, P01 HL34343, R01 AI28928, and R55 AR40734.

REFERENCES

Anantharamaiah GM (1986): *Methods Enzymol* 128:627–647.
Anantharamaiah GM, Venkatachalapathi YV, Brouillette CG, Segrest JP (1989): *Arteriosclerosis* 10:95–105.

Anantharamaiah GM, Brouillette CG, Engler JA, de Loof H, Venkatachalapathi YV, Boogaerts J, Segrest JP (1990): *Adv Exp Med Biol* 285:131–140.

Anantharamaiah GM, Jones JL, Brouillette CG, Schmidt CF, Chung BH, Hughes TA, Bhown AS, Segrest JP (1985): *J Biol Chem* 260:10248–10255.

Argiolas A, Pisano JJ (1983): *J Biol Chem* 258:13697–13702.

Argiolas A, Pisano JJ (1984): *J Biol Chem* 259:10106–10111.

Argiolas A, Pisano JJ (1985): *J Biol Chem* 260:1437–1444.

Bevins CL, Zasloff M (1990): *Annu Rev Biochem* 59:395–414.

Blackburn WD, Jr., Dohlman JG, Venkatachalapathi YV, Pillion DJ, Koopman WJ, Segrest JP, Anantharamaiah GM (1991): *J Lipid Res* 32:1911–1918.

Cornette JL, Cease KB, Margalit H, Spouge JL, Berzofsky JA, DeLisi C (1987): *J Mol Biol* 195:659–685.

Cullis PR, de Kruijff B (1979): *Biochim Biophys Acta* 559:339–420.

Eisenberg D, Wesson M (1990): *Biopolymers* 29:171–177.

Eisenberg D, Weiss RM, Terwilliger TC (1982): *Nature (London)* 229:371–374.

Ellens H, Siegel DP, Alford D, Yeagle PL, Boni L, Lis LJ, Quinn PJ, Bentz J (1989): *Biochemistry* 28:3692–3703.

Epand RM, Epand RF, McKenzie RC (1987): *J Biol Chem* 262:1526–1529.

Epand RM, Jones AJS, Schreier S (1977): *Biochim Biophys Acta* 491:296–304.

Gallaher WR (1987): *Cell* 50:327–328.

Heldenberg D, Caspi D, Levtov O, Werbin B, Fishel B, Yarn M (1983): *Clin Rheumatol* 2:387–391.

Higashijima T, Uzu S, Nakajima T, Ross EM (1988): *J Biol Chem* 263:6491–6494.

Hirai Y, Yashuhara T, Yoshida H, Nakajima T, Fujino M, Kitanda C (1979): *Chem & Pharm Bull (Tokyo)* 27:1942–1944.

Ishida BY, Frolich J, Fielding CJ (1987): *J Lipid Res* 28:778–786.

Janoff A (1975): *Ann NY Acad Sci* 256:402–408.

Jones M, Antharamaiah GM, Segrest JP (1992): *J Lipid Res* 33:287–296.

Kaiser ET, Kizdy FJ (1984): *Science* 223:249–255.

Liu D, Huang L, Moore MA, Anantharamaiah GM, Segrest JP (1990): *Biochemistry* 29:3637–3643.

Luo CC, Li WH, Moore MN, Chan L (1986): *J Mol Biol* 187:325–340.

Maciejko JJ, Holmes DR, Kotte BA, Zinsmeister AR, Dinh DM, Mao SJ (1983): *N Engl J Med* 309:385–389.

Mahley RW, Innerarity TL, Rall SC, Jr., Weisgraber KL (1984): *J Lipid Res* 25:1277–1294.

Owens RJ, Anantharamaiah GM, Kahlon JB, Srinivas RV, Compans RW, Segrest JP (1990): *J Clin Invest* 6:1142–1150.

Perainin A, Snyderman R (1989): *J Immunol* 143:1669–1673.

Popovic M, Sarngadharan MG, Read E, Gallo RC (1984): *Science* 224:497–500.

Segrest JP, Jackson RL, Morrisett JD, Gotto AM, Jr. (1974): *FEBS Lett* 38:247–253.

Segrest JP, de Loof H, Dohlman JG, Brouillette CG, Anantharamaiah GM (1990): *Proteins Struct Funct Genet* 8:103–117.

Segrest JP, Jackson RL, Marchesi VT, Guyer RB, Terry W (1972): *Biochem Biophys Res Commun* 49:964–969.

Singer SJ, Nicolson GL (1972): *Science* 175:720–731.

Sodroski J, Goh C, Rosen C, Campbell K, Haseltine WA (1986): *Nature (London)* 322:470–474.

Soutar AK, Garner CW, Baker HN, Sparrow JT, Jackson RL, Gotto AM, Jr., Smith

LC (1975): *Biochemistry* 14:3057–3064.

Srinivas RV, Birkedal B, Owens RJ, Anantharamaiah GM, Segrest JP, Compans RW (1990): *Virology* 176:48–57.

Srinivas RV, Venkatachalapathi YV, Rui Z, Owens RJ, Gupta KB, Anantharamaiah GM, Segrest JP, Compans RW (1991): *J Cell Biochem* 45:224-237.

Starkey PM, Barrett AJ, Burleigh MC (1977): *Biochim Biophys Acta* 483:386–397.

Tytler EM, Segrest JP, Venkatachalapathi YV, Gupta KB, Anantharamaiah GM (1991): *Arterioscler Thromb* 11:1445a.

Tytler EM, Segrest JP, Epand RM, Nei S-Q, Epand RF, Mishra VK, Venkatachalapathi YV, Anantharamaiah GM (1993): *J Biol Chem* 268:22112–22118.

Venkatachalapathi YV, Phillips MC, Epand RM, Epand RF, Tytler EM, Segrest JP, Anantharamaiah GM (1993): *PROTEINS: Structure, Function, and Genetics* 15:349–359.

Weissman G (1977): *Arthritis Rheum* (Suppl) 20:S193-S204.

Zasloff M, Martin B, Chen H-C (1988): *Proc Natl Acad Sci USA* 85:910–913.

9

"DE NOVO" ENGINEERING OF PEPTIDE IMMUNOGENIC AND ANTIGENIC DETERMINANTS AS POTENTIAL VACCINES

Pravin T. P. Kaumaya, Susan Kobs-Conrad,
Ann M. DiGeorge, and Vernon C. Stevens

Introduction

In this chapter, we summarize some current approaches to the de novo design of structurally defined polypeptides with emphasis on their application to synthetic peptide vaccine development and review our attempts at engineering conformational peptides for vaccines. The purpose of this review is twofold:

1. to briefly enumerate strategies of synthetic peptide design as it pertains to elucidating and mapping B-cell antigenic determinants, and

2. to view this field, and specifically synthetic vaccines from design principles and perspectives, as it relates to the topographic nature of antigenic sites recognized by B cells.

Despite the success of inactivated and attenuated vaccines in eradicating many of the important infectious diseases, current vaccines have several crucial drawbacks (Brown, 1990). There are numerous and pressing incentives, both medical and economical, to develop novel strategies for the production of vaccines. Many diseases remain for which no vaccine exist—notably malaria, herpes, and the autoimmunodeficiency syndrome

Peptides: Design, Synthesis, and Biological Activity
Channa Basava and G. M. Anantharamaiah, Editors
©1994 *Birkhäuser Boston*

(AIDS). The idea of using synthetic peptides as antigens or immunogens is not new, and there are immediate and potential applications in medicine for their use as biochemical probes and more importantly as potential synthetic vaccines. Peptide-based vaccines are attractive because they may be safe, cheap, and stable, with minimal side effects. They would eliminate the need to assemble vaccines from inactivated preparations of α virulent strains of pathogenic organisms. They would avoid the necessity of a source of biological material (the blood of infected patients, for example) from which antigenic proteins are prepared as the basis of a subunit vaccine.

Although the molecular basis of immunological recognition remains by and large unclear, our understanding of the immune components and their interaction in producing successful antibody responses has recently been greatly advanced. A wealth of information concerning the rules that govern the binding of peptides to the major histocompatibility complex (MHC) molecules (Allen, 1987; Babbitt et al., 1985; Parham, 1988; Unanue, 1984), crystallographic studies of antigen–antibody complexes (Amit et al., 1986; Colman et al., 1987; Padlan et al., 1989; Sheriff et al, 1987) and MHC class I (Bjorkman et al., 1987a, 1987b; Fremont et al., 1992) have provided considerable insight into our understanding of the processes of immune recognition. A central issue relating to the size and topographical nature of antigenic sites is now resolved: B cells recognize antigens in their native form in solution via specific receptors on the B-cell surface, in a highly conformation-dependent fashion involving residues that may be far apart (discontinuous epitopes) in the primary structure but proximal in the three-dimensional structure because of protein folding. The practical consequences of these findings in terms of peptide vaccines is that an effective immune response to an antigen, resulting in optimal B-cell proliferation and differentiation into antibody-secreting cells, requires the design of peptides that can mimic conformational regions of the protein made up of mostly discontinuous epitopes (Hogrefe et al., 1989; Kaumaya et al., 1990a, 1990b, 1992a). The ability of an antibody molecule to effectively neutralize a virus or a protein antigen depends in part on its affinity for the corresponding sequence, which is a direct consequence of attaining shape complementarity. Examination of the six known antigen–antibody complexes demonstrates that the interacting surfaces between antigen and antibody spans approximately 750 Å^2, which represents some 16–18 amino acid residues on either molecule. Similar examples are evident in other protein–protein, enzyme–inhibitor, and ligand–receptor interactions. Thus, in principle it should be possible to design an antibody that will bind to a predetermined region on the surface of a protein or virus with known three-dimensional structure. Although this is not a simple undertaking, a variety of strategies and approaches can be used to design peptides that embody the conformational and molecular characteristics important for immunological recognition.

De novo design of peptides and proteins can be used to unravel the complexities that exist in the primary sequence and secondary or tertiary structure relationships in proteins as well as to substantiate current views on protein structural organization. While many instances of successful de novo design of polypeptides can be found (Anthony-Cahill, 1992; DeGrado and Lear, 1985; Engel et al., 1991; Fedorov et al., 1992; Ghadiri et al., 1992; Gutte et al., 1979; Hahn et al., 1990; Hecht et al., 1990; Hodges et al., 1988, 1990; Karle and Balaram, 1990; Kaumaya et al., 1990a, 1990b, 1991, 1992a; Kobs-Conrad et al., 1992, 1993a; Krizek et al., 1991; Lau et al., 1984; Lear et al., 1988; Lee and Kaumaya, 1992; Michael et al., 1992; Moser et al., 1987; Mutter and Vuilleumier, 1989; Mutter et al., 1986a, 1988a, 1988b, 1992; Osterhout et al., 1992; Regan and DeGrado, 1988; Zhou et al., 1992; Zhu et al., 1992), there are few examples of a biologically relevant functional protein obtained that way. Any of the strategies rely on the design of artificial polypeptides that bear no resemblance to specific functional protein molecules but which mimic certain known protein structural motifs (as revealed by crystallographic analysis of a large number of proteins). If the basic premise of de novo design of peptides and proteins is to produce novel and artificial molecules with unprecedented properties, an equally strong case exists for the design of preselected antigenic peptide fragments that can adopt a three-dimensional architecture. This reasoning stems from the intriguing ability of some antibodies raised against a short peptide fragment to cross-react with the intact native antigen. Although this phenomenon has generated much interest, and offers a powerful approach to developing a new generation of synthetic peptide vaccines (Milich, 1990; Steward and Howard, 1987; Van Regenmortel, 1989), the underlying principle governing whether a short peptide is able to act as a good antigenic mimic of a protein epitope is poorly understood at present. In practice, there are many problems to be solved, and the considerable promise to developing peptides suitable for vaccination has not yet been realized because the B-cell response elicited by a peptide antigen is governed by a number of poorly understood events such as epitope structure, T-cell dependence, adjuvancy, route of immunization, immunogen stability, etc. New approaches to the development of peptide vaccines will require the rational manipulation of the in vivo immune response in such a way that optimal B-cell and T-cell specificities are obtained (Berzofsky, 1991a, 1991b; Milich, 1989, 1990).

The principal aim of our studies, and as part of a long-term study in our laboratories, is to develop strategies for the design of peptide vaccines that can provide optimal B-cell, T-helper-cell, and cytotoxic T-cell responses for native protein antigens. One of our objectives is based on the general hypothesis relating to the topographical nature of antigenic sites that we have developed and tested in a series of novel experiments (Kaumaya et al., 1990a, 1990b, 1991, 1992a, 1992b). Our strategy was founded on the knowledge that B cells recognize antigens in their native form in solution via specific receptors on the B-cell surface. Our approach to the de novo design of topographic determinants has focused on preserving maximal sequence homology to the native sequence to preserve the functional specificity (without abrogating antibody binding) and introducing rational sequence mutations to faciltate overall folding to maintain conformational mimicry. Our initial approach was based on the premise that an α-helix on the surface of a protein will only have a fraction of the residues exposed because of a helical pitch of 3.6 residues per turn. Such an antigenic site (sequence 310–327) would be conformation dependent, not involving all the contiguous residues of the helical segment. To simulate a native-like conformation, the α-helical segment of 18 residues was idealized and further stabilized into an $\alpha\alpha$-supersecondary structural motif ($\alpha\alpha$-fold). In our incremental strategy, antigenic regions displaying certain secondary structural motifs such as the α-helix and β-turns and loops are iteratively engineered to fit an appropriate host such as a variety of supersecondary structural motifs ($\alpha\alpha$, $\alpha\beta$, $\beta\alpha\beta$, $\beta\alpha\beta\alpha$, 4–α-helical bundles, α-coiled coils, leucine zipper, zinc-finger, and helix-turn-helix).

The model protein selected for these studies is the C_4 isozyme of LDH. Several features of LDH-C_4 make it attractive for the synthesis of antigenic conformational peptides. The primary amino acid sequence of mouse LDH-C_4 had been determined as well as its three-dimensional structure to a 2.9-Å level (Hogrefe et al., 1987). LDH-C_4, which differs from the A and B isozyme by 25%–35%, is expressed only in sperm and testis and thus is immunogenic in female mice. Antibodies specific for LDH-C_4 do not cross-react with LDH-A and LDH-B (Lerum and Goldberg, 1974). Moreover, immunization with LDH-C_4 has been demonstrated to reduce fertility in mice (Goldberg, 1973), rabbits, and baboons (Goldberg et al., 1981) and appears to be a promising candidate for a contraceptive vaccine. Linear continuous determinants of LDH-C_4 have been extensively mapped with short peptides encompassing the entire antigenic structure (Hogrefe et al., 1989).

Structural Correlates of B-Cell Antigenic Determinants

It is important at this juncture to distinguish between peptide antigenicity and immunogenicity. The term B-cell antigenicity refers to the ability of a protein or peptide sequence to bind specifically to an antibody in vitro, whereas immunogenicity refers to the ability of an antigenic site to elicit antibody production. Antigenicity is primarily an intrinsic characteristic of a peptide while immunogencity depends in large part on the quality of T-helper activity, immunization protocol, the nature of T–B interactions, and the genetics of the immunized animal. Many studies aimed at elucidating the antigenic sites on globular protein antigens have involved a determination of the ability of peptide segments of a protein to elicit antibodies to the native structure (Crumpton, 1974; Sela, 1966). The classical approach has been to synthesize a panel of candidate peptides, immunize, and test the antipeptide antisera for reactivity with the immunizing peptide or the corresponding native protein (Lerner, 1984). Initially, this led to the belief that proteins contain only a small number of discrete epitopes that are situated in highly accessible surface areas of the molecule and which could be either continuous or discontinuous in character (reviewed by Atassi, 1984; Benjamin et al., 1984). Another approach, namely the study of antigenic cross-reactivities between related proteins, led to the opposing view that virtually the entire accessible surface of a protein is potentially able to combine with appropriate antibodies (Benjamin el al., 1984). Because only a small part of the surface of globular proteins corresponds to a linear array of residues in direct peptide linkage, this view implies that a considerable number, if not the majority, of epitopes are discontinuous in nature (Barlow et al., 1986; Benjamin et al., 1984). In such a case, many protein epitopes would escape detection when they are analyzed by means of linear synthetic peptides. As pointed out by Van Regenmortel (1989), the method chosen for antigenicity studies largely determines the results obtained. These alternative, and often conflicting, interpretations of antigenicity reflect conceptual difficulties confronted by workers in the field.

Recent studies intended to unravel the nature of protein antigenicity have been significantly advanced by the crystal structure determinations of complexes of antibody Fabs with their protein antigens (Amit et al., 1986; Colman et al., 1987; Padlan et al., 1989; Sheriff et al., 1987) and the phenomenon of cross-reactive antigenicity between proteins and short peptides. It is clear from the x-ray studies that the binding of antibodies to antigens is highly specific and exquisitely sensitive to the three-dimensional structure of the protein. The degree of surface complementarily between interfaces extends over a large area, 750 Å^2, and none of the antibodies are directed to a single continuous epitope but instead bind to discontinuous segments of the protein. The studies of peptide cross-reactivities are, however, less clear, and the mechanism by which an antibody raised against a short peptide can react with the native protein is poorly understood.

The only exact way to identify antigenic determinants is resolution of the x-ray structure of the antigen–antibody complex. As yet there are unfortunately only crystallographic data for one cross-reactive antipeptide-antibody complex (Stanfield et al., 1990). In this 2.8-Å structure, only 9 residues of the putative 19-residue peptide could be unambiguously delineated while the remainder of the peptide is presumably in random-coil conformation. The complete identification of the B-cell antigenic sites for even the well-characterized models is incomplete because they are based on the identification of continuous epitopes. It can be concluded from these results that short peptides could not preserve the conformational and topological features contributing to a discontinuous antigenic determinant because of their high chain flexibility. Thus, a priori they represent a tool of only limited value for mimicking the complex conformational and dynamic properties of antigenic epitopes on the protein surface.

Other methods for elucidating continuous epitopes involve the rapid synthesis of large numbers of small peptides on spacer molecules linked to small plastic pins (Geysen et al., 1984) or synthesis in tea bags (Houghten, 1985). In the "Pepscan" approach the peptides are not cleaved from the pins but instead are tested for reactivity with antibodies by an enzyme-linked immunosorbent assay (ELISA). Again, this method is confined to the identification of linear continuous epitopes. Alternatively, a mimotope approach (Geysen et al., 1987) in which no idea of the epitope structure or sequence is required has been put forward to identify conformational epitopes. This method is based on the progressive synthesis of randomized peptides and relies on an incremental reactivity with a defined monoclonal antibody for identifying the best-fitting candidate. Various techniques have been described for the production of large numbers (10^6–10^9) of random short peptides that can easily be surveyed for binding to a ligand or antibody (Devlin et al., 1990; Scott and Smith, 1990). Although these techniques are extremely powerful, their applicability to a wide range of interactions has yet to be demonstrated.

Prediction of Antigenic Sites in Proteins

Crystallographic studies are limited by difficulties in obtaining suitable crystals for either the antibody Fab or its complex with peptide antigen, and so various methods have been developed for predicting antigenic determinants in a protein by analyzing its hydrophilicity, flexibility, mobility, solvent exposure, amphiphilicity, reverse turns, α-helical propensities, and protrusion. These algorithms do not predict native antigenic determinants, but only a subset of B-cell determinants that have a high chance of producing protein-reactive antipeptide antibodies. During the past several years we have had considerable experience and success in selecting potential peptide immunogens for a diverse set of proteins with varying applications. Three different ordered structures are known in proteins: the α-helix, the β-turn/loop, and the β-sheet (Chothia, 1984). These structures should consequently be highly relevant to the modulation of the humoral immune response. By combining these methods with the conformational predispositions of protein segments such as amphiphilic α-helices, reverse turns or β-turns, and loops, we have increased the reliability and confidence in selecting potential peptide immunogens.

The selection of peptide candidates by computer-aided analysis using the various correlates of protein antigenicity and secondary structural predictions can be easily performed. The profiles of chain flexibility and mobility of individual sequences can be calculated according to Karplus and Schultz (1985). Hydropathy profiles are calculated using the scale of Kyte and Doolittle (1982) over a 7-residue span setting and are finally smoothed with a 3-residue span. Hydrophilicity profiles are generated using the program by Hopp and Woods (1981) using a 6-residue window. Analysis of the exposure of an amino acid residue to water (1.4-Å probe) can be carried out by the Rose solvent exposure algorithm (Rose et al., 1985). Protrusion indices are calculated by the method of Thornton et al. (1986), which predicts portions of proteins that are accessible and protrude out into the solvent. Jemmerson and Patterson (1986) developed a method to identify conformation-dependent epitopes by proteolysis of antigen–antibody complexes. The probability that a 5-residue sequence is an antigenic epitope can be determined by the method of Welling et al. (1985). Computer programs by Chou and Fasman (1978), Novotny et al. (1986), Eisenberg et al. (1984), Kaiser and Kedzy (1984), and Schiffer and Edmunson (1967) can be used to predict the secondary structure: α-helix, β-strand/sheet, β-turn/loop, random coil, and helical amphiphilic moment. Selection of the best vaccine candidates can be deduced as follows:

1. Computer-generated profiles for individual algorithms are analyzed, and sequences are scored on their respective index values and are assigned a priority value from 1 to 6.

2. Sequences can be ranked by comparing the joint predictions involving the combination of several different empirical predictive algorithms (flexibility, mobility, hydrophilicity, solvent exposure, protusion, and antigenicity). The highest ranking sequences will have the highest individual score for the maximum number of analyses examined (6/6), and successive candidates would have the next highest score (5/6), and so on.

3. The best-scoring epitopes can further be ranked by correlation with their secondary structural attributes. For example, an amphiphilic α-helical sequence or a β-turn/loop region is preferred over a random coil fragment.

4. Finally, consideration can be given to the individual amino acid sequence (e.g., hydrophobic/hydrophilic balance, aromaticity). Electrostatic ion pairs and helix dipole interaction in helical segments can also be taken into account.

De Novo Engineering of Topographic B-Cell Determinants

A few attempts relating to the design of conformational peptides with respect to elucidating discontinuous epitopes are mainly confined to cyclizations or additions of cysteines for intrachain disulfide bridges of loop sequences. In an attempt to mimic an Ω-loop in cytochrome c and to examine the effects of various alterations in peptide structure on antibody binding, Jemmerson and Hutchinson (1990) showed that the affinty of the antibodies could be increased by relaxing the loop structure by inclusion of appropriate Gly spacers. Other approaches have relied on linking two contiguous sequences of the α- and β-subunit of human choriogonadotropin (Bidart et al., 1990) to form a construct that elicited antibodies that recognize the native protein. Atassi (1984) described surface simulation peptides in which spatially adjacent residues were linked via appropriately spaced glycine residues to mimic the surface of the corresponding epitope and which were claimed to encompass the total antibody response. Conformational protein-specific antipeptide antibodies were elicited in a strategy that linked an unrelated amphiphilic peptide sequence to a B-cell epitope (Gras-Masse et al., 1988). Schulze-Gammen et al. (1986) proposed methods to mimic helical sequence as well as β-turn mimics in which antibodies were elicted to recognize the respective immunogens.

Examination of the rules governing the topology (Chothia, 1984; Cohen and Parry, 1986, 1990; Efimov, 1991; Levitt and Chothia, 1976; Milner-White and Poet, 1986; Segrest et al., 1990) of protein chains suggests that by combining different secondary structural units within a single peptide chain it may be possible to design and synthesize supersecondary structures which can be assembled so as to fold in a globular structure such as an $\alpha\alpha$, two antiparallel packed α-helices, or $\beta\alpha\beta$, a helix packed against two adjacent parallel β-sheet strands. For instance, de novo design has been reported of peptides with predetermined structures such as amphiphilic helices (Eisenberg et al., 1986; Kaumaya et al., 1990a; Regan and DeGrado, 1988), β-sheets and β-turns (Schultze-Gammen et al., 1985), α-helical coiled coils (Engel et al., 1991; Hodges et al., 1988, 1990; Zhou et al., 1992; Zhu et al., 1992), $\beta\alpha\beta$ topology (Kobs-Conrad et al., 1993b; Kaumaya et al., 1990b; Mutter et al., 1986b), 4-helix bundles (Ghadiri et al., 1992; Ho and DeGrado, 1987; Kaumaya et al., 1990a; Mutter et al., 1992; Osterhout et al., 1992), and antiparallel β barrels (Daniels et al., 1988).

During the past several years we have been conducting a systematic and comprehensive study of antipeptide antibody responses to well-defined epitopes of the protein antigen LDH-C$_4$ in an attempt to develop a contraceptive vaccine (Kaumaya et al., 1990a, 1990b, 1991, 1992a, 1992b). The design of peptide vaccines with improved binding affinities and titers and enhanced immunity must a priori rely on the engineering of structured peptides that mimic antibody recognition sites. Such epitope design, with the relevant molecular mimicry, is considerably more difficult than synthesizing linear sequential epitopes. We have proposed a strategy for engineering peptide vaccines (Kaumaya et al., 1990a, 1992a) that has its origin in our current knowledge of how proteins fold. This approach relied on the design of supersecondary structural motifs and factors known to stabilize globular proteins such as hydrophobic interactions, helix dipole, electrostatic interactions, etc., which resulted in the design of a three-dimensional epitope that elicited high-affinity antibodies specific for the native protein (Kaumaya et al., 1992a). A large panel of peptides has been designed, synthesized, purified, and extensively characterized by various biophysical measurements [circular dichroism (CD); Fourier-transform infrared spectroscopy (FTIR); small-angle x-ray scattering (SAXS)]. Their immunochemical properties have been studied by direct and competitive ELISA. A wide range of experimental results obtained have been integrated to show the validity of our general hypothesis and demonstrate our success in unification of several sets of experimental results by a common hypothesis. The following subsections summarize our various approaches to the design of topographic determinants that mimic discontinuous regions of a protein antigen.

α-Helical Topological Designs

Protein structural motifs such as αα-folding units, 4-α-helical bundles, α-coiled coils, and leucine zippers are found in a variety of biological systems, and their common building block is the α-helix. A key point is that in most cases an isolated α-helix (<15 residues) is marginally stable in an aqueous environment. Additional interactions are required to stabilize the helix in proteins. The supersecondary structural motifs, which can be considered as intermediates in the folding process, can provide the necessary medium- and long-range interactions for stabilization. A theme common to all these motifs is the amphiphilic α-helix in which opposing hydrophobic and hydrophilic residues tend to segregate on opposite faces of the helix, with the net result being the interdigitation of the nonpolar residues to form an hydrophobic core. The α-helix bundle consisting of parallel and antiparallel aligned α-helices is a widely recognized supersecondary structural motif in natural proteins such as cytochrome c, tobacco mosaic virus, and myohemerythrin. The amphiphilicity and heptad sequence repeat in their primary structures are considered to be key features. The heptad repeat consisting of a 7-residue pattern (a-b-c-d-e-f-g) where a and d are generally occupied by hydrophobic residues is also characteristic of the two-stranded coiled-coil motifs found in fibrous proteins such as tropomyosin and in DNA-binding proteins that contain the leucine zipper motif (Landschultz et al, 1988; O'Shea et al., 1989, 1991; Vinson et al., 1989). Such patterns are exemplified by two or three right-handed α-helices wrapping around one another in a left-handed manner, in parallel and in register, to generate the two-stranded α-helical coiled-coil motif stabilized by hydrophobic interaction between the apolar residues in the a and d positions.

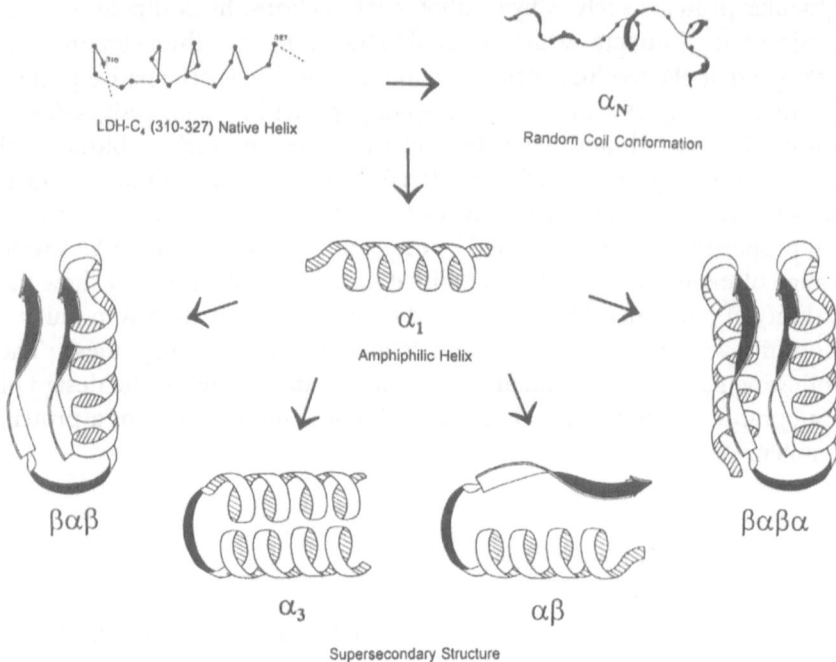

Figure 9–1. Schematic illustration of designed peptides with various topologies: α_N is shown in random coil conformation; α_1 is idealized amphiphilic structure that was further engineered into $\alpha\alpha$-supersecondary structure α_3, $\alpha\beta$, $\beta\alpha\beta$, and $\beta\alpha\beta\alpha$ topologies.

Topographic Determinants: Theoretical Design Considerations

Our strategy to produce an antigenic peptide that assumes the conformation of the corresponding segment of the native protein is based on general concepts of protein folding. A linear, accessible antigenic sequence that displays certain structural features (α-helix, β-sheet, β-turn, hairpin-loop) and which incorporates favorable interactions known to enhance peptide and protein stability (electrostatic interactions, salt bridges, helix dipole, amphiphilicity, etc.) is selected (Figure 9–1). The structural features of the antigenic site are then stabilized by design features that will allow their incorporation into a framework consisting of supersecondary structures (Levitt and Chothia, 1976). The amphiphilic nature of the peptide acts as a major driving force for the adoption of a folded conformation, resulting in a hydrophobic core and a hydrophilic surface. Basic to the concept is that hydrophobic residues tend to cluster into the apolar interior of the globular protein where they are shielded from the surrounding solvent, a process which is thermodynamically very favorable because of the hydrophobic effect. On the other hand, hydrophilic residues occupy sol-vent-accessible exteriors where they enhance solubility. Intramolecular hydrophobic interaction within the helices or sheets are responsible for the overall stability of the structure. Natural globular proteins are believed to fold by a similar mechanism.

To test whether a predetermined structure could be designed and synthesized, sequence 310–327 (designated α_N) of mouse LDH-C_4 was selected as the conformational target antigenic peptide (Figure 9-2) because sequences 304–316 and 318–330 of LDH-C_4 bound antibodies to the native protein. The three-dimensional structure of LDH-C_4 confirmed that this sequence (α_N) was located on the surface and forms part of an extended α-helical structure. Thus, it would be possible to engineer this sequence by incorporation into a stable supersecondary structure (e.g., $\alpha\alpha$, $\alpha\beta$, and $\beta\alpha\beta$). Fourier analysis (Eisenberg et al., 1984) and helical wheel representation (Schiffer and Edmundson, 1967) (Figure 9-3) showed the sequence to be amphiphilic. We hypothesized that if the amphiphilicity of sequence 310–327 could be idealized without affecting the spatial orientation of the accessible hydrophilic residues, it could be stabilized by hydrophobic interaction. To achieve this in a rational way we measured the surface accessibility of each amino acid using a spherical probe of radius 10 Å (Hogrefe et al., 1987; Novotny et al., 1986), indicating that residues Glu^{311}, Ser^{318}, Ala^{319}, and Glu^{326} were buried in the three-dimensional structure of the protein and therefore did not represent important contact residues for antibody binding or recognition (see Figure 9-3). These residues were substituted by Leu, and Trp^{323} was replaced by Glu. The idealized amphiphilic sequence, designated α_1, exhibited two very important properties that were shown to stabilize α-helical structures in solution: (a) an α-helix dipole (Shoemaker et al., 1987) whereby the negative charge (Glu^{310}) at the N terminus and a positive charge (Lys^{327}) at the C terminus stabilized the helix by position-dependent electrostatic interaction, and (b) appropriate distribution of ion pairs (Sundaralingam et al., 1987), where Glu^{312} and Lys^{316}, Glu^{323} and Lys^{327} form ion pairs in position (i, i + 4), and Lys^{317} and Asp^{320} form ion pairs in position (i, i + 3). This ion pairing of hydrophilic side chains should contribute to the stability of the solvent-exposed, α-helical secondary structure; α_1 is amphiphilic and therefore could represent a potential helper T-cell epitope (Berzofsky, 1991a, 1991b). Sequence 313–320 of α_1 is a glycine followed by 2 or 3 hydrophobic residues ending with Asp, and conforms to the Rothbard algorithm, which is a sequence motif present in a number of known T-cell epitopes.

From the foregoing it seemed likely that sequence 310–327 had the promise of being a potent antigenic determinant capable of being recognized by both the B-cell and T-cell repertoires. We modeled that sequence to ensure that it had the minimal structural requirements necessary for further stabilization of the secondary structure. Thus, the coordinates of that peptide

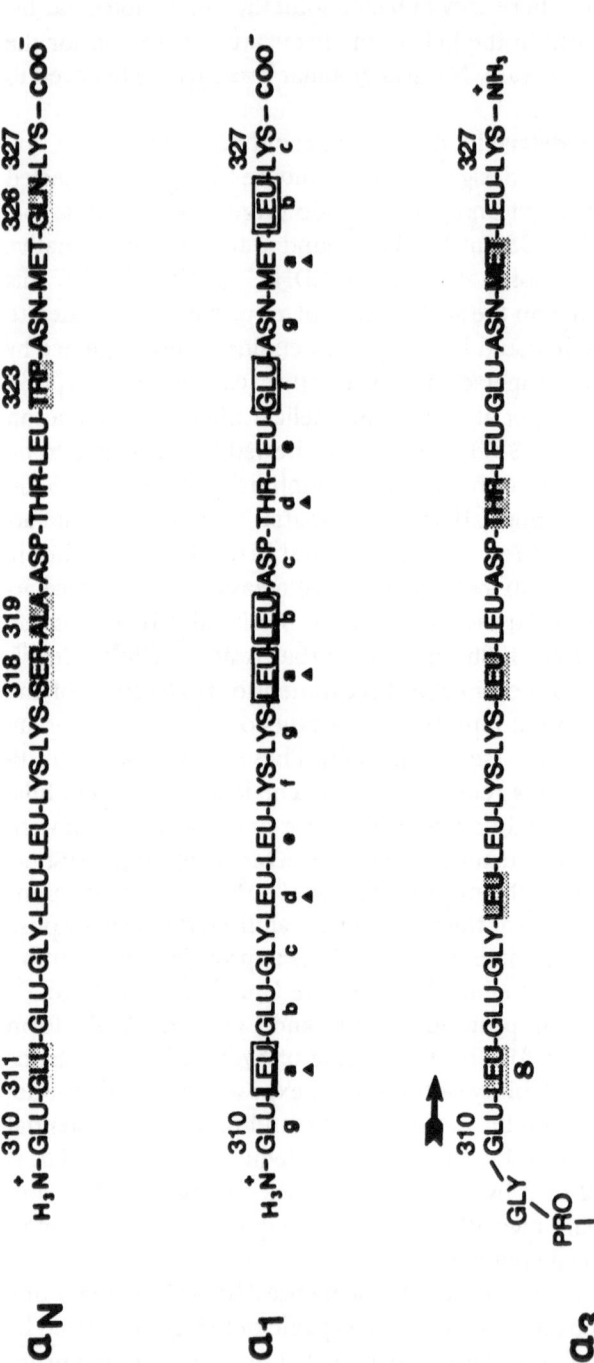

Figure 9-2. Amino acid sequences of LDH-C$_4$ sequence 310–327 (α_N) and engineered sequences α_1 and α_3. Shaded residues in α_N did not contact 10-Å probe; boxed residues in α_1 represent mutated residues to idealize amphiphilic properties; α_3 is engineered conformational epitope.

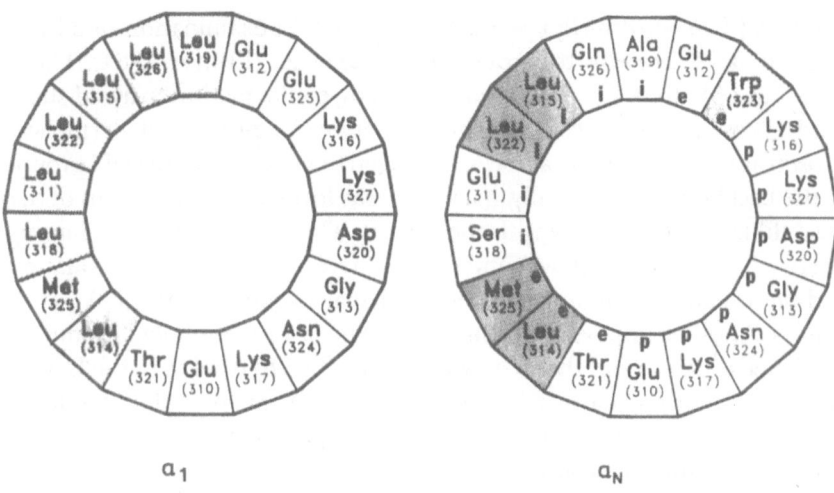

Figure 9-3. Helical wheel representation of α_1 and α_N. In α_N wheel: p, protruding; e, external; i, internal, based on 10-Å probe measurements.

segment obtained from the refinement of the LDH-C_4 structure from the Brookhaven Protein Data Bank were used to refine sequence 310–327 on a computer graphics system using Frodo, and was transformed to coincide with the known α-helices of a four-α-helix bundle. The superimposition on the hemerythrin structure resulted in a satisfactory match of the critical residues. At this stage, we were satisfied that sequence 310–327 could be modeled into an $\alpha\alpha$-fold and further stabilized by association into an α-helical bundle. The amphiphilic nature of 310–327 does not guarantee association into an α-helical bundle because the helices should pack with their helical axes nearly antiparallel to one another (being inclined by just 20°) in this highly symmetrical fold. This arrangement allows tight packing of the side chains protruding from the apolar face of the helices, which is favored by electrostatic interactions between the helices caused by the dipole moment of the α-helices. Thus, if the amino acid sequence of 310–327 displays a 7-residue "heptad" repeat in which a and d are apolar residues, it would give rise to an apolar surface stripe inclined around the axis of each α-helix at about 18° to each other. This pattern of packing of the helices and interdigitation of the hydrophobic residues would result in a four-helical bundle, thus stabilizing this structure more than other possible aggregates.

Having satisfied ourselves that this indeed would be the case, we proceeded to the next stage of the design, namely the $\alpha\alpha$-fold. We opted to use the same sequence for the antiparallel helix and had to decide on a connecting piece for joining the two helices. A 4-residue β-turn consisting of residues (-Leu-Ser-Pro-Gly), was selected based on examination of 33 patterns in native proteins that code for an $\alpha\alpha$-corner (Efimov, 1984). The C terminus of helix A Glu^{310} should have an α_L conformation to avoid steric hindrances; thus, massive hydrophobic residues are prohibited. Serine was chosen as the first residue as it can hydrogen bond with the free NH groups of the backbone. Additionally, if a β-turn was formed, the side chain of Ser 4 would interact favorably with the solvent. The short connection joining the two helices (denoted by A and B) must have an extended conformation and be oriented approximately perpendicular to the axes of the A and B helices. Another important feature is that the last hydrophobic residue of the A-helix (Leu-1) and the first hydrophobic (Leu 8) residue of the B-helix must cluster to form a pair in position 1–8. Leu was placed at residue 3 because its side chain in that position is completely buried in the hydrophobic core and a hydrophobic residue is required.

Validity of Structural Designs: Biophysical Characterization

A variety of independent biophysical techniques (CD, peptide monolayers, FTIR, and SAXS) were used to fully characterize the model peptides (Kaumaya et al., 1990a). We showed by CD that α_1 and α_3 behaved as typical α-helices: minima at 222 nm (n-π^*) and 208 nm (π-π^*) and a maximum at 200 nm (π-π^*). As predicted, α_N showed a characteristic random coil minimum at 200 nm (Figure 9–4). The mean residue molar ellipticities at 222 nm were -20,310 degree cm^2/dmole for α_1 and -22485 degree cm^2/dmol for α_3. We investigated the concentration dependencies of peptide solutions (1–400 μM, 0.01 M Tris HCl/0.16 M KCl, pH 7.4). Spectra typical of random coil conformations were obtained at low concentrations, and spectra typical of α-helices were obtained as the concentrations were increased. The spectra for α_1 and α_3 were sharply dependent on peptide concentration, in contrast to α_N, which showed no tendency for secondary structure formation. The concentration dependence of the mean residue molar ellipticity (222 nm), for α_1 when analyzed as a co-operative monomer–oligomer equilibrium, can be optimally described by a monomer–tetramer with an equilibrium constant of 7.42×10^{-16} M^3 and a free energy of tetramerization of -20.9 kcal/mol. α_3 was optimally fit to a monomer–dimer equilibrium with a dissociation constant of 1.18×10^{-18} M^3 and a free energy of dimerization of -7.8 kcal/mol.

The abilities of the peptides to form stable monolayers at the air–water interfaces were determined to test whether the peptides form amphiphilic secondary structures. Analysis of the force area (π/A) curves obtained on compression of these monolayers yields information concerning the molecular cross-sectional areas and thus the degree of association of the peptides. The data indicated that α_1 is tetrameric (3.6 molecules/aggregate) and α_3 is dimeric (1.5 molecules/aggregate).

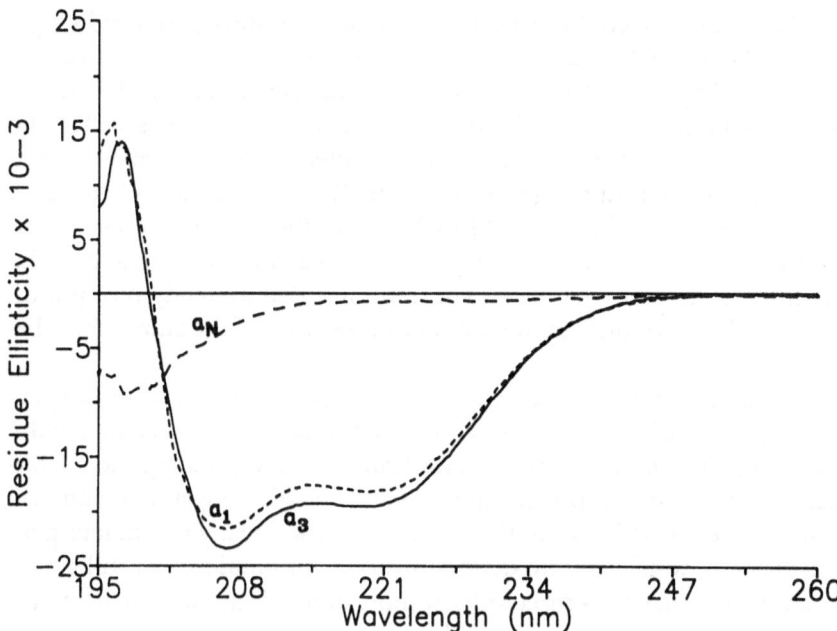

Figure 9-4. CD spectra of α_N, α_1, and α_3 in 0.01 M Tris-HCl/0.16 M KCL, pH 7.4.

The FTIR data confirmed that both α_1 and α_3 have high helical content (50% for α_3 and 44% for α_1). In contrast, α_N exhibits low helix content (14%). The 1660 cm^{-1} assignment for α_3 is consistent with the fact that a β-turn is present while this feature is absent in α_1. Shape analysis by SAXS for α_1 gives a molecular weight of 10,570, confirming that α_1 exists as a tetramer. Guinier analysis for α_3 gave a molecular weight for α_3 of 8660 and a radius of gyration of 17.3, supporting the fact that α_3 exists as a dimer (calculated MW, 9075). P(r) curves and the Rg values indicated that α_3 and α_1 have a similar overall shape. The SAXS data for α_N could not be analyzed because of the formation of large nonspecific aggregates.

Immunogenicity and Antigenicity of Engineered Constructs

The validity of the proposed strategy was initially tested by first determining whether the synthetic peptides α_N, α_1, and α_3 are immunogenic in vivo and whether they elicit antibodies that bind the native protein. We raised antisera to the various peptides in inbred and outbred mice as well as in rabbits. For immunizations, the synthetic immunogens were used as free peptides and were purposefully not coupled to any carrier protein. The presence of antigenic activity was evaluated by direct binding in an enzyme-linked immunosorbent assay (ELISA) and specificity was evaluated by competitive ELISA and capture methods.

The engineered conformational 40-residue peptide (α_3) induced a high-titer/high-affinity IgG antibody response much more effectively than the corresponding linear α_1 or α_N peptide (Kaumaya et al., 1992a). The resulting α_3 antibodies were specific for the anticipated structure as well as the sequence in the native protein and thus pointed to the importance of tertiary conformation in antigen recognition. The stabilization of α_1 into a supersecondary $\alpha\alpha$ folding motif (α_3) exposes the antibody-accessible hydrophilic residues of the peptide sequence in a manner comparable to the structure in the native protein. This indicates that antibody recognition indeed is directed solely to the solvent-exposed side of the amphiphilic helix.

Mutation of buried residues in the native protein (to idealize the peptide sequence) did not result in abrogation of antibodies specific for the native protein. These results are significant for understanding the conformation dependency of protein epitopes and peptide antigenicity, and may provide an explanation as to the paradox of how linearly continuous peptide epitopes, which have no defined structure in solution, can still generate antibodies that cross-react with the more ordered structure in the native protein. That such cross-reactivity is the rule rather than an exception is easily understood if one considers that the antibodies raised are generally of low affinity because only a few residues are in the right conformation at the time. From these results we concluded that the immune response against α_3 was almost entirely directed to the solvent-exposed surface of the stabilized amphiphilic α-helix (α_3). The immune response to α_3 (as determined by ELISA against both the peptide and native LDH-C_4) progressed in parallel, indicating the specificities of the antigen–antibody interaction. We propose that the relatively high immunogenicity exhibited by α_3 partly results from the native-like conformation that it adopts. The lower immune response to α_1 can be easily rationalized in structural terms. α_1 is an 18-residue amphiphilic sequence and considerably less stable than α_3 (40-residue stabilized $\alpha\alpha$ fold) and thus would not be able to mimic the native sequence as closely as would α_3; that is, the sequence is without structural stability. The low immunogenicity exhibited by α_N reflects its lack of structure in solution, which is consistent with immunization results obtained by others with free peptides.

$\alpha\beta$, $\beta\alpha\beta$, and $\beta\alpha\beta\alpha$ Topological Designs

$\alpha\beta$ proteins have mixed or alternating segments of α-helical and β-strand secondary structures with the α-helices able to pack on both sides or in some cases on the same side of the β-sheet. For example, the $\beta\alpha\beta$ unit consists of a β-sheet with two parallel strands in Van der Waals' contact with an α-helix antiparallel to these strands. The folded conformations of these structural motifs have been analyzed extensively (Edwards et al., 1987;

Fedorov et al., 1992; Mutter et al., 1986b), and two underlying factors are important. First, residues in the protein motif interior pack closely, and second, packed secondary structures have a conformation close to the minimum free-energy conformation of the isolated secondary structure. There is also a strong tendency for the helices to pack onto sheets with their axes nearly parallel to the sheet strands for optimal surface complementarity. Other attempts at the design and synthesis of peptides displaying mixed α-helical and β-strand/sheet topologies have been made. These include a 34-residue $\beta\beta\alpha$ designed to bind nucleic acids (Gutte et al., 1979), a 32- to 35-residue folding unit with $\beta\alpha\beta$ packing (Mutter et al., 1986b), and a twice-repeated, 73-residue $\alpha\beta\beta$ unit consisting of a four-stranded antiparallel β-sheet with one side screened by two α-helices (Fedorov et al., 1992).

We extended our incremental approach to the de novo design of protein antigenic sites, as well as the study of the folding properties of these immunogenic peptides, by engineering peptide sequences with other topologies such as $\alpha\beta$, $\beta\alpha\beta$, and $\beta\alpha\beta\alpha$ (Kaumaya et al., 1991; Kobs-Conrad et al., 1993b). The α_1 idealized amphiphilic sequence 310–327 was stabilized into a 27-residue $\alpha\beta$, a 41-residue $\beta\alpha\beta$, and a 62-residue $\beta\alpha\beta\alpha$ folding unit. The design principles included several considerations. First, could these peptides have a compact structure that is stabilized by medium- and long-range interactions of the type found in globular proteins? A recognized factor in the folding of proteins is the burying of hydrophobic side chains. Packing of α-helices on α-helices ($\alpha\alpha$, $\alpha\alpha\alpha$), α-helices on β-sheets ($\beta\alpha$, $\alpha\beta$, $\beta\alpha\beta$), and β-sheets on β-sheets ($\beta\beta$, $\beta\beta\beta$) are classical examples of interdigitation of nonpolar side chains. Second, in the de novo protein design it is equally important to understand the nature of loops that connect secondary structures (Milner-White and Poet, 1986; Pabo and Suchanek, 1986). The connecting piece for joining the two helices into a β-hairpin turn (Leu-Ser-Pro-Gly) was based on the examination of patterns in native proteins that code for $\alpha\alpha$ corners (Edwards et al., 1987; Efimov, 1984, 1991). The hairpin turn was designed to yield a stereochemically sensible conformation in which there were no disallowed close contacts; tight packing of the hydrophobic core residues and exposure of polar charged groups to solvent were examined. There is at present no direct evidence on the strengths and specificities of these interactions.

For the $\alpha\beta$ construct, a 3-residue linker sequence consisting of Gly-Ala-Gly was chosen to link the 18-residue α-helix to the 10-residue β-strand consisting of alternating Ser-Leu. The first Gly with a positive ϕ is necessary to allow very tight reversal of the main chain direction; the second residue is an Ala in β conformation, and the third residue was Gly. The design of this construct was based on an analysis of four families of loops with distinct conformation and sequence patterns (Edwards et al., 1987) that indicated that such a sequence would allow the polypeptide chain hydrophobic residue to closely pack into the core for stabilizing the structure.

For the βαβ construct, an 8-residue β-strand (alternating Leu-Ser) was linked to the C-terminal end of the 18-residue α-helix via a 4-residue β-turn (Leu-Ser-Pro-Gly). The amino end of the α-helix was extended with a 3-residue Gly-Ala-Gly into the amino-terminal 8-residue β-strand. The βαβα construct was designed similarly to this peptide by extension of the amino-terminal strand.

These model peptides were synthesized and purified, and their folding properties were studied by CD. All three peptides showed high α-helical content intermixed with β-strand/sheet structures. Rabbits were immunized with each of the constructs, and their antisera were analyzed by direct and competitive ELISA. Our results demonstrated that these engineered conformational peptides are highly immunogenic, eliciting high titers of antipeptide antibodies. The competitive ELISA data are consistent with our general hypothesis that antibodies raised to these constructs have a higher affinity for the native protein than the respective immunogenic sequences and are mimicking the α-helical region of the protein antigen LDH-C_4 with accuracy (Kobs-Conrad et al., 1993b).

Loop-Structured Peptides/Zinc Finger Motifs

A loop region is defined as a continuous segment of a polypeptide chain that connects two segments of a regular secondary structure which adopts a "loop-shaped" conformation. The term loop also describes regions that are disulfide bonded. Most loop regions in proteins serve an important function and play an important role in macromolecular recognition processes as exemplified by the exquisite specificity of the antigen-combining sites in immunoglobulins that are constructed from six loops formed by the six hypervariable regions. In many DNA-binding proteins, the helix-loop-helix motif sequences are responsible for recognition of the double helical structure, as are the leucine zipper and zinc finger motifs. Loops are generally more flexible and mobile than helix or sheet structures or β-hairpins. Although we have shown the importance of amphiphilic α-helical regions as determinants of antigenicity, not all B-cell antigenic epitopes occur in α-helices. The β-turn/hairpins and loop regions of proteins, which by virtue of their location are prime candidates for recognition by antibodies, have been implicated as major immunogenic epitopes (Beyreuther et al., 1987; Dorow et al., 1985; Fourquet et al., 1988; Jemmerson and Hutchinson, 1990). Approaches to mimicking these structures have relied on either cyclization or intrachain disulfide bridging, which unavoidably imposes undesirable steric constraints and results in nonnative conformations. These cyclizations impart rigidity to an otherwise flexible loop, and as a result these constructs do not adequately mimic the conformational nature of the epitope and are poorly immunogenic.

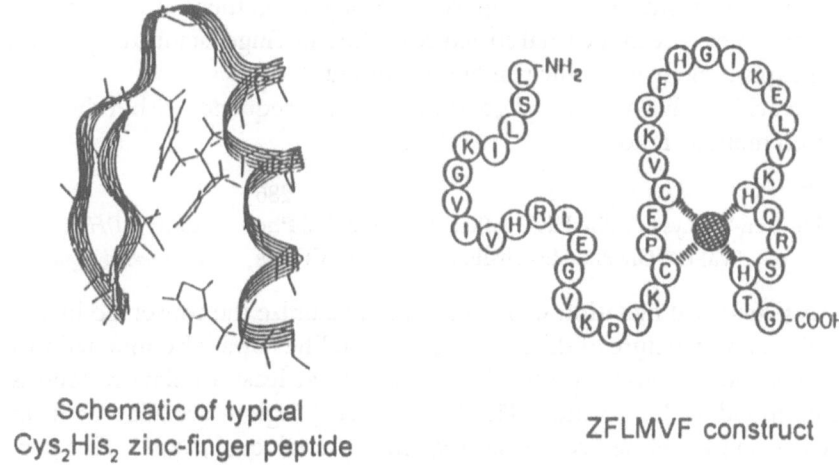

Schematic of typical
Cys₂His₂ zinc-finger peptide

ZFLMVF construct

Figure 9–5. Sequence and conformation of LDH-C$_4$ zinc finger peptide.

Successful introduction of metal-binding activity into model peptides encoding "zinc finger" domains has been reported (Krizek et al., 1991; Lee et al., 1989; Merkle et al., 1991; Michael et al., 1992; Xu et al., 1991). These constructs are largely unfolded in the absence of appropriate metal ions but adopt unique three-dimensional structures in their presence. The use of the "zinc finger" supersecondary structure motif offers the advantage that it is a well-characterized structure consisting of a β-strand region at the amino terminus (which includes the cysteinyl zinc ligands) and an α-helical region (containing the histidyl zinc ligands) at the carboxyl terminus; these are linked by a loop region of somewhat variable topology. The spacing sequence between the carboxyl-terminal cysteine ligand and the amino-terminal histidine ligand residue (the "loop") is always composed of 12 residues. Two hydrophobic residues are present at conserved positions of this sequence; these stabilize the structure via hydrophobic interactions and also may modulate the mode of liganding of Zn^{2+} to the appropriate residues. The most common zinc finger is the Cys$_2$ His$_2$ type, found in many transcriptionally active proteins (Berg, 1990). A survey of about 200 sequences of this type has revealed a basic structural pattern (Krizek et al., 1991), which has been verified by nuclear magnetic resonance (NMR) spectroscopy of numerous zinc finger peptides (Kochoyan et al., 1991; Omichinski et al., 1990; Xu et al., 1991).

To determine whether the zinc finger motif could provide a template for engineering an immunogenic loop-structured region that would elicit an immune response highly focused on the corresponding region in the native protein, we chose a sequence from the antigen LDH-C$_4$ (Figure 9–5). Molecular modeling of the 274–286 loop region of LDH-C$_4$ suggested that hydrophobic residues in the loop will be brought together to form a hydrophobic inner core in the final structure of the zinc finger-stabilized peptide and expose the hydrophilic residues to solvent.

To achieve this, we have aligned the 274–286 sequence within the conserved motif as follows:

274   286
Thr-Leu-Val-Lys-Gly-Phe-His-Gly-Ile-Lys-Glu-**Glu**-Val-**Phe**   *native LDH-C*$_4$
Val-Lys-Gly-Phe-His-Gly-Ile-Lys-Glu-**Leu**-Val-**Lys**   *engineered sequence*

A Glu-to-Leu mutation was required to maximize the conserved hydrophobic core structure of the zinc finger motif. Phe[287] was also mutated to a Lys residue, because a positively charged (or at least a polar) residue is often found at this position. The Cys_2 and His_2 regions are adapted from the previously defined consensus sequence (Krizek et al., 1991). This peptide binds Co^{2+} in a 1:1 fashion (as determined by absorption spectroscopy), indicating that the appropriate zinc finger structure has been successfully achieved. To elicit the relevant T-cell help for antibody production to the B-cell epitope, the "promiscuous" T-cell epitope from measles virus MVF was linked to the amino terminus. The purified chimeric peptide forms the zinc finger structure as determined by spectroscopy of its Co^{2+} complex. The chimeric construct of the zinc finger loop B-cell epitope with a "promiscuous" T-cell peptide produced high-titered antibodies for the immunogen with moderate reactivity against the native protein (Kobs-Conrad et al., 1993). We have demonstrated that the cyclized disulfide loop 38-57 of the β-subunit of human chorionic gonadotropin (hCG), when coupled to the carrier protein DT (diptheria toxoid), is more immunogenic than the uncyclized peptide, albeit with low levels of cross-reactivity for hLH (Stevens et al., 1986). Thus, to develop an effective and efficacious antifertility hCG vaccine to this discontinuous epitope, three immediate problems must be elaborated and circumvented: (1) the effect of carrier protein versus measles virus "promiscuous" T-cell epitope (MVF) on immunogenicity; (2) the effect of chemical cyclization on cross-reactivity; and (3) adequate conformational mimicry (zinc finger stabilization) with regard to antigenic reactivity. The immediate aim of this ongoing study is to compare the antigenicity and immunogenicity of three constructs: DT-β-(38–57) disulfide loop, MVF-β-(3857) disulfide loop, and MVF-β-(38–57) zinc finger loop. We have designed and synthesized these constructs and presently are evaluating their immune responses in mice and rabbits.

Chimeric B-Cell and "Promiscuous" T-Cell Epitope Design

The most common approach for raising an effective immune response when short peptides are used as immunogens requires immunization of experimental animals with a conjugate consisting of the peptide coupled to a carrier protein. Covalent conjugation of antigenic determinants to large carrier molecules is undesirable in vaccine design becauses this often results in hypersensitivity, conformational change, loss of epitopes, appearance of undefined structures, batch-to-batch conjugate irreproducibility, and inappropriate presentation of epitopes. Consequently, the use of peptides in this context for human vaccines is severely restricted. More fundamentally, the role of carrier obscures efforts to elucidate the physical basis for the induction of protein-reactive antipeptide antibodies because the conformation of the peptide immunogen in these constructs is not verifiable.

Because it is generally accepted that, in a given haplotype, specific T-cell stimulation is a necessary prerequisite to B-cell proliferation (Roy et al., 1989), a strategy that is finding increasing use in the design of synthetic vaccines consists of co-linear synthesis of B- and T-cell epitopes (Borras-Cuesta et al., 1987; Clarke et al., 1987; Francis et al., 1987; Leclerc et al., 1987; Milich et al., 1987). T cells provide "help" to B cells displaying the same processed, MHC-restricted form of the antigen, demonstrating that the T-cell response to a protein antigen is under genetic control (Benacerraf and McDevitt, 1972; Buus et al., 1987). Most T-cell epitopes defined thus far have had limited activity across divergent MHC class II haplotypes; that is, different mouse strains appear to preserve and present different regions of proteins for stimulation of T cells and no single site has been stimulatory for all MHC types (Buus et al., 1987; Sette et al., 1989). This genetic restriction results in a T-cell epitope that binds an MHC molecule of only one individual but not the MHC molecule of another individual of the same species, and therefore elicits immune responses that are in most cases restricted to only one or a few alleles of the MHC with limited activity across divergent MHC class II haplotypes. This genetically restricted T-cell stimulatory activity of peptides is a serious obstacle, and consequently such constructs incorporating "helper" T cells would be of limited practical value as a universal vaccine effective in the majority of an outbred population. A solution to this problem could be of use to the so-called permissive interaction of some T-cell antigenic peptides with a wide range of MHC haplotype (O'Sullivan et al., 1991).

Reports have described T-cell epitopes that are broadly reactive in multiple haplotypes (Brett et al., 1989; Sinigaglia et al., 1988), thus providing a significant advance in the characterization of epitopes which bind multiple H-2 alleles. A number of so-called promiscuous T-cell epitopes from tetanus toxin (Ho et al., 1990; Panina-Bordignon et al., 1989), measles virus (Partidos and Steward, 1990), and malaria peptide (Fern and Good, 1992) have been reported to be universally immunogenic. These epitopes shown below, which bind several isotypic and allotypic forms of human MHC molecules in a permissive way, can be recognized by a single T-cell clone, imply-

CHIMERIC CONSTRUCTS

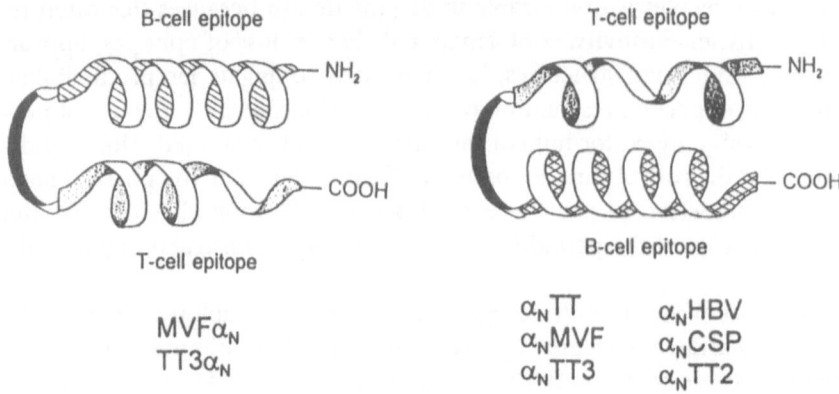

Figure 9-6. Chimeric B-cell and "promiscuous" T-cell constructs.

ing that some peptide sequences are not restricted to only one allele. T-cell epitopes capable of binding to the majority of immune response gene product motifs are preferred in strategies to overcome genetic restriction in the context of vaccine design.

1. [TT] N-S-V-D-D-A-L-I-N-S-T-I-Y-S-Y-F-P-S-V   (TT12)   580-599
2. [TT1] P-G-I-N-G-K-A-I-H-L-V-N-N-Q-S-S-E   (TT21)   916-932
3. [TT2] Q-Y-I-K-A-N-S-K-F-I-G-I-T-E-L   (P2)   830-844
4. [TT3] F-N-N-F-T-V-S-F-W-L-R-V-P-K-V-S-A-S-H-L-E   (P30)   947-967
5. [MVF] L-S-E-I-K-G-V-I-V-H-R-L-E-G-V   (MVF)   288-302
6. [HBV] F-F-L-L-T-R-I-L-T-I-P-Q-S-L-N   (HBsAg)   19-33
7. [CSP] T-C-G-V-G-V-R-V-R-S-R-V-N-A-A-N-K-K-P-E   (*P. vivax* CSP)   317-336

We have engineered the α_N sequence into chimeric constructs with each of the promiscuous T-cell epitopes. These peptides (Figure 9-6) are approximately 40 residues in length [an 18-residue B-cell epitope, a 4-residue linker sequence (-Leu-Ser-Pro-Gly-), and an 18- to 22-residue T-cell epitope]. Our initial studies consisted of two model peptides incorporating a conformational B-cell epitope of LDH-C_4 and a promiscuous T-cell epitope of tetanus toxin (Ho et al., 1990) (sequence 582–599, designated TT), as reported by Kaumaya et al. (1992b, 1993b). The solution structures (by CD) of α_1-TT and α_N-TT indicate that they fold into defined α-helical conformation as originally anticipated. Therefore, they are mimicking the topography of the corresponding region in the native LDH-C_4. The α_1-TT and α_N-TT constructs were highly immunogenic, producing high titers of antibodies in rabbits as early as in the primary + 2-week sera. These constructs were effective in producing antibodies in four of the six inbred/congenic mouse strains (BALB/c and B10.D2, H-2^d; C3H/HeJ and B10.BR, H-2^k; C57BL/6 and C57BL/10, H-2^b) of different H-2 haplotypes tested (Kaumaya et al., 1993b). There appears to be a strong correlation between the capacity for the hybrid peptides to be stimulatory for the corresponding T cells and their ability to be immunogenic. This correlation appears to break down in H-2^d strains of mice, as no antibodies were elicited in BALB/c and B10.D2 strains although T-cell activation was detectable. Conversely, high titers of antibodies are elicited in some strains (B10.BR and C57BL/10) without detectable IL-2 responses. Finally, we showed that a determinant that was previously restricted to the H-2^k could be rendered immunogenic in H-2^b with the promiscuous TT epitope.

To further understand the nature of the "promiscuous" T-cell epitopes, and to uncover ground rules for selection of T-cell epitopes that would activate T cells to provide help to B cells, we extended our studies to two other "promiscuous" T-cell epitopes, one from tetanus toxoid (sequence 830–844), designated TT2, and the other from the measles virus (sequence 288–302), designated MVF (Partidos and Steward, 1990). Similar design principles as detailed (Seo et al., 1993) were applied for the syntheses of three peptide immunogens incorporating the promiscuous T-cell epitopes (designated α_N-MVF, MVF-α_N, and α_N-TT2). Our initial studies in rabbits showed that high titers of antipeptide antibodies specific for the native protein were elicited, and further studies are in progress to assess relative affinities for the native protein.

We have also conducted limited experiments in mice, and preliminary results obtained in six strains of mice bearing three different haplotyopes show that the measles virus T-cell epitope, when coupled to α_N (as in α_NMVF), as well as the TT2 T-cell epitope (as in α_NTT2) can be used to bypass the MHC restriction in the H-2^d strains of mice, a restriction which was not overcome by α_NTT. The MVF T-cell epitope is not as effective as the TT and TT2 epitopes in inducing help in the H-2^b strains of mice (see Table 9-1). The differential orientation of the T-cell and B-cell epitopes is also under investigation.

Table 9-1. Antibody Responses to Chimeric B-cell and "Promiscuous" T-cell Epitopes

	H-2b		H-2k		H-2d	
Immunogens	C57BL/6	C57BL/10	C3H/HeJ	B10.BR	B10.D2	BALB/c
α_1TT	++[a]	+++[b]	+++	+++	+[c]	---[d]
α_NTT	+++	+++	+++	+++	+	---
α_NTT2	+++	---	+++	+++	+++	++
α_NMVF	++	+	+++	+++	+++	+++
MVFα_N	---	*	+++	*	*	+++

[a–d] Symbols: ++, Medium titers[a]; +++, high titers[b]; +, low titers[c]; —, negative[d]; *, not tested.

Additional peptides with the α_N restricted epitope of LDH-C_4 have been synthesized with human hepatitis B surface antigen (HBV, sequence 19–33), *P. vivax* (CSP, sequence 317–336), and tetanus toxoid (TT$_3$, sequence 947–967); the immune responses to these constructs in mice and rabbits are currently being evaluated (DiGeorge et al., 1993).

The mechanisms of directional help in such T-cell-dependent, B-cell responses by chimeric constructs are poorly understood and are dependent on a number of factors: peptide processing by APC (antigen presenting cell), presence of T cells of appropriate specificity, affinity of the T-cell epitope for MHC class II molecules, and antigen mimicry. To delineate the mechanisms of the interplay between the pairing of B and T epitopes in a single epitope, a B-cell epitope (α_N) derived from the protein antigen mouse lactate dehydrogenase C_4(LDH-C_4) was co-synthesized with a promiscuous T-cell epitope either from tetanus toxoid (TT3, sequence 947–967) or from the fusion protein of measles virus (MVF, sequence 288–302). Four constructs were synthesized in a way that the T-cell epitope was amino terminal (α_NTT3 and α_NMVF) or C terminal (TT3α_N and MVFα_N) to the B-cell epitope. Immunization of inbred and outbred mice as well as rabbits with these constructs elicited high titers of anti-chimera antibodies, which also bound strongly to the native protein LDH-C_4. Cross-reactivity studies within each set showed extensive overlapping specificities among the various immunogens when assayed by direct ELISA. The antisera reactivities for the native protein indicate that highly specific LDH-C_4 antibodies are generated in either orientation. There were cross-reactivities between the peptides with defined epitope orientation and the antisera induced by the peptides with the reverse orientation. Competitive ELISA with rabbit antisera showed that peptides with either orientation competed strongly with LDH-C_4 for the corresponding antisera. Preliminary results (Wang et al., 1993) indicated that the orientation of the T-cell epitope relative to the B-cell epitope does not influence the immunogenicity of the synthetic peptides to the native protein in our LDH-C_4 model.

These current studies are providing several leads in defining the necessary T-cell epitopes, or combinations thereof, that may represent the best method for ensuring adequate T-cell-stimulating activity in an outbred population with a heterogeneous MHC make-up. We expect to pinpoint several sequences that could serve as optimal T-cell determinants (DiGeorge et al., 1993). The extended studies described here will allow us to characterize in detail the specificity of these various T-cell epitopes, which in turn may provide information for the design of peptides that bind in an allele-specific manner or bind a variety of divergent histocompatibility types. Correlating peptide structure with antibody reponse and T-cell activation will enable us to identify the optimal immunodominant T-cell epitopes for incorporation into our universal template vaccine strategy. We hope to gain considerable information as to the isotypes being produced when different promiscuous T-cell epitopes are used because peptide antigen (B-cell epitope) structures are known to influence the expression of antibody variable and constant region structure. For example, when the conformational epitope in either orientation$_3$ of LDH-C$_4$ (no promiscuous epitope) was used as an immunogen in the responder H-2^k strains of mice, predominantly IgG2a antibodies were secreted. On the other hand, when the same α epitope was colinearly synthesized with the TT "promiscuous" epitope, only IgG1 and IgG2b antibodies were abundantly produced (Wang et al., 1993).

Multivalent B-Cell and T-Cell Vaccines

Improvements in immunogenicity of peptides is generally achieved by increasing their effective size and the number of copies by coupling to carrier proteins or a multibranched carrier core (Tam, 1988) to prevent their rapid clearance from the bloodstream by glomerular filtration. The high-density, multimeric presentation of epitopes, as has been shown for carrier protein, results in high titers of low-affinity antibodies (low cross-reactivity to the cognate sequence in the native protein). More importantly, any such design must allow the incorporation of stabilized conformational determinants such as those described that mimic the shape of the sequence in the native protein. However, if the latter criterion is not met, simply increasing the number of epitopes will not yield antibodies of high affinity or specificity. At present there is no acceptable carrier for use in humans, which in itself argues strongly in favor of replacing such an approach with strategies utilizing carrier-free moieties to improve immunogenicity.

We have designed a β-sheet template on which multiple B- and T-cell sites can be grafted in any combination and orientation. We have reported (Kobs-Conrad et al., 1992) the synthesis of a β-sheet template that allowed simultaneous dual copies of a B-cell and a T-cell epitope to be constructed sequentially (Figure 9–7). A combinatorial Fmoc/t-butyl, Fmoc/benzyl, Boc/benzyl approach as well as a fourth level of protecting group strategy was used to achieve the synthesis of a template bearing multiple individual epitopes. The synthetic peptide can be unambiguously characterized by peptide sequencing to fully ascertain its chemical composition. The assembly of different epitopes within a single folding unit may exhibit the highest potential for the construction of synthetic vaccines. Model template-peptides onto which duplicate copies of a tetanus toxoid epitope (TT) and duplicate copies of LDH-C$_4$ B cell determinants (α_N and α_1) were assembled into two peptides designated α_1TT-template and α_NTT-template. These constructs generated enhanced immune responses in outbred rabbits as early as 1 week after the primary immunization as compared to the colinear constructs α_1TT and α_NTT. We demonstrated that this type of construct could also be used to incorporate conformational epitopes, because

α_1,TT-Template

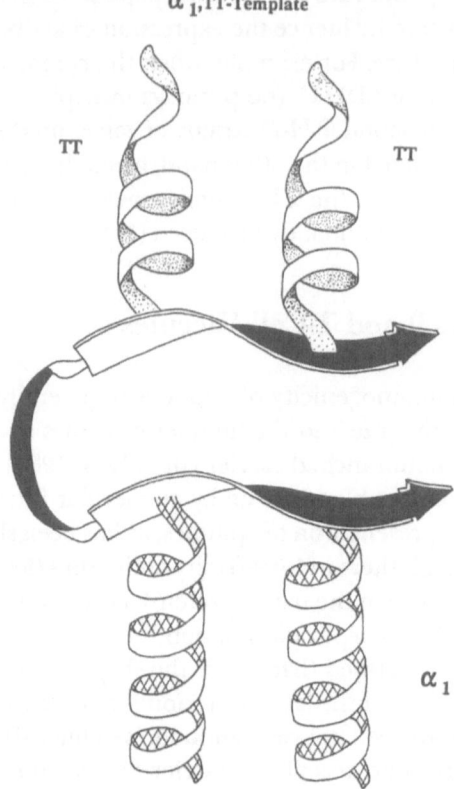

TT   TT

α_1

Figure 9–7. Schematic representation of multivalent template vaccine construct α_1TT template.

the α_1TT-template antibodies cross-reacted with the conformational α_3 construct in direct and competitive ELISA. Limited studies to date in three strains of mice and outbred mice have recently been completed. These constructs are extremely immunogenic, inducing high-titered antibodies (titers >12,800) specific for the native protein in all three strains of mice tested (as shown next); all individual outbred mice responded equally well. An unexpected and surprising finding in these studies is that we were able, by grafting dual copies of the B-cell determinant α_1 or α_N onto the template with dual copies of the TT promiscuous epitope, to raise protein-reactive antibodies in the nonresponder to α_1TT, α_NTT (BALB/c) strains, thereby bypassing the haplotype restriction associated with the B-cell epitope of LDH-C_4.

We have extended our previous studies to a systematic investigation involving four novel peptide vaccine constructs incorporating one T-cell site–

one B-cell epitope; one T-cell site–two B-cell epitopes; two T-cell sites–one B-cell epitope; and two T-cell sites–two B-cell epitopes (Kaumaya et al., 1993a). The study was initiated to explore whether haplotype-restricted immune responses to peptide antigens could be bypassed and whether immunogenicity and T-cell activation (peptide-driven IL-2 bioassay) could be correlated. Antibody responses in three strains of inbred mice, outbred mice, and rabbits, and our preliminary results, are summarized here:

   i.   High-titered IgG antibodies specific for the immunogen and the native protein are readily obtained (as early as primary + 1 week), indicating that isotype switch can occur fairly soon after immunization.

   ii. Lymphocytes from peptide immunized mice from all strains produced IL-2 in response to in vitro stimulation with the respective immunogen.

   iii. T-cell activation and antibody responses are well correlated.

   iv. Multiple B-cell epitopes consisting of LDH residues 1–18 and 310–327 produced higher titers of antibodies than the respective individual epitopes.

   v.   High-level, long-lasting response up to primary + 16 weeks is generally observed.

Thus, we have established the basis of our template peptide approach to modulate the appropriate immune response, and further studies are required to determine whether the template immunogens can be used to bypass haplotype-restricted immune responses in several inbred strains of mice. The biological significance of this approach is manyfold and could be used: (1) to construct epitopes in defined orientation and conformation, thus preserving the appropriate molecular mimicry of the B-cell epitope and enabling characterization of each construct; (2) to incorporate a number of different epitopes that could be used to bypass MHC restriction and thus overcome the problem of antigenic shift and drift that occurs in viral systems, and (3) to substitute for carrier proteins by increasing stability and size to prevent rapid clearance from the bloodstream by glomerular filtration, thereby avoiding the phenomenon of carrier-induced epitopic suppression.

Conclusions and Prospects

We have shown that it is possible (1) to design peptides with predetermined conformational properties, (2) to structurally characterize these properties by a variety of biophysical techniques, (3) to generate antibodies with high titers without coupling to a carrier protein, and (4) to generate protein-reactive antipeptide antibodies despite sequence changes and as long as the alterations are restricted to buried residues in the native protein.

Although these results are significant in understanding the conformational nature of protein epitopes and protein folding, there are still flaws in the present design, and many more questions remain that we hope to address in future designs. One of the major limitations in our present design is that we are still unaware of what constitutes an immunodominant epitope. When an antigen and antibody interact, they do so over a large surface area. Although an α-helix (e.g., 310–327) may be regarded as a discontinuous segment in that not all residues are located on the surface, it is conceivable that residues surrounding the helix but not part of the helix constitute part of the determinant. Only examination of antigen–antibody complexes by x-ray crystallography can accurately discern the exact boundaries of such an epitope. Despite these reservations, we are confident that the present approach and those from other laboratories will provide a basis for peptide engineering studies, the results of which will, in turn, permit further alterations that modulate specificity toward a predetermined structure.

These investigations can now be used to address a number of important questions in terms of a universal peptide vaccine strategy: How much molecular mimicry of an epitope must be preserved for enhanced immunogenicity? What is the most adequate synthetic preparation that will allow several B- and T-cell epitopes to be incorporated in a single construct? Is it sufficient to employ a single dominant determinant? Could multiple epitopes confer enhanced immunogenicity? Is MHC polymorphism really a stumbling block or can the challenge of polymorphism be met with relatively few promiscuous T-cell peptides binding to the most frequent MHC class II alleles? What patterns of cytokines are being secreted at the time of T-cell and B-cell interaction? What is the nature of the link between antibody isotypes, T-cell epitopes, and B-cell epitope structure? Can isotype patterns be governed by selection of T-cell epitopes?

REFERENCES

Allen PM (1987): *Immunol Today* 8:270.

Amit AG, Mariuzza RA, Phillips SEV, Poljak RJ (1986): *Science* 233:747–753.

Anthony-Cahill SJ, Benfield PA, Fairman R, Wasserman ZR, Brenner SL, Stafford WF, Altenbach C, Hubbell WL, DeGrado WF (1992): *Science* 255:979–983.

Atassi MZ (1984): *Eur J Biochem* 145:1–20.

Babbit B, Allen P, Matsueda G, Haber E, Unanue E (1985): *Nature (London)* 317:359.

Barlow DJ, Edwards MS, Thornton JM (1986): *Nature (London)* 322:747–748.

Benacerraf B, McDevitt H (1972): *Science* 175:273.

Benjamin DC, Berzofsky JA, East IJ, Gurd FRN, Hannum C, Leach SJ, Margoliash E, Michael JG, Miller A, Prager EM, Reichlin M, Sercaz EE, Smith-Gill SJ, Todd PE, Wilson AC (1984): *Annu Rev Immunol* 2:67–101.

Berg JM (1990): *Annu Rev Biophys Chem* 19:405–421.

Berzofsky JA (1991a): *Semin Immunol* 3:203–216.

Berzofsky JA (1991b): *Mol Immunol* 28:217–223.

Beyreuther K, Schulze-Gahmen U, Bieseler B, Prinz H (1987): In: *Chemical Synthesis in Molecular Biology*, GBF Monographs, Vol. 8, pp. 199–222. Weinheim: VCH Verlag.

Bidart J, Troalen F, Ghillani P, Rouas N, Razafindratsita A, Bohuon C, Bellet D (1990): *Science* 248:736–739.

Bjorkman PJ, Saper MA, Samraoui B, Bennett WS, Strominger JL, Wiley DC (1987a): *Nature (London)* 329:506.

Bjorkman, PJ, Saper MA, Samraoui B, Bennett WS, Strominger JL, Wiley DC (1987b): *Nature (London)* 329:512.

Borras-Cuesta F, Petit-Camurdan A, Fedon Y (1987): *Eur J Immunol* 17:1213–1215.

Brett SJ, Cease KB, Ouyang CS, Berzofsky JA (1989): *J Immunol* 143:771.

Brown F (1990): *Lancet* 335:587–590.

Buus S, Sette A, Colon S, Miles C, Grey HM (1987): *Science* 235:1353.

Chothia C (1984): *Annu Rev Biochem* 53:537–572.

Chou PY, Fasman GD (1978): *Adv Enzymol Relat Subj Biochem* 47:45–148.

Clarke BE, Newton SE, Carroll AR, Francis MJ, Appleyard G, Syred AD, Highfield PE, Rowlands DJ, Brown F (1987): *Nature (London)* 330:381–384.

Cohen C, Parry DAD (1986): *Trends Biol Sci* 11:245–248.

Cohen C, Parry DAD (1990): *Proteins Struct Funct Genet* 7:1–15.

Colman PM, Laver WG, Varghese JN, Baker AT, Tulloch PA, Air GM, Webster RG (1987): *Nature (London)* 326:358–363.

Crumpton MJ (1974): In: *The Antigens*, Vol. 2, pp. 1–78. New York: Academic Press.

Daniels SB, Reddy PA, Albrecht E, Richardson JC (1988): In: *Peptides: Chemistry and Biology*, Proceedings of the 10th American Peptide Symposium, Marshall GR, ed., p. 383. Escom, Leiden.

DeGrado WF, Lear JD (1985): *J Am Chem Soc* 107:7684–7689.

Devlin JJ, Panganiban LC, Devlin PE (1990): *Science* 249:404–406.

DiGeorge AM, Wang B, Kobs-Conrad S, Kaumaya PTP (1994). In: *Peptides: Chemistry, Structure, and Biology*. Hodges RS, Smith JA eds., Escom, Leiden (in press).

Dorrow DS, Shi PT, Carbone FR, Minasian E, Todd PEE, Leach SJ (1985): *Mol Immunol* 22:1255–1264.

Edwards MS, Sternberg MJE, Thornton JM (1987): *Protein Eng* 1:173–181.

Efimov AV (1984): *FEBS* 166:33–38.

Efimov AV (1991): *Protein Eng* 4:245–250.

Eisenberg D, Weiss RM, Terwilliger TC (1984): *Proc Natl Acad Sci USA* 81:140–144.

Eisenberg D, Wilcox W, Eshita SM, Pryciak PM, Ho SP, DeGrado WF (1986): *Proteins Struct Funct Genet* 1:16–22.

Engel M, Williams RW, Erickson BW (1991): *Biochemistry* 30:3161–3169.

Fedorov AN, Dolgikh DA, Chemeris VV, Chernov BK, Finkelstein AV, Schulga AA, Alakhov YB, Kirpichnikov MP, Ptitsyn OB (1992): *J Mol Biol* 225:927–931.

Fern J, Good MF (1992): *J Immunol* 148:907–913.

Fourquet P, Bahraoui E, Fontecilla-Camps JC, Van Rietschoten J, Rochat H, Granier C (1988): *Int J Pept Protein Res* 32:81–88.

Francis MJ, Hastings GZ, Syred AD, McGinn B, Brown F, Rowlands DJ (1987): *Nature (London)* 330:168.

Fremont DH, Matsumura M, Stura EA, Peterson PA, Wlison IA (1992): *Science* 257:919–927.

Geysen HM, Meloen RH, Barteling SJ (1984): *Proc Natl Acad Sci USA* 81:3998–4002.

Geysen HM, Rodda SJ, Mason TJ, Tribbick G, Schoofs PA (1987): *J Immunol Methods* 102:259-274.

Ghadiri MR, Soares C, Choi C (1992): *J Am Chem Soc* 114:4000-4002.

Goldberg E (1973): *Science* 181:458-459.

Goldberg E, Wheat TE, Powell JE, Stevens VC (1981): *Fert Steril* 35:214-217.

Gras-Masse H, Jolivet M, Drobecq H, Aubert JP, Beachey EH, Audibert F, Chedid L, Tartar A (1988): *Mol Immunol* 25:673-678.

Gutte B, Daumigen M, Wittschieber E (1979): *Nature (London)* 81:650-655.

Hahn KW, Klis WA, Stewart JM (1990): *Science* 248:1544-1547.

Hecht MH, Richardson JS, Richardson DC, Ogden RC (1990): *Science* 249:884-891.

Ho SP, DeGrado WF (1987): *J Am Chem Soc* 109:6751-6758.

Ho PC, Mutch DA, Winkel KD, Saul AJ, Jones GL, Doran TJ, Rezepczyk CM (1990): *Eur J Immunol* 20:477-483.

Hodges RS, Zhou NE, Kay CM, Semchuk PD (1990): *Pept Res* 3:123-137.

Hodges RS, Semchuk PD, Taneja AK, Kay CM, Parker JMR, Mant CT (1988): *Pept Res* 1:19-30.

Hogrefe HH, Kaumaya PTP, Goldberg E (1989): *J Biol Chem* 264:10513-10519.

Hogrefe HH, Griffith JP, Rossmann MG, Goldberg E (1987): *J Biol Chem* 262:13155-13162.

Hopp TP, Woods KR (1981): *Proc Natl Acad Sci USA* 78:3824-3828.

Houghten RA (1985):. *Proc Natl Acad Sci USA* 82:5131-5135.

Jemmerson R, Hutchinson RM (1990): *Eur J Immunol* 20:579-585.

Jemmerson R, Paterson Y (1986): *BioTechniques* 4(1):18-31.

Kaiser ET, Kezdy FJ (1984): *Science* 249-255.

Karle IL, Balaram P (1990): *Biochemistry* 29:6747-6756.

Karplus PA, Schulz GE 1985): *Naturwissenschaften* 72:212-213.

Kaumaya PTP, Berndt K, Heindorn D, Trewhella J, Kezdy FJ, Goldberg E (1990a): *Biochemistry* 29:13-23.

Kaumaya PTP, VanBuskirk AM, Goldberg E, Pierce SK (1990b): In: *Peptides: Chemistry, Structure and Biology*, Smith JA, Rivier J, eds., pp. 709-713. Leiden: ESCOM.

Kaumaya PTP, VanBuskirk A, Kobs S, Goldberg E, Pierce SK (1991): In: *Peptides 1990*, Giralt E, Andreu D, eds., pp. 611-613. Leiden: ESCOM.

Kaumaya PTP, VanBuskirk A, Goldberg E, Pierce SK (1992a): *J Biol Chem* 267:6338-6346.

Kaumaya PTP, Feng N, Kobs-Conrad S, Seo YH, VanBuskirk AM, Sheridan JF (1992b): In: *Peptides: Chemistry, Structure and Biology*, Smith JA, Rivier J, eds., pp. 883-885. Leiden: ESCOM.

Kaumaya PTP, Kobs-Conrad S, Seo YH, DiGeorge AM (1993a): In: *Peptides 1992*, Schneider CH, Eberle AN, eds. Leiden: ESCOM 139-141.

Kaumaya PTP, Seo YH, Kobs S, Feng N, Lee H, VanBuskirk AM, Sheridan J, Stevens V (1993b): *J Mol Recog* 6:81-94.

Kobs-Conrad S, Gerdau A, Kaumaya PTP (1992): In: *Peptides: Chemistry, Structure and Biology*, Smith JA, Rivier J, eds., pp. 886-888. Leiden: ESCOM.

Kobs-Conrad S, Lee H, DiGeorge AM, Kaumaya PTP (1993a): In: *Peptides 1992*, Schneider CH, Eberle AN, eds. Leiden: ESCOM 561-562.

Kobs-Conrad S, Lee H, DiGeorge AM, Kaumaya PTP (1993b): *J Biol Chem* 268(34):25285-25295.

Kourlisky P, Claverie J (1989): *Adv Immunol* 45:107-193.

Kochoyan M, Havel TF, Nguyen DT, Dahl CE, Keutmann HT, Weiss MA (1991):

Biochemistry 30:3371–3386.

Krizek BA, Amann BT, Kilfoil VJ, Merkle DL, Berg JM (1991): *J Am Chem Soc* 113:4518–4523.

Kyte J, Doolittle RF (1982): *J Mol Biol* 157:105–132.

Landschulz WH, Johnson PF, McKnight SL (1988): *Science* 240:1759.

Lau SYM, Taneja AK, Hodges RS (1984): *J Biol Chem* 259:13253–13261.

Lear JD, Wasserman ZR, DeGrado WF (1988): *Science* 240:1177–1181.

LeClerc G, Przewlocki G, Schutze MP, Chedid L (1987): *Eur J Immunol* 17:1213.

Lee H, Kaumaya PTP (1992): In: *Peptides: Chemistry and Biology*, Smith JA, Rivier J, eds., pp. 368–370. Leiden: ESCOM.

Lee MS, Gippert GP, Soman KV, Case DA, Wright PE (1989): *Science* 245:635–637.

Lerner RA (1984): *Adv Immunol* 36:1–4.

Lerum J, Goldberg E (1974): *Biol Reprod* 11:108–115.

Levitt M, Chothia C (1976): *Nature (London)* 261:552–558.

Merkle DL, Schmidt MH, Berg JM (1991): *J Am Chem Soc* 113:5450–5451.

Michael SF, Kilfoil VJ, Schmidt MH, Amann BT, Berg JM (1992): *Proc Natl Acad Sci USA* 89:4796–4800.

Milich DR (1989): *Adv Immunol* 45:195–282.

Milich DR (1990): *Semin Immunol* 2:307–315.

Milich DR, McLachlan A, Thornton GB, Hughes J (1987): *Nature (London)* 329:547.

Milner-White EJ, Poet R (1986): *Biochem J* 240:289–292.

Moser R, Frey S, Munger K, Hehlgans T, Klauser S, Langen H, Winnacker E, Mertz R, Gutte B (1987): *Protein Eng* 1:339–343.

Mutter M, Vuilleumier S (1989): *Angew Chem* 101:551–571.

Mutter M, Altmann K-H, Vorherr T (1986a): *Z Naturforsch* 41B:1315–1322.

Mutter M, Altmann K, Florsheimer A, Herbert J (1986b): *Helv Chim Acta* 69:786–792.

Mutter M, Altmann K, Tuchscherer G, Vuilleumier S (1988a): *Tetrahedron* 44:771–785.

Mutter M, Altmann E, Altmann K, Hersperger R, Koziej P, Nebel K, Tuchscherer G, Vuilleumier S, Gremlich H, Muller K (1988b): *Helv Chim Acta* 71:835–847.

Mutter M, Tuchscherer GG, Miller C, Altmann K-H, Carey RI, Wyss DF, Labhardt AM, Rivier JE (1992): *J Am Chem Soc* 114:1463–1470.

Novotny J, Handschumacher M, Haber E, Bruccoleri RE, Carlson WB, Fanning DW, Smith JA, Rose GD (1986): *Proc Natl Acad Sci USA* 83:226–230.

Omichinski JG, Clore GM, Appella E, Sakaguchi K, Gronenborn AM (1990): *Biochemistry* 29:9324–9334.

O'Shea EK, Rutkoski R, Kim PS (1989): *Science* 243:538–542.

O'Shea EK, Klemm JD, Kim PS, Alber T (1991): *Science* 254:539–544.

Osterhout JJ, Jr., Handel T, Na G, Toumadje A, Long RC, Connolly PJ, Hoch JC, Johnson WC, Jr., Live D, DeGrado WF (1992): *J Am Chem Soc* 114:331–337.

O'Sullivan D, Arrhenius T, Sidney J, Del Guercio M, Ablertson M, Wall M, Oseroff C, Southwood S, Colon SM, Gaeta FCA, Sette A (1991): *J Immunol* 147:2663–2669.

Pabo CO, Suchanek EG (1986): *Biochemistry* 25:5987–5991.

Padlan EA, Silverton EW, Sheriff S, Cohen GH (1989): *Proc Natl Acad Sci USA* 86:5938–5942.

Panina-Bordignon P, Tan A, Termijtelen A, Demotz S, Corradin G, Lanzavecchia A (1989): *Eur J Immunol* 19:2237–2242.

Parham P (1988): *Immunol Today* 9:65.

Partidos CD, Steward MW (1990): *J Gen Virol* 71:2099–2105.

Regan L, DeGrado WF (1988): *Science* 241:976–978.

Rose GD, Geselowitz AR, Lesser GJ, Lee RH, Zehfus MH (1985): *Science* 229:834–838.

Roy S, Scherer MT, Briner TJ, Smith JA, Gefter ML (1989): *Science* 244:572.

Schiffer M, Edmundson AB (1967): *Biophys J* 2(7):121–135.

Schulze-Gahmen U, Klenk HD, Beyreuther K (1986): *Eur J Biochem* 159:283–289.

Schulze-Gahmen U, Prinz H, Glatter U, Beyreuther K (1985): *EMBO J* 4:1731–1737.

Scott JK, Smith GP (1990): *Science* 249:386–390.

Sela M (1966): *Adv Immunol* 5:29–129.

Sela M 1990): *Proteins* 8:103–117.

Seo YH, Kobs-Conrad S, Kaumaya PTP (1993): In: *Peptides 1992*, Schneider CH, Eberle AN, eds. Leiden: ESCOM 866–867.

Segrest JP, De Loof H, Dohlman JG, Brouillette CG, Anantharamaiah GM (1990): *Proteins* 8:103–117.

Sette A, Buus S, Appella E, Smith JA, Chesnut R, Miles C, Colon SM, Grey HM (1989): *Proc Natl Acad Sci USA* 86:3296.

Sheriff S, Silverton EW, Padlan EA, Cohen GH, Smith-Gill S, Finzel BC, Davies DR (1987): *Proc Natl Acad Sci USA* 84:8075–8079.

Shoemaker KR, Kim PS, York EJ, Stewart JM, Baldwin RL (1987): *Nature (London)* 326:563–567.

Sinigaglia F, Guttinger M, Kilgus J, Doran DM, Matlie H, Etlinger H, Trzeciak A, Gillessen D, Pink R (1988): *Nature (London)* 336:778.

Stanfield RL, Fieser TM, Lerner RA, Wilson IA (1990): *Science* 248:712–719.

Stevens VC, Chou W, Powell JE, Lee AC, Smoot J (1986): *Immunol Lett* 12:11.

Steward MW, Howard CR (1987): *Immunol Today* 8:51-58.

Sundaralingam M, Sekharudu YC, Yathindra N, Ravichandran V (1987): *Proteins Struct Funct Genet* 2:64–71.

Tam JP (1988): *Proc Natl Acad Sci USA* 85,:5409–5413.

Thornton JM, Edwards MS, Taylor WR, Barlow DJ (1986): *EMBO J* 5:409–413.

Unanue ER (1984): *Annu Rev Immunol* 2:395.

Van Regenmortel MHV (1989): *Immunol Today* 10:266–272.

Vinson CR, Sigler PB, McKnight SL (1989): *Science* 246:911–916.

Wang B, Kobs-Conrad S, Kaumaya PTP (1994): In: *Peptides: Chemistry, Structure, and Biology*, Hodges RS, Smith JA, eds., Leiden: ESCOM (in press).

Welling GW, Weijer WJ, Van der Zee R, Welling-Wester S (1985): *FEBS Lett* 188:215–218.

Xu RX, Horvath SJ, Klevit RE (1991): *Biochemistry* 30:3365–3371.

Zhou NE, Kay CM, Hodges RS (1992): *J Biol Chem* 267:2664–2670.

Zhu BY, Zhou NE, Semchuk PD, Kay CM, Hodges RS (1992): *Int J Pept Protein Res* 40:171–179.

10

COMPLEMENTARY PEPTIDES: APPLICATIONS OF THE MOLECULAR RECOGNITION THEORY TO PEPTIDE AND PROTEIN PURIFICATION AND DESIGN

Michael A. Jarpe and J. Edwin Blalock

Introduction

Molecular recognition, the process by which two molecules recognize one another in a specific manner, is a fundamental requirement for most if not all biological reactions. However, the mechanism(s) by which molecules interact specifically is/are poorly understood. At present, our knowledge of bonding interactions and structure is not sufficient to accurately and frequently predict how or which peptide or protein pairs will bind one another. In the past decade, a novel approach has been proposed that has succeeded in predicting the interactions of proteinaceous molecules with high frequency. This method, based on the molecular recognition theory (MRT), has proven useful in designing interactive peptides, isolating receptors, and producing antireceptor and antiidiotypic antibodies (Blalock, 1990; Clarke and Blalock, 1991). Although the exact mechanism by which these peptides interact is not known, a growing body of work has accumulated that successfully applies this technique and supports the usefulness of this novel method. An overview of this methodology and its applications are the subject of the following chapter.

Peptides: Design, Synthesis, and Biological Activity
Channa Basava and G. M. Anantharamaiah, Editors
©1994 *Birkhäuser Boston*

Theory

It was observed by Blalock and Smith (1984) that complementary strands of DNA encode amino acid residues that are characterized by an inversion of hydropathy of their R groups. Specifically, a codon that specifies a hydrophilic residue has a complementary codon that specifies a hydrophobic residue and vice versa. In contrast, slightly hydrophilic amino acids have complementary codons for slightly hydrophilic amino acids. This relationship was shown to exist when codons are read either from the conventional 5'-3' direction or from the 3'-5' direction (Blalock and Bost, 1986). The independence of this relationship from reading direction occurs because the middle base of the codon, which does not change when read in either direction, is responsible for the hydropathy of the amino acid. Inverted hydropathy encoded on the two nucleic acid strands then occurs as a result of most hydrophilic amino acids having a second base A that is complemented by the second base U of most hydrophobic amino acids. Slightly hydrophilic amino acids tend to have a second base G or C and complement themselves.

If the hydropathy of amino acids specified by the coding strand is plotted against the hydropathy of amino acids encoded by the complementary strand, a correlation of −0.77 exists (Blalock and Bost, 1986; Blalock and Smith, 1984). Taken further, each segment of double-stranded DNA can be deciphered to four potential peptide sequences, all hydropathically related (Clarke and Blalock, 1991); Figure 10-1 outlines this relationship. According to our terminology, the peptide derived from the coding strand read in the 5'-3' direction is termed the sense peptide. The same strand read 3'-5' yields the antisense peptide. These two peptides will have similar hydropathic profiles. Likewise, the complementary strand can be decoded to two peptides. The sense complementary peptide is read 5'-3' while the antisense complementary peptide is read 3'-5'. These two peptides have similar hydropathic profiles compared to one another but are hydropathically inverted compared to the peptides derived from the coding strand.

The finding that the same linear array of hydropathy of a peptide is encoded on a single strand of nucleic acid in either reading direction suggests this property is an important component of the organization of the genetic code and one that may have preceded directionality to the handling of genetic information. Further, it suggests that the linear array of hydropathy as is symmetrically encoded may be an important component of structure and function. Thus, a single nucleotide sequence may specify two structurally and perhaps functionally related peptides when read in the sense or antisense direction. In fact, we have provided evidence that the genetically encoded linear pattern of hydropathy of amino acids rather than the amino acid sequence per se defines gross secondary and tertiary structure and function (Clarke and Blalock, 1990). If one assumes that the

A. Amino acid sequences

Antisense (3'-5')	HOOC- G	V	Q	L -NH₂
Sense (5'-3')	H₂N- W	M	D	F -COOH

Coding strand	5' UGG	AUG	GAC	UUC 3'
Non-coding strand	3' ACC	UAC	CUG	AAG 5'

Sense Complementary (5'-3')	HOOC- P	H	V	E -NH₂
Antisense Complementary (3'-5')	H₂N- T	Y	L	K -COOH

B. Hydropathy

Antisense (3'-5')	HOOC- G	V	Q	L -NH₂
	-0.4	4.2	-3.5	3.7
Sense (5'-3')	H₂N- W	M	D	F -COOH
	-0.9	1.9	-3.5	2.7

Sense Complementary (5'-3')	HOOC- P	H	V	E -NH₂
	-1.6	-3.2	4.2	-3.5
Antisense Complementary (3'-5')	H₂N- T	Y	L	K -COOH
	-0.7	-1.3	3.7	-3.9

Figure 10-1. Relationship of sequences derived from both strands of DNA for carboxyl-terminal tetrapeptide of gastrin (McGuigan and Campbell-Thompson, 1992). **A.** Amino acid sequences derived from coding and noncoding strands translated in the 5'-3' direction and the 3'-5' direction. **B.** Hydropathic values for the four amino acid sequences (Blalock and Bost, 1986; Blalock and Smith, 1984).

linear array of hydropathy of amino acids is a key to the gross shape of a peptide or protein, then a complete inversion of the hydropathy may be a key to inverted or complementary shape.

The foregoing is the essence of the MRT, which proposes that complementary nucleotide sequences encode peptides which interact as a result of a genetically determined inversion of their respective hydropathic profiles (Bost et al., 1985b). This was first tested with the peptide hormone corticotropin (ACTH). A peptide was synthesized corresponding to the noncoding strand of ACTH mRNA and tested for its ability to bind to ACTH. In a solid-phase binding assay, ACTH was found to specifically bind to its complementary peptide, termed HTCA, with nanomolar affinity (Bost et al., 1985b). Further, equivalent binding was observed with HTCA peptides based on a sense or antisense reading of ACTH complementary RNA (Blalock and Bost, 1986). The observation that these peptides had different amino acid sequences but the same linear array of hydropathy suggested that this latter property was responsible for the interaction. Additional support for the idea that inverted hydropathy is the driving force for the interaction comes from the observation that peptides derived from computer-assisted, as well as nucleotide sequence-directed, inversion also interact (Fassina et al., 1989a). The similarity of structure of 5'-3' and 3'-5' complementary petpides, as is suggested by these studies, is also implied by the finding that the peptides are antigenically related (Pascual et al., 1988; Torres and Johnson, 1990). An up-to-date list of the many interacting complementary peptides designed by at least one of these two methods is provided in Table 10–1.

Applications

Various aspects of the MRT have now been used successfully by a number of different laboratories for a variety of applications. For the purpose of this chapter, these applications are divided into five categories: purification and diagnostic procedures, enzyme inhibitors, antibodies to complementary peptides, and therapeutic applications.

Purification Procedures

Purification of proteins expressed with recombinant methodologies is a major and expensive hurdle in the production of large quantities of protein. Existing methods include gel filtration, ion exchange, HPLC, and immunoaffinity chromatography. Aside from immunoaffinity chromatography, these techniques lack the specificity that is crucial to purification. Immunoaffinity purification has the advantage of specificity, although the affinity is often too high. Also, it is not always cost effective in large-scale purification applications and can result in immunoglobulin bleeding into the sample. Fassina and colleagues have developed purification protocols utilizing the complementary peptide approach for the purification of recombinant proteins (Chaiken et al., 1989; Fassina and Cassani, 1992; Fassina et al., 1987, 1989a, 1989b, 1992a, 1992b, 1992c, 1993). This method can be specific, of tailor-made affinity, and cost effective on very stable supports. The successful uses to date of complementary peptides for purification of proteins and peptides include c-raf (Fassina et al., 1989a), tumor necrosis factor-α (Fassina et al., 1992a), interleukin-1 (IL-1) (Fassina and Cassani, 1992), endothelin (Fassina et al., 1992b), interferon-β (Scapol et al., 1992), and bradykinin (Fassina et al., 1993). For example, recombinant tumor necrosis factor α (rTNF-α) has been purified using a complementary peptide that was designed to recognize rTNF-α residues (144–157). This peptide immobilized to a solid support was able to purify rTNF-α from crude *E. coli* lysates (Fassina et al., 1992a). Additionally, the peptide affinity column was able to selectively bind the targeted peptide fragment, TNF-α (144–157), to the exclusion of peptides representing all other rTNF-α sequences.

Another example is the purification of recombinant interferon-beta (IFNβ) (Scapol et al., 1992). Three peptides were synthesized that were

Table 10-1. Interactive Complementary Peptide Pairs

Complementary peptide to:	Number of amino acids	K(M)	References
ACTH	24	3×10^{-10}	Bost et al., 1985a
Ribonuclease S peptide	20	1.3×10^{-6}	Shai et al., 1987
c-raf oncogene product	20	3.8×10^{-4}	Fassina et al., 1989a
Arginine vasopressin, neurophysin fragment	20	Not determined	Fassina et al., 1989b; Shai et al., 1987,1989
Endothelin	18	$25–55\times 10^{-6}$	Fassina et al. 1992b; Zamai et al., 1992
Endothelin	14(tetrameric)	10×10^{-6}	Fassina and Cassani, 1993
γ-endorphin	17	2×10^{-5}	Bost et al, 1985b
Tumor necrosis factor α	14 (octameric)	1×10^{8}	Fassina et al., 1992a
Interferon-β	14,13	Not determined	Scapol et al., 1992
Prolactin	13	5×10^{-6}	Ebner et al., 1989; Bajpai et al., 1991
Acetylcholine receptor	13	9×10^{-5}	Radding et al., 1992
Interleukin-1β	9, 12, 13, or 14	2×10^{-5} (12-mer)	Fassina and Cassani, 1992; Sisto, 1992
LHRH	10	1×10^{-4}	Mulchahey et al., 1986; Gorcs et al., 1986
Substance P	9	6×10^{-6}	Bost and Blalock, 1989
Myelin basic protein	9	Not determined	Maier and Blalock, unpublished data
Bradykinin	9 (tetrameric)	Not determined	Fassina et al., 1993
Angiotensin II	8	1×10^{-6}	Elton et al., 1988; Budisavlijevic et al., 1992
Calmodulin/troponin C	8	1×10^{-6}	Dillon et al., 1991
Collagen	7	5×10^{-5}	DeSouza and Brentani, 1992
Interleuken-2	6, 13, or 14	6×10^{-5} (6-mer)	Fassina, 1993; Weigent et al.,1986
Fibronectin	6	Not determined	Brentani et al., 1988
Insulin	6	3×10^{-9}	Knutson, 1988
Arginine vasopressin	9	Not determined	Johnson and Torres, 1988
Cystatin C fragment	5	Not determined	Ghiso et al., 1990
Fibrinogen	5	2.5×10^{-4}	Gartner and Taylor, 1991
Dopamine receptor	5	Not determined	Nagy and Frawley, 1991
Laminin	5	Not determined	Nomizu et al., 1991
α-Melanocyte-stimulating hormone	5	Not determined	Al-Obeidi et al., 1989; Hruby et al., 1992
β-Melanocyte-stimulating hormone	5	Not determined	Al-Obeidi et al., 1989; Hruby et al.,1992
Enkephalin	5	Not determined	Misra et al., 1993
HIV protease	5–15	0.1 to 1×10^{-3}	Roller et al., 1991
Gastrin	4	7×10^{-8}	McGuigan and Campbell-Thompson, 1991

complementary to three predicted surface-exposed areas of Chinese hamster ovary cell-derived recombinant IFNβ (CHO-rIFNβ). The peptides were synthesized on solid resin supports and used attached as the affinity matrix. All three peptides purified the CHO-IFNβ in a manner comparable to a monoclonal antibody affinity column. No purification was seen with resin support alone. Although not yet studied, such complementary peptide columns in tandem could be used to markedly increase the degree of purification. It is likely that such optimization will yield appropriate specificity, capacity, and increased efficiency of purification that would be useful in large-scale purification such as is required in an industrial setting. Thus, this method allows for the production of site-specific binding peptides that can be targeted at will to the purification of biologically important proteins and peptides.

Diagnostic Procedures

A related use of complementary peptides is the design of specific peptides that can be used to identify and quantify protein in a diagnostic manner. The advantage of this methodology over the existing use of antibodies is the time and cost of producing and purifying antibodies. One drawback has been the lack of consistent high-affinity binding, which is essential for the development of sensitive assays. This problem has been recently overcome with the use of multimeric complementary peptides that increase the avidity of complementary peptide binding. Multimeric peptides are produced by synthesizing a peptide on a branched support. Much like a multiple antigenic peptide (Posnett and Tam, 1989), the end result is a peptide that has two, four, or eight identical branches (Fassina et al., 1992a). Such multimeric complementary peptides have been used in a sandwich-type assay developed for the quantitation of IL-2 (Fassina, in press). Three sites of IL-2 were selected, and complementary peptides were designed and synthesized in multimeric form. One of these peptides was immobilized to a microtiter plate. IL-2 was then captured on the plate and detected with a biotinylated complementary peptide directed to another region of IL-2. As little as 10 ng/ml could be detected with this assay even in the presence of bovine serum albumin (BSA) or 10% goat serum. A modification of this assay was used to measure low concentrations of TNF-α (Fassina et al., 1992a). In this study, TNF-α was measured using a competition assay with a multimeric complementary peptide bound to a microtiter plate.

   In principle, this method could be extended beyond the assay of proteins in vitro and used for any application for which antibodies are now used. For instance, cell-surface markers on various tissues, including tumor cells, could be targeted with complementary peptides. These peptides coupled to the appropriate agents could be used in imaging or fluorescent techniques. One need only know the amino acid sequence of the target protein to produce a specific probe.

Enzyme Inhibitors

There is currently great interest in potentially controlling disease by development of inhibitors of the activity of specific enzymes. Traditional methods of isolating enzyme inhibitors involve the screening of hundreds or thousands of compounds until an inhibitor is found. The inhibitor is then modified to optimize its activity. A recent advancement in this field has been made through the use of structural analysis of the enzyme–inhibitor complex in an effort to rationally design inhibitory molecules. This process is hampered by the initial identification of potential drug leads with inhibitory activity that can be optimized. As a more rational approach, a complementary peptide can now be used to interact with and modify enzyme activity. A group of inhibitors has been designed and tested for the inhibition of HIV-1 protease (Roller et al., 1992). Forty-two complementary peptides were synthesized that were designed to interact with different functional domains of HIV-1 protease. It was found that peptides directed toward the flap and α-helical regions of the protease were the best inhibitors, with inhibitory constants between 100 and 300 μM. Although this affinity is low, the peptides are potential drug leads that can provide a basis for further drug design to increase the inhibitor activity.

A second approach to modifying enzyme activity is to essentially deplete the substrate by directing the complementary peptide to the proteolytic cleavage site in the substrate protein or peptide. The feasibility of this approach was initially demonstrated by Fassina et al. (1989a) through the observation that a complementary peptide to a fragment of c-raf could complex with the c-raf peptide and protect it from tryptic degradation. More recently, this same technique was successfully applied to block the activity of collagenase on collagen (DeSouza and Brentani, 1992) as well as chymotrypsin-catalyzed hydrolysis of big endothelin (Zamai et al., 1992). In these latter two instances, the complementary peptide encompassed only the cleavage site and not the entire substrate molecule. A third approach was to identify the active site (five amino acids) of the protease inhibitor, cystatin C, and search a database for a complementary peptide sequence (Ghiso et al., 1990). This sequence was located in the fourth component of complement (C4). Cystatin C was then shown to bind C4 through the complementary peptide sequences as well as to block the complement cascade. C4 and cystatin C were not known to interact before this work was done. In theory, this approach could be used in reverse to search databases for sequences complementary to an enzyme active site to identify potential inhibitors. Thus, simple sequence analysis for complementarity could be used to ascertain novel peptide inhibitors or enzymes that might be acted on by known inhibitors.

A complementary peptide was used as the basis for the development of an assay for endothelin-converting enzyme activity as well as its possible inhibition (Fassina and Cassani, 1993). This complementary peptide bound a biotinylated peptide substrate sequence from endothelin before but not after cleavage. Thus, noncleaved residual peptide bound the solid-phase complementary peptide and was detected by streptavidin conjugated to peroxidase. The complementary peptide in this assay was rendered insusceptible to hydrolysis by synthesis in the all-D configuration, which has equal binding affinity to an all-L form (Fassina et al., 1989a, 1992a, 1992b; Roller et al., 1992).

Antibodies to Complementary Peptides

When the MRT was initially proposed, the mechanism by which complementary peptides recognized one another was postulated to be driven by complementary shapes that resulted from an inverted linear pattern of hydropathy. This was first tested by using antibodies to complementary peptides. We reasoned that if a complementary peptide were recognizing a peptide ligand in a shape-dependent manner, the complementary peptide could have conformation similar to that of the binding site of the receptor for the ligand. Therefore, antibodies to the complementary peptide should interact with the receptor. This was first shown with the hormone ACTH and its complement HTCA (Bost et al., 1985b); antibodies to HTCA recognized a receptor for ACTH on adrenal cells that harbor this receptor. These studies suggested that complementary peptide recognition may be shape- or conformation dependent. Together with the aforementioned studies (Clarke and Blalock, 1990), these results also suggested that the shape or conformation of a peptide may depend in large measure on the linear array of hydropathy as encoded by the DNA sequence. Because a peptide was the immunogen, however, these studies do not rule out the possibility that a linear rather than conformational epitope is being recognized by the antibodies to the complementary peptide. In all likelihood, both cases occur.

From these early experiments with antibodies to complementary peptides, it was obvious that the ability to raise receptor-specific antibodies would be a valuable tool in the isolation of receptors. A number of successful receptor isolations have been carried out thus far (Table 10–2). It is clear that with this technique antibodies can be raised and used to purify receptors of many different types. In the future, these antibodies or their induction may have enzyme inhibitor activity (DeSouza and Brentani, 1992) and utility as receptor agonists or antagonists as well as immunoconjugates

Table 10-2. Anticomplementary Peptide Antibodies That Recognize Receptors

Antibody to the complementary peptide of	Receptor size (Daltons)	Reference
ACTH	83,000	Bost et al., 1985; Bost and Blalock, 1986; Clarke and Bost, 1990; Jones et al., 1991
δ-opiate	58,000	Carr et al., 1986, 1989
LHRH	60,000 + 51,000	Costa et al., 1990; Gorcs et al., 1986; Mulchahey et al., 1986; Neri et al., 1991
Fibronectin	140,000	Brentani et al., 1988
Fibrinogen	108,000	Pasqualini et al., 1989
AVP	62,000 + 55,000 76,000 + 70,000	Abood et al., 1989 Swords et al., 1990
Angiotensin II	66,000	Elton et al., 1988
Substance P	58,000	Pascual et al., 1989
Prolactin	Not determined	Ebner et al., 1989
Gastrin	Not determined	McGuigan and Campbell-Thompson, 1992
β-endorphin caroxyterminus	56,000 + 58,000 + 64,000	Shahabi et al., 1992

targeted to specific cells as therapeutic or imaging reagents. Indeed, active immunization with a complementary peptide has been reported to block the in vivo activity of a hypothalamic-releasing factor (Gorcs et al., 1986).

A related application involves antibodies, raised against complementary peptides, that bind other antibodies at their antigen-binding site (Blalock et al., 1989). These antibodies are termed antiidiotypic. Antibodies, in a broader sense, can be considered receptors whose ligands are the antigens to which they bind. Theoretically, complementary peptides that interact with peptide antigens by mimicking an antibody-combining site could be used to raise antiidiotype antibodies that bear an "internal image" of the peptide antigen. These antibodies would bind the original antibody in a manner similar to that of the antigen. This idea was first demonstrated with antibodies to ACTH, endorphins, and their complementary peptides (Smith et al., 1987). A number of other studies have also shown similar results (Table 10-3).

Autoreactive antibodies have been shown to be involved in a number of autoimmune diseases. In the case of myasthenia gravis, autoantibodies bind to the acetylcholine receptor and block neuromuscular transmission, causing fatigue and muscle weakness. If the binding of the disease-causing antibody could be specifically inhibited, the disease might be prevented or reversed with few side effects. This theory was tested on an experimental model of myasthenia gravis in rats (Araga et al., 1993). Immunization of rats with the disease-causing epitope of the acetylcholine receptor (AChR 61-76) produces symptoms of myasthenia gravis. When rats were immunized with a complementary peptide to the acetylcholine receptor (RhCA 67-16) before being challenged with an AChR, antiidiotypic antibody re-

Table 10-3. Idiotypic and Antiidiotypic Antibodies Induced by Immunization with Complementary Peptides

Antigen	Antibodies		Reference
	Polyclonal	Monoclonal	
ACTH	+		Smith et al., 1987
β-endorphin	+		Smith et al., 1987
Phosphorycholine		+	Kang et al., 1988
Myelin basic protein 80–89		+	Blalock et al., 1989; Whitaker et al., 1989; Zhou and Whitaker, 1990
Substance P	+		Pascual and Bost, 1989
Myelin basic protein 1–9		+	Zhou and Whitaker, 1990, 1992

sulted. After challenge with AChR, only 25% of the animals showed signs of disease compared to 90% in a control group that was not immunized with RhCA 67-16. This demonstrates the potential for this type of therapy in the treatment of antibody-mediated autoimmune diseases.

Cell-mediated or T-lymphocyte-associated autoimmune diseases such as multiple sclerosis (MS) may also be amenable to complementary peptide antibody therapy as such antibodies have been shown to bind T-cell receptors as well as autoantibodies against a disease-causing epitope (Zhou and Whitaker, 1993). In fact, a monoclonal antibody to a complementary peptide of myelin basic protein blocked the development of disease in an animal model of MS (Zhou and Whitaker, 1993).

Therapeutic Applications

A final diverse and exciting application of the MRT is the generation of therapeutic agents that may be used to treat disease. There is a constant need for novel pharmaceutical compounds that can approach the problem of drug design from different directions. The complementary peptide represents a method that can be used to design agonists and antagonists of many receptors and ligands in ways very different than those conventionally used. Examples of these new possible therapeutics are shown in Table 10-4.

As previously mentioned, one approach is to synthesize peptide ligands that have the same linear pattern of hydropathy as the ligand of interest yet different amino acid sequences. This method has been used to design an agonist of the ACTH receptor (Clarke and Blalock, 1990) and an antagonist of the growth hormone-releasing hormone receptor (unpublished data). Second, complementary peptides can be designed that specifically bind and alter the ligand of interest. For instance, a complementary peptide that bound angiotensin II (AII) in vitro was shown to function as a relatively

Table 10-4. Possible Therapeutic Uses of Complementary Peptides

Target	Action on		Result		Reference
	Ligand	Receptor	Agonist	Antagonist	
Angiotensin II	+			+	Budisavligevic et al., 1992
Arginine vasopressin	+			+	Johnson and Torres, 1988
Enkephalin	+		+		Misra et al., in press
Melanocyte-stimulating hormone	+		+	+	Al Obeidi et al., 1989; Hruby et al., 1992
Luteinizing hormone-releasing hormone	+			+	Mulchahey et al., 1986
Fibrinogen	+			+	Gartner and Taylor, 1990, 1991
Laminin	+			+	Nomizu et al., 1992
Endothelin	+			+	Zamai et al., 1992
Calcium		+	+		Dillon et al., 1991
Acetylcholine		+		+	Radding et al., 1992
Dopamine		+		+	Nagy and Frawley, 1991

potent AII antagonist in vivo (Budisavlijevic et al., 1992), and peptides complementary to fibrinogen blocked platelet aggregation (Gartner and Taylor, 1991; Gartner et al., 1991). The complex of arginine vasopressin (AVP) and its complementary peptide was a receptor antagonist (Johnson and Torres, 1988). In contrast, complementary peptides for methionine (Met-Enk) or leucine (Leu-Enk) enkephalin were designed to interact with Met–Enk and Leu–Enk, respectively. These peptides were shown to enhance the agonist activity of enkephalin in a peptide-specific manner with the complement to Met–Enk acting only on Met–Enk and the Leu–Enk complement acting only on Leu–Enk (D. N. Dhawan, personal communication; Misra et al., 1993). Thus, in theory these drugs can target the ligand itself rather than the receptor and create peptide complexes that are either antagonists or superagonists, as has been described for melanocyte-stimulating hormone (Al-Obeidi et al., 1989; Hruby et al., 1992). In some instances, this approach could be more specific than conventionally made receptor agonists and antagonists if two different ligands bound the same receptor and the complementary peptide bound only one of the ligands. Additionally, the complementary peptides could be synthesized in an all-D form for increased stability.

If on the other hand one makes complementary peptides to the binding sites of receptors, one can create novel ligands that are agonists or antagonists. This is the case even if the receptor of interest is for a nonpeptide ligand. Thus, peptide mimetics of nonpeptides can be rationally designed. For example, a peptide mimetic of calcium that was designed to bind the calcium-coordinating sites of calmodulin was found to bind calmodulin and induce a calmodulin-dependent contraction of smooth muscle (Dillon et al., 1991). Similarly, using this approach, peptide mimetics have been constructed for acetylcholine (Radding et al., 1992), dopamine (Nagy and Frawley, 1991), and ouabain (J. D. Neill, personal communication).

Future Directions

As with any new discovery, there are always failures to verify certain aspects of the findings. Complementary peptides are no exception and have failed to work in a very limited number of instances (Blalock, 1990). Although most of these failures are explainable by technique or design (Blalock, 1990), it will be important in the future to understand the true generality of the theory. However, considering the very large number of successful applications that are covered in this chapter, it seems safe to say that the procedure probably works far more often than would be expected by chance alone. With this assumption, it appears that peptides derived from the MRT, with optimization of design and procedure or technique, have a bright future with regard to pharmaceutical application. More theoretically, a complete understanding of this idea may shed light on the evolution of interacting proteins (Bost and Blalock, 1985b), the problem of protein folding and shape (Dillon et al., 1991; Draper, 1989), and the facile identification of sites of protein interaction (Ghiso et al., 1990; Palla et al., 1993). With regard to the latter, the Human Genome project will undoubtedly yield many protein sequences of unknown function. Thus, the ability to identify possible interaction sites with known proteins may help to decipher the puzzle. Such an application of the MRT seems particularly likely because complementary nucleotide sequences have been found in the known binding sites of interacting proteins (Bost et al., 1985a; Brown et al., 1992; Campbell and Hidechika, 1991; Djabali et al., 1991; Slootstra and Roubos, 1991a, 1991b). In other cases, they have been used to identify the previously unknown binding sites of interleukins 1 and 2 and their receptors as well as cystatin C and the fourth component of complement (Ghiso et al., 1990; Palla et al., 1993; Weigent et al., 1986).

Acknowledgments

The authors thank Diane Weigent for excellent editorial assistance. This work was supported in part by RO1 DK38024, PO1 NS29719, and a grant from the Council for Tobacco Research #2222. M.A.J. is supported by Hypertension Training Program grant HL07457.

REFERENCES

Abood LG, Michael GJ, Xin L, Knigge KM (1989): *J Recept Res* 9:19–25.
Al-Obeidi FA, Hruby VJ, Sharma SD, Hadley ME, De Castrucci AML (1989): In: *Peptides 89*, Rivier JE, Marshall GR, eds., pp. 530–532. ESCOM.
Araga S, LeBoeuf RD, Blalock JE (1993): *Proc Natl Acad Sci USA* 90:8747–8751.
Bajpai A, Hooper KP, Ebner KE (1991): *Biochem Biophys Res Commun* 180:1312–1317.

Blalock JE (1990): *Trends Biotechnol* 8:140–144.

Blalock JE, Bost KL (1986): *Biochem J* 234:679–683.

Blalock JE, Smith EM (1984): *Biochem Biophys Res Commun* 121:203–207.

Blalock JE, Whitaker JN, Benveniste EN, Bost KL (1989): *Methods Enzymol* 178:63–74.

Bost KL, Blalock JE (1986): *Mol Cell Endocrinol* 44:1–9.

Bost KL, Blalock JE (1989): *Methods Enzymol* 168:16–28.

Bost KL, Smith EM, Blalock JE (1985a): *Biochem Biophys Res Commun* 128:1373–1380.

Bost KL, Smith EM, Blalock JE (1985b): *Proc Natl Acad Sci USA* 82:1372–1375.

Brentani RR, Ribeiro SF, Potocnjak P, Pasqualini R, Lopes JD, Nakaie CR (1988): *Proc Natl Acad Sci USA* 85:364–367.

Brown R, Meldrum C, Cousins S (1992): *Med Hypotheses* 38:322–324.

Budisavlijevic M, Bea ML, Bensoussan M, Laubie M, Pham Van Chuong P, Dussaule J, Verroust P, Ronco P (1992): *J Hypertension* 19:345–353.

Campbell W, Hidechika O (1991): *Biochem Biophys Res Commun* 175:207–214.

Carr DJJ, Blalock JE, Bost KL (1989): *Immunol Lett* 20:181–186.

Carr DJJ, Bost KL, Blalock JE (1986): *J Neuroimmunol* 12:329–337.

Chaiken I, Fassina G, Shai Y (1989): In: *Protein Recognition of Immobilized Ligands*, Hutchens W, ed. New York: Liss.

Clarke BL, Blalock JE (1990): *Proc Natl Acad Sci USA* 87:9708–9711.

Clarke BL, Blalock, JE (1991): In: *Antisense Nucleic Acids and Proteins: Fundamentals and Applications*, van der Krol AR, Mol JNM, eds., pp. 169–186. New York: Dekker.

Clarke BL, Bost KL (1990): *Biochem Biophys Res Commun* 168:1020–1026.

Costa O, Mulchahey JJ, Blalock JE (1990): *Prog NeuroEndocrinImmunol* 3:55–60.

DeSouza SJ, Brentani R (1992): *J Biol Chem* 267:13763–13767.

Dillon J, Woods WT, Guarcello V, LeBoeuf RD, Blalock JE (1991): *Proc Natl Acad Sci USA* 88:9726–9729.

Djabali K, Portier M-M, Gros F, Blobel G, Georgatos SD (1991): *Cell* 64:109–121.

Draper KG (1989): *Biochem Biophys Res Commun* 163:466–470.

Ebner KE, Varma S, Bajpai A (1989): Abstract #814, p. 226, 71st Annual Meeting of the Endocrine Society. Endocrine Society Press.

Elton TS, Dion LD, Bost KL, Oparil S, Blalock JE (1988): *Proc Natl Acad Sci USA* 85:2518–2522.

Fassina G (1993): In: *Peptides 1992*, Proceedings of the 22d Symposium of the European Peptide Society, Schneider CH, Eberle AN, eds., pp 907–908. ESCOM Science Publishers B.V.

Fassina G, Cassani G (1992): *Biochem J* 282:773–779.

Fassina G, Cassani G (1993): *Pept Res* 6:73–78.

Fassina G, Cassani G, Corti A (1992a): *Arch Biochem Biophy* 296:137–143.

Fassina G, Consonni R, Zetta L, Cassani G (1992b): *Int J Pept Protein Res* 39:540–548.

Fassina G, Corti A, Cassani G (1992c): *Int J Peptide Protein Res* 39:549–556.

Fassina G, Germani S, Cassani G (In Press): In: *Peptides 91*, Proceedings of the 22d Symposium of the European Peptide Society, Schneider CH, Eberle AN, eds., pp 627–628. ESCOM Science Publishers B.V.

Fassina G, Zamai M, Chaiken I (1987): *J Cell Biochem* 35:9.

Fassina G, Roller PP, Olson AD, Thorgeirsson SS, Omichinski JG (1989a): *J Biol Chem* 264:11252–11257.

Fassina G, Zamai M, Brigham-Burke M, Chaiken IM (1989b): *Biochemistry* 28:8811–8818.

Gartner TK, Taylor DB (1990): *Thromb Res* 60:291–309.

Gartner TK, Taylor DB (1991): *Proc Soc Exp Biol Med* 198:649–655.

Gartner TK, Loudon R, Taylor DB (1991): *Biochem Biophys Res Commun* 180:1446–1452.

Ghiso J, Saball E, Leoni J, Rostagno A, Frangione B (1990): *Proc Natl Acad Sci USA* 87:1288–1291.

Gorcs TJ, Gottschall PE, Coy DH, Arimura A (1986): *Peptides (Orlando)* 7:1137–1145.

Hruby VJ, Sharma SD, Collins N, Matsunaga TO, Russel KC (1992): In: *Synthetic Peptides: A User's Guide*, Grant GA, ed., pp. 289–345. New York: Freeman.

Johnson HM, Torres BA (1988): *J Immunol* 141:2420–2423.

Jones MR, Bassett JM, Hoskinson RM, Wynn PC (1991): In: *16th Lorne Protein Conference, 1991* (abstract).

Kang C-Y, Brunck TK, Kieber-Emmons T, Blalock JE, Kohler H (1988): *Science* 240:1034–1036.

Knutson VP (1988): *J Biol Chem* 263:14146–14151.

McGuigan JE, Campbell-Thompson M (1992): *Gastroenterology* 103:749–758.

Misra PK, Hage W, Katti SB, Mathur KB, Raghubir R, Patnaik GK, Dhawan BN (1993): *Pharm Res (NY)* 10:660–661.

Mulchahey JJ, Neill JD, Dion LD, Bost KL, Blalock JE (1986): *Proc Natl Acad Sci USA* 83:9714–9718.

Nagy GM, Frawley LS (1991): Abstract #716, p 209, 73rd Annual Meeting of the Endocrine Society. The Endocrine Society Press.

Neri C, Ban E, Taragnat C, Caldani M, Haour F, Calas B, Martin PM (1991): *Pept Res* 4:26–31.

Nomizu M, Shiraishi N, Yamada Y, Roller PP (1991): In: *12th American Peptide Symposium*, June 16-21, 1991, Cambridge, Massachusetts, p. 502. ESCOM.

Palla E, Bensi G, Solito E, Buonamassa DT, Fassina G, Raugei G, Spano F, Galeotti M, Mora M, Domenighini M, Rossini M, Gallo E, Carinci V, Bugnoli M, Bertini F, Parente L, Melli M (1993): *J Biol Chem* 268:13486–13492.

Pascual DW, Blalock JE, Bost KL (1989): *J Immunol* 143:3697–3702.

Pascual DW, McBurnett RT, Blalock JE, Bost KL (1988): *FASEB J* 2:A1044, Abstr. 4345.

Posnett DN, Tam JP (1989): *Methods Enzymol* 178:739–746.

Pasqualini R, Chamone DF, Brentani RR (1989): *Biol Chem* 264:14566–14570.

Radding W, Hageman GR, Gantenberg NS, Bradley RJ, Liu Y, Kemp G (1992): *J Autonom Nerv System* 40:161–170.

Roller PP, M Nomizu, Snyder SW, Oroszian S, McMahon JB (1991): In: *12th American Peptide Symposium*, June 16-21, 1991, Cambridge, Massachusetts, p. 436. ESCOM.

Roller PP, Nomizu M, Snyder SW, Oroslan S, McMahon JB (1992): In: *Peptides 1991*, Schneider CH, Eberle AN, eds., pp 709–710. ESCOM.

Scapol L, Rappuoli P, Viscomi GC (1992): *J Chromatogr* 600:235–242.

Shahabi NA, Bost KL, Madhok TC, Sharp BM (1992): *J Pharmacol Exp Ther* 263:876–883.

Shai Y, Brunck TK, Chaiken IM (1989): *Biochemistry* 28:8804–8811.

Shai Y, Flashner M, Chaiken IM (1987): *Biochemistry* 26:669–675.

Sisto A (1993): In: *Peptides 1992*, Schneider CH, Eberle AN, eds., pp 747–748. ESCOM Science Publishers B.V.

Slootstra JW, Roubos EW (1991a): In: *Antisense Nucleic Acids and Proteins: Fundamentals and Applications*, van der Krol AR, Mol JNM, eds., pp. 205–228. New York: Dekker.

Slootstra JW, Roubos EW (1991b): *Biochem Biophys Res Commun* 179:266–271.

Smith LR, Bost KL, Blalock JE (1987): *J Immunol* 138:7–9.

Swords BH, Carr DJJ, Blalock JE, Berecek KH (1990): *Neuroendocrinology* 51:487–492.

Torres BA, Johnson HM (1990): *J Neuroimmunol* 27:191–199.

Weigent DA, Hoeprich PD, Bost KL, Brunck TK, Reiher WE III, Blalock JE (1986): *Biochem Biophys Res Commun* 139:367–374.

Whitaker JN, Sparks BE, Walker DP, Goodin R, Benveniste EN (1989): *J Neuroimmunol* 22:157–166.

Zamai M, Menziani MC, De Benedetti PG, Patrono C, Caiolfa VR (1992): *Med Chem Res* 2:208–216.

Zhou S-R, Whitaker JN (1990): *J Immunol* 145:2554–2560.

Zhou S-R, Whitaker JN (1992): *Clin Immunol Immunopathol* 63:74–83.

Zhou S-R, Whitaker JN (1993): *J Immunol* 150:1629–1642.

11

CONFORMATIONAL STUDIES ON MODEL PEPTIDES AND PEPTIDOMIMETICS

Shashidhar N. Rao, K. Ramnarayan, and V. N. Balaji

Introduction

Peptides are one of the most widely studied classes of compounds in the course of drug discovery. A number of endogenous peptides (e.g., endorphins and enkephalins) have been recognized as vital biological effectors such as hormones and neurotransmitters (Dutta, 1989). Short peptide segments (e.g., Arg-Gly-Asp) in large adhesion proteins such as fibrinogen, fibronectin, and vitronectin play a crucial role in mediating their interactions with the glycoprotein receptor complexes on the surfaces of activated platelets (Ruoslahti and Pierschbacher, 1986, 1987). The physiological receptors for many endogenous peptide ligands have been well characterized and employed in identifying potent synthetic peptides. However, peptide-based drugs suffer from the disadvantage of poor oral bioavailability (Fauchere, 1986) because they are subjected to metabolic degradation by proteolytic enzymes. Consequently, compounds that are very potent in vitro tend to exhibit a weaker effect in the physiological medium. Also, some of the metabolic products could be potentially toxic. In light of this, a variety of strategies to design peptidomimetics have evolved to provide enhanced metabolic stability without any loss of biological activity (Meek et al., 1990;

Peptides: Design, Synthesis, and Biological Activity
Channa Basava and G. M. Anantharamaiah, Editors
©1994 *Birkhäuser Boston*

Milner-White, 1989; Morgan and Gainor, 1990; Roberts et al., 1990). These strategies include chemical modification of peptide bonds susceptible to metabolism and synthesis of small organic molecules with functional groups essential for the biological activity of the peptide leads. Synthetic analogs of somatostatin and luteinizing hormone releasing hormone (LHRH) are examples in point of recently marketed drugs developed using such strategies (Freidinger, 1989).

Concurrent with experimental studies on peptidomimetics, recent years have seen a number of theoretical studies aimed toward the elucidation of their structures and understanding of their structure–activity relationships. The structures of unmodified peptides form an important key to such an understanding, because it is often necessary, in designing a peptidomimetic, to retain the three-dimensional attributes of the native peptide (Balaji and Ramnarayan, 1991). Since the proposal of the α-helix (Pauling et al., 1951), significant efforts have been devoted toward the analyses of structures and conformation of peptides, starting with the pioneering work of Ramachandran and co-workers (see Ramachandran and Sasisekharan, 1968). A number of reviews describing such studies have appeared in the literature (Krimm and Bandekar, 1986; Ramachandran and Sasisekharan, 1968; Scheraga, 1968).

The conformational profiles of various peptides have been studied using the methods of molecular mechanics, molecular dynamics, quantum mechanics, and Monte Carlo simulations (Jorgensen and Tirado-Rives, 1988; Ravishankar et al., 1986; Weiner et al., 1984). While major attention has been focussed on peptides with *trans* amides, theoretical investigations on the role of *cis* amide bonds in peptides have also been reported (Jorgensen and Gao, 1988; Nagarajaram et al., 1992; Ramakrishnan et al., 1985; Ramnarayan and Ramakrishnan, 1987). Conformational analyses in terms of the torsions $\phi(C-N-C^\alpha-C)$ and $\psi(N-C^\alpha-C-N)$ (Figure 11–1) have been typically reported with fixed bond lengths and bond angles (see Ramachandran and Sasisekharan, 1968; Scheraga, 1968). Similar methods have also been employed in studying model compounds with amino acid derivatives (e.g., 1-amino-1-carboxylic acid cyclopropane, ACC) (Crisma et al., 1989). The models obtained are, in general, qualitatively consistent with experimental data both in the solution phase [high-resolution nuclear magnetic resonance (NMR), IR, UV, Raman spectroscopy, etc.) and in the solid phase (x-ray crystallography). However, many of the experimental results are not completely rationalized by the existing theoretical models for the peptide structures. For example, some of the x-ray data on Aib (α-aminoisobutyric acid-) containing residues (Karle et al., 1988) cannot be satisfactorily accounted for by the earlier reported conformational energy calculations (Smith et al., 1981; Venkatarama Prasad and Sasisekharan, 1979). Also, the barriers to conformational transitions were predicted to be much higher than those observed experimentally.

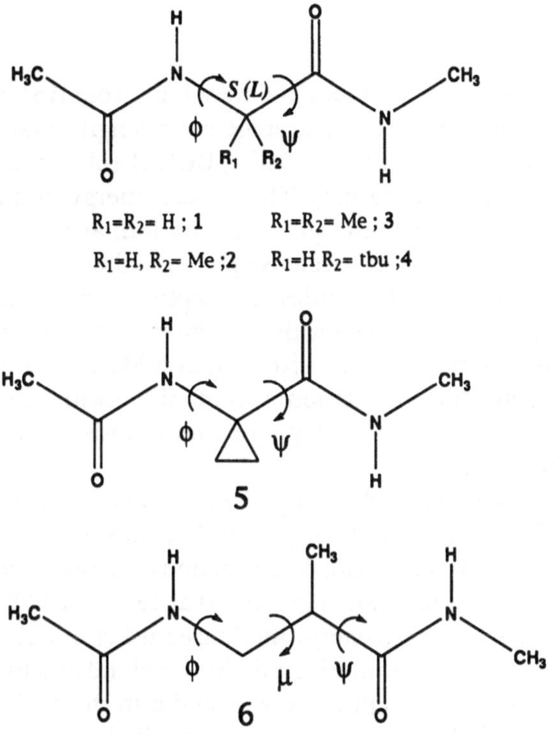

Figure 11-1. Schematic representation of model compounds **1** –**6** and definition of conformational parameters φ, ψ, and μ.

In this chapter, we revisit the conformational spaces of a few model peptides with a view to understand the impact of incorporating bond length and bond angle flexibility, observed in the x-ray crystal structure database of oligopeptides. The main goal of our investigations is to characterize the changes in the (φ, ψ) space in modified peptide systems with a view to deriving the structural basis for the design of peptidomimetics. Toward this goal, we specifically describe here our studies on (a) the refinement of the conformational maps for L-alanyl, glycyl, and Aib dipeptide systems using improved force field parameters, (b) the effect of bulk at the Cα atom through the conformational analyses of L-*tert*-butyl glycine and ACC-containing dipeptides, and (c) modifications to peptide structures by replacing an α-amino acid by a β-amino acid (specifically, α-methyl-β-alanine). These studies have been carried out using the methods of molecular mechanics. The salient features obtained in the models for the peptides and peptidomimetics are significantly improved over those reported previously and are in good qualitative agreement with the experimental data.

Methods

Preliminary models of compounds **1–5** were built from first principles using crystallographically observed average bond lengths and bond angles and the model building program MOL_BUILD (obtained courtesy of MOLARK, Encinitas, California). These were energy minimized using MM2IBM (Balaji et al., manuscript in preparation) at a dielectric of 4.0. This value of the dielectric has been used by a number of previous investigations of the structures of peptides and peptidomimetics and is important in deriving results consistent with experimental observations (Balaji et al., 1987). The program MM2IBM [version of MM2 force field (Allinger, 1977) ported to an IBM workstation] was modified with dihedral drivers and parameters to provide geometry of peptides consistent with their x-ray structure analyses.

   Conformations of the model compounds **1–5** were generated as a function of $\phi(C\text{-}N\text{-}C^{\alpha}\text{-}C)$ and $\psi(N\text{-}C^{\alpha}\text{-}C\text{-}N)$ at 10° intervals. In the case of **6**, the pseudopeptide with β-amino acid, conformations were generated as a function of the torsions ϕ and μ, while keeping ψ at 180° and 300°. The collections of conformations were energy minimized using MM2IBM (Balaji et al., manuscript in preparation) with a dielectric of 4.0 and by allowing all the degrees of freedom except ϕ and ψ (ϕ and μ in the case of **6**). A constraint weight of 1000 kcal/mole/degree was applied to these torsions during the minimizations.

   Isoenergy contours were then drawn in the ϕ–ψ space at 1-kcal/mole intervals using CONFS (MOLARK) executing on a network of hardware platforms. Contour thickness decreases as its value relative to the global minimum increases. Contours with values to 5 kcal/mole relative to the global minimum are shown (Figure 11–1). High-energy conformational spaces (characterized by energies >6 kcal/mole relative to the global minimum) are shown either by blocked areas or hatched lines. The global minimum is marked "1", while the secondary minima are marked "2", "3", etc. The positions and energies of the minima in each of the plots are tabulated. The structures corresponding to the minima are called M1_1, M2_1, etc., with suffixes indicating the molecule number (see Figure 11–1). The percentages of the conformational space enclosed by the 1- to 5-kcal/mole contours are also listed.

Results

α-Amino Acid Dipeptides (Gly, L-Ala, Aib, and L-tert-Butyl-Gly)

The conformational energy plot for glycyl dipeptide **1** in the ϕ–ψ space is shown in Figure 11–2. This plot has a near-inversion symmetry about

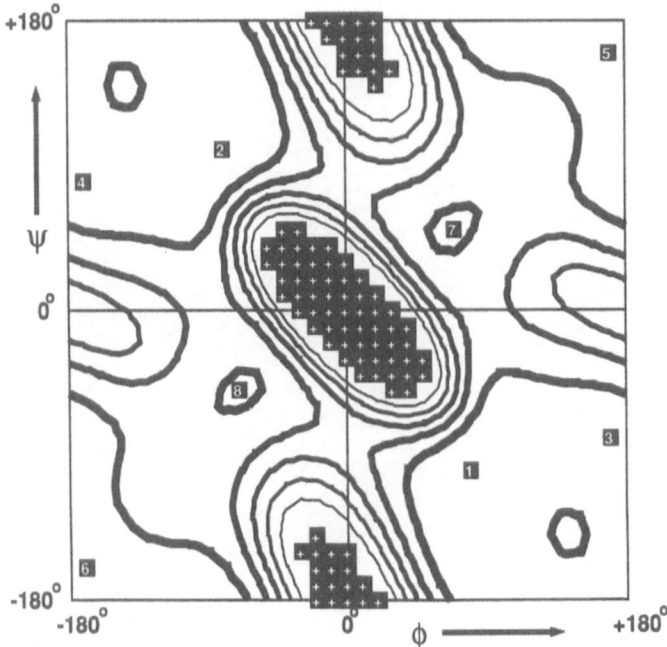

Figure 11-2. Energy plot for **1** in (ϕ,ψ) space (minima in Table 11-1).

(ϕ,ψ) = (0°,0°). The global minimum is seen at the (ϕ,ψ) combination of (80°, −100°), which corresponds to the 2_7 helical structure or the γ-turn. The symmetrically situated secondary minimum M2 at (ϕ,ψ) = (−80°, 100°) has almost the same energy value as M1 (0.03 kcal/mole). Six other minima were observed (Table 11-1), including those corresponding to left-and right-handed α-helices (M7 and M8). All eight minima lie within 1 kcal/mole of M1, consistent with the significant conformational flexibility afforded by glycine. The barriers to transition between the global minima (M1 and M2) via either the left- or right-handed α-helical regions are about 2.25 kcal/mole. The corresponding barrier between M1 and M8 is about 1.7 kcal/mole. The 3-kcal/mole contour encloses nearly 77% of the total conformational space (Table 11-2).

A methyl group in L-alanyl dipeptide **2** introduces conformational restrictions (Figure 11-3) as compared to **1** as revealed by the reduction in the percentages of the conformational spaces enclosed by isoenergy contours to 5 kcal/mole (see Table 11-2). The global minimum corresponds to a threefold helical structure, while the minimum in the α-helical region is a secondary minimum, destabilized by 0.75 kcal/mole relative to M1. The left-handed α-helical region is further destabilized (by 1.13 kcal/mole

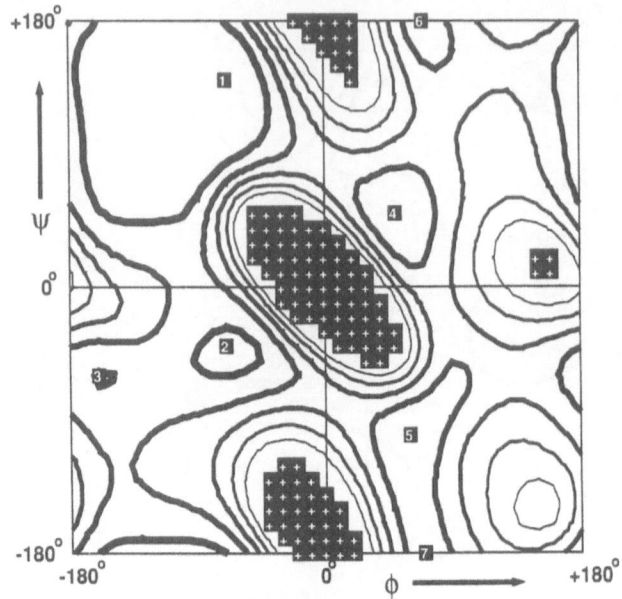

Figure 11-3. Energy plot for **2** in (ϕ,ψ) space (minima in Table 11-3).

Table 11-1. Energy Minima of 1 in the Conformational Space (ϕ, Ψ)

Minimum Number	ϕ	Ψ	Relative Energy	Map Mark
1	80.0	-100.0	0.00	1
2	-80.0	100.0	0.03	2
3	170.0	-80.0	0.62	3
4	-170.0	80.0	0.62	4
5	170.0	160.0	0.76	5
6	-170.0	-160.0	0.76	6
7	70.0	50.0	0.88	7
8	-70.0	-50.0	0.91	8

Table 11-2. Percentages of the Total Conformational Space Enclosed by Isoenergy Contours (1–5 kcal/mole) for Compounds 1–6

Countour Level (kcal/mole)	1 Fig. 2	2 Fig. 3	3 Fig. 4	4 Fig. 5	5 Fig. 6	6 Fig. 7a ($\mu = 60$)	6 Fig. 7b ($\mu = 180$)
1	31	12	5	4	5	5	5
2	63	33	24	10	20	21	18
3	77	59	54	17	39	36	31
4	85	75	77	25	54	52	42
5	88	84	87	34	71	66	55

Table 11-3. Energy Minima of 2 in the Conformational Space (ϕ, Ψ)

Minimum Number	ϕ	Ψ	Relative Energy	Map Mark
1	-70.0	140.0	0.00	1
2	-70.0	-40.0	0.75	2
3	-160.0	-60.0	0.95	3
4	50.0	50.0	1.13	4
5	60.0	-100.0	1.19	5
6	70.0	180.0	1.51	6,7

relative to M1). Two other minima occur in the lower right-hand quadrant; these are destabilized by 1.2 and 1.5 kcal/mole, respectively, relative to the global minimum (Table 11-3). The barriers to conformational transitions between M1 and M2 are about 1.8 kcal/mole and those between M1 and M4 about 2.5 kcal/mole. The barriers between the minima in the α-helical region and M5 are at least 2.6 kcal/mole.

Further conformational restriction is seen for **3**, containing the Aib residue (Figure 11-4). The global minima correspond to the centers of the left- and right-handed α-helical regions. However, a larger number of secondary minima, all within 2 kcal/mole of M1, are seen (Table 11-4). By contrast with the case of L-alanyl dipeptide, the (ϕ,ψ) plot of **3** shows a minimum in the lower right-hand quadrant, destabilized relative to M1 by less than 0.5 kcal/mole. The barriers to transitions between the α-helical region and the β-region are about 2.3 kcal/mole.

The (ϕ,ψ) plot of L-*tert*-butyl glycyl dipeptide, **4**, shows global minima in the β-sheet and collagen-like regions (Figure 11-5). The right- and left-handed α-helical regions are destabilized by 0.92 and 2.57 kcal/mole, respectively, relative to the global minima. The lower right-hand quadrant minima (M5 and M6) are destabilized by nearly 4 kcal/mole. The barriers to transitions between the right- and left-handed α-helical region and the β-region are about 2.8 and 3.8 kcal/mole, respectively (Table 11-5).

1-Amino-1-Carboxylic Acid Cyclopropane (ACC) Dipeptide, 5

In the conformational energy plot for **5**, the global minimum occurs at (ϕ,ψ) = (-80°,100°) with M2 (destabilized by <0.1 kcal/mole) occurring at (80°,-100°) (Figure 11-6). In addition, four local minima, two of which are within 1.2 kcal/mole of M1, are found (Table 11-6). A number of conformations with either of the two torsions near 0° have an energy of at least 10 kcal/mole above the global minimum. The barriers to transition between the global minimum and local minima are about 2 kcal/mole via pathways excluding (ϕ,ψ) = (0°,0°). Because the positions of M1 and M2 are related by inversion symmetry, the conformational transitions between these two

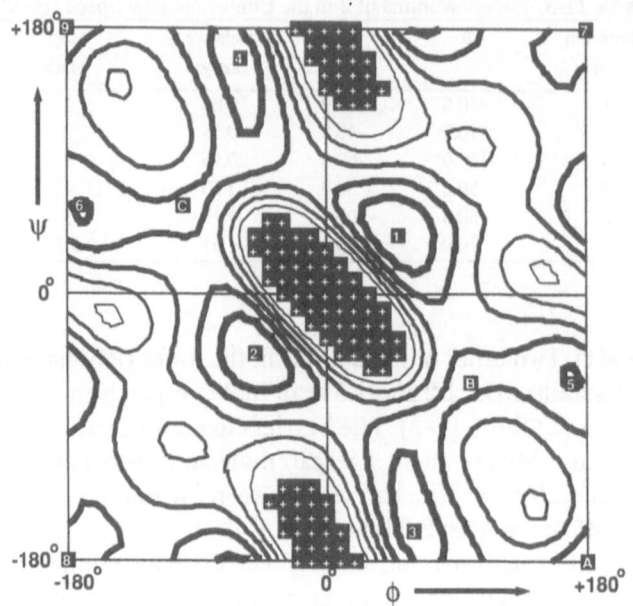

Figure 11–4. Energy plot for **3** in (ϕ,ψ) space (minima in Table 11–4).

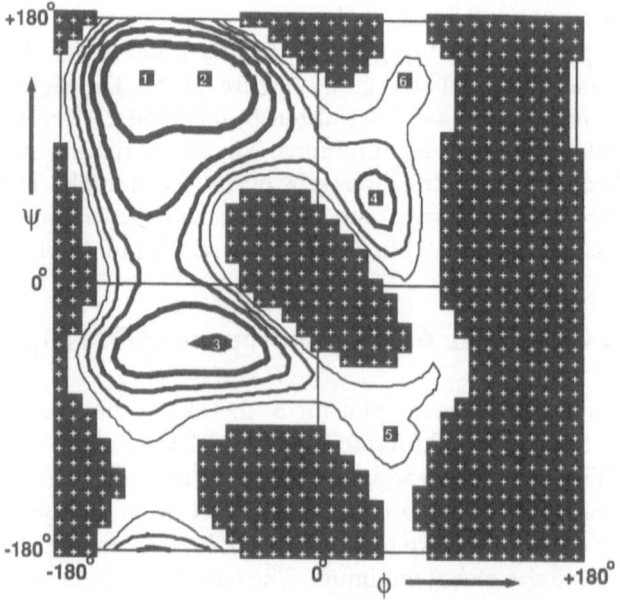

Figure 11–5. Energy plot for **4** in (ϕ,ψ) space (minima in Table 11–5).

Table 11-4. Energy Minima of 3 in the Conformational Space (ϕ, Ψ)

Minimum Number	ϕ	Ψ	Relative Energy	Map Mark
1	50.0	40.0	0.00	1
2	-50.0	-40.0	0.01	2
3	60.0	-160.0	0.48	3
4	-60.0	160.0	0.48	4
5	170.0	-60.0	0.91	5
6	-170.0	60.0	0.91	6
7	180.0	180.0	1.38	7,8,9,A
8	100.0	-60.0	1.73	B
9	-100.0	60.0	1.75	C

minima take place in pathways that necessarily include structures similar to the α-helix, the 3_{10} helix, and those structures related to them. Nearly 71% of the conformational space is enclosed by the 5-kcal/mole contour (see Table 11-2).

α-Methyl-β-Alanine, 6

A complete conformational analysis of **6** as a function of ϕ, μ, and ψ shows that ψ is mainly confined to about $-60°$ and $180°$. Thus, the conformational energy calculations on **6** were carried out as a function of ϕ and μ while keeping ψ about $-60°$ and $180°$ (Figures 11-7A and 11-7B, respectively). In Figure 11-7A, the global minimum occurs at $\phi = 100$ and $\mu = -60°$. The plot shows an almost mirror symmetry about the $\phi = 0°$ and $\mu = 0°$ lines. Five other minima (Table 11-7A) have values relative to the global minimum that lie within 1 kcal/mole. The transition to barriers between various minima is significantly higher (~6 kcal/mole) via the $\phi = 0°$ pathway than via the $\phi = 180°$ pathway (~1-3 kcal/mole). In Figure 11-7B, the global minimum occurs at $\phi = -110°$ and $\mu = -60°$, while eight other minima are found within 2.6 kcal/mole of the global minimum (Table 11-7B). The barrier to transition between M1_6 and M2_6 is about 6 kcal/mole via the $\phi = 0°$ and $\phi = 180°$ pathways, with a barrier of more than 10 kcal/mole for any path involving $\phi = 0°$.

Table 11-5. Energy Minima of 4 in the Conformational Space (ϕ, Ψ)

Minimum Number	ϕ	Ψ	Relative Energy	Map Mark
1	-120.0	140.0	0.00	1
2	-80.0	140.0	0.01	2
3	-70.0	-40.0	0.92	3
4	40.0	60.0	2.57	4
5	50.0	-100.0	3.94	5
6	60.0	140.0	4.60	6

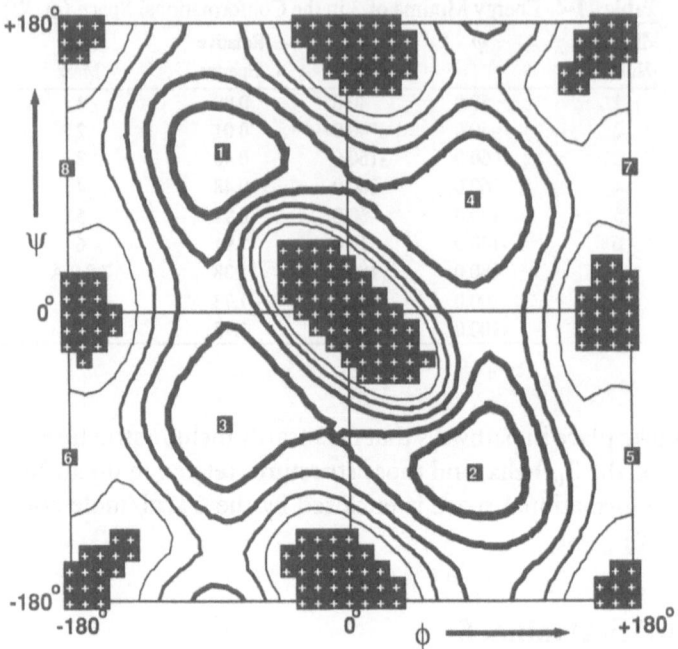

Figure 11-6. Energy plot for 5 in (ϕ,ψ) space (minima in Table 11-6).

Discussion

Conformational energy calculations on dipeptides of glycine, L-alanine, and Aib are generally consistent with those reported in the literature reviewed here (see following). However, our energy plots do differ in some of the details from those previously reported. The right-handed α-helical conformation is a secondary minimum for L-Ala dipeptide destabilized by less than 1 kcal/mole relative to the global minimum, which lies in the β-region (see Table 11-7). In the latter region, the 1-kcal/mole contour covers a large number of commonly observed structural motifs such as extended β-strand, β-pleated sheet, collagen conformation, β-turn, γ-turn, and threefold and fourfold helical conformations. The counterpart to this region in the lower right-hand quadrant is relatively restricted with the local minima being at least 1.2 kcal/mole greater than the global minimum. The left-handed α-helical conformation is destabilized relative to the right-handed α-helical conformation by about 0.4 kcal/mole. Although this difference is not large, it is qualitatively consistent with the commonly observed right-handed α-helices in the structures of proteins and oligopeptides as seen by x-ray crystallography.

Table 11-6. Energy Minima of 5 in the Conformal Space (ϕ, Ψ)

Minimum Number	ϕ	Ψ	Relative Energy	Map Mark
1	-80.0	100.0	0.00	1
2	80.0	-100.0	0.08	2
3	-80.0	-70.0	1.10	3
4	80.0	70.0	1.12	4
5	180.0	-90.0	4.03	5,6
6	180.0	90.0	4.11	7,8

The conformational energy profile of the Aib dipeptide, **3**, is quite interesting and differs from that reported earlier (Smith et al., 1981; Venkataram Prasad and Sasisekharan, 1979) in a number of ways. While the plot in Figure 11-4 is symmetrical, as is to be expected, in addition to the global minima in the a-helical region, in the lower right-hand and upper left-hand quadrants there are low-energy minima (destabilized by less than 0.5 kcal/mole) that correspond to left- and right-handed polyproline structures (Balaji, 1981; Sasisekharan and Balaji, 1979). Earlier calculations had predicted these conformations to be energetically destabilized by more than 2 kcal/mole relative to the α-helical conformation. Thus, our calculations better account for the x-ray crystal structure occurrence of the (ϕ, ψ) ~ (-50°, 131°) (Karle et al., 1988) because this point lies within 1 kcal/mole of the global minimum. Further, the number of secondary minima obtained for **3** are larger than those obtained earlier.

To the best of our knowledge, no previous studies have been reported on the conformational analyses of L-*tert*-butyl-glycyl dipeptide. Based on the accessible conformational space in its (ϕ,ψ) plot, it is clear that **4** can be accommodated in a variety of conformations in the β-region including three-fold, fourfold, PPI, and PPII structures (Balaji, 1981; Sasisekharan and Balaji, 1979). The right-handed α-helical conformation is not as favored energetically as the low-energy structures in the β-region, while the left-handed α-helical conformation is energetically expensive. In this light, L-*tert*-butyl-glycine can be employed to force a conformation in the β-region of the (ϕ,ψ) space.

The global minimum of **5** corresponds to a left-handed γ-turn, consistent with the results of earlier studies on a model compound with ACC (Crisma et al., 1989; Varughese et al., 1985). Our calculations have been carried out incorporating full conformational flexibility, while the earlier ones used fixed bond lengths and bond angles. This difference reflects on the barriers to conformational transitions between various minima. In our studies, transitions are feasible between various minima with barriers of about 1–3 kcal/mole in contrast to more than 20 kcal/mole as reported earlier (Crisma et al., 1989). Further, the previous calculations did not find minima in the lower left and upper right quadrants of the plot as we have

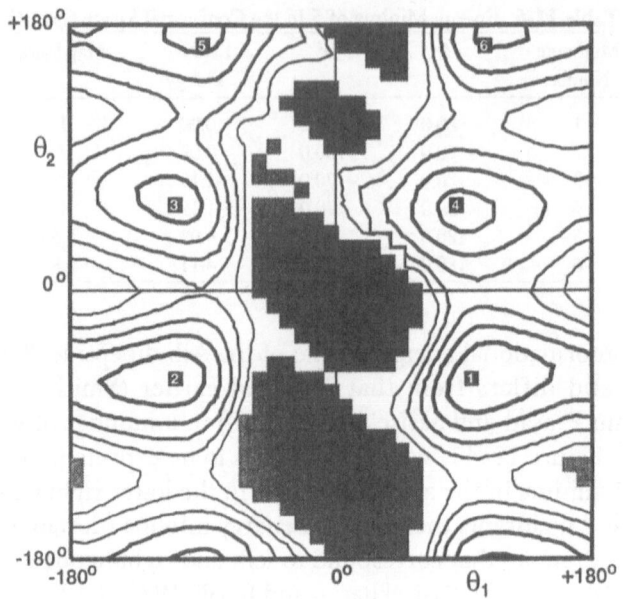

Figure 11–7A. Energy plot for **6** in (φ,μ) space (minima in Table 11–7) at ψ = –60°.

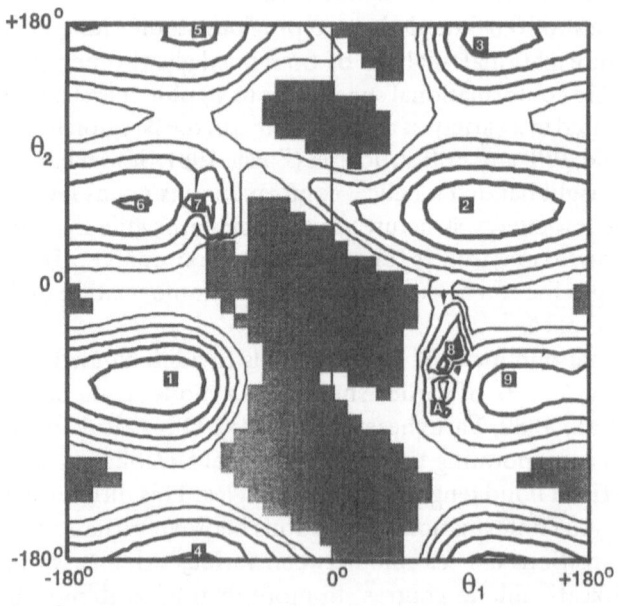

Figure 11–7B. Energy plot for **6** in (φ,μ) space (minima in Table 11–7) at ψ = 180°.

Table 11-7A. Energy Minima of 6 in the Conformational Space (ϕ, μ) at $\Psi \sim -60°$.

The Global Minimum (minimum #1) Energy is 0.32 kcal/mole

Minimum Number	ϕ	μ	Relative Energy	Map Mark
1	100.0	-60.0	0.00	1
2	-110.0	-60.0	0.37	2
3	-110.0	60.0	0.53	3
4	90.0	60.0	0.67	4
5	-90.0	170.0	0.72	5
6	110.0	170.0	0.80	6

done. The left- and right-handed α-helical structures are destabilized by less than 2 kcal/mole relative to the global minimum, instead of 5 kcal/mole as was reported earlier (Crisma et al., 1989); Varughese et al., 1985).

Our results on 5 are also in qualitative agreement with the solution-phase studies (IR and proton NMR) on oligomers of ACC. The IR data on model compounds were interpreted in terms of intramolecular hydrogen bonds, while the NMR spectra studied at varying concentrations predicted structures amenable to both inter- and intramolecular hydrogen bonds (Crisma et al., 1989).

How do the results of our investigations compare with the x-ray crystal-lographic analyses of ACC-containing compounds? In the energy-refined models of 5, the bond angle $\tau(N-C^{\alpha}-C)$ is considerably larger (~123°) compared to the standard value of 110° in a normal peptide because of the strain introduced by the cyclopropyl ring at C^{α}. This value is comparable to the average of 121.7° in the crystal structures of ACC-containing compounds (Valle et al., 1989) where it varies from 116° to 124°. The torsion angles reported for ACC residues in single crystals lie within the conformational space enclosed by the 4-kcal/mole contour seen in Figure 11–5. It is inter-

Table 11-7B. Energy Minima of 6 in the Conformational Space (ϕ, μ) at $\Psi \sim 180°$.

The Global Minimum (minimum #1) Energy is 0.3 kcal/mole

Minimum Number	ϕ	μ	Relative Energy	Map Mark
1	-110.0	-60.0	0.00	1
2	100.0	60.0	0.15	2
3	110.0	170.0	0.54	3
4	-90.0	180.0	0.78	4,5
5	-130.0	60.0	0.90	6
6	-90.0	60.0	0.99	7
7	90.0	-40.0	1.24	8
8	130.0	-60.0	1.36	9
9	80.0	-80.0	2.59	A

esting that our investigations do find some crystal conformations with ψ values around $0°$ in the energetically favorable domains. On the other hand, previous studies predicted such conformations be destabilized by more than 20 kcal/mole. This emphasizes the significance of bond length and bond flexibility taken into account in our calculations.

The energy-refined models of 6 are characterized by the lack of intramolecular hydrogen bonding interactions. Only M2_6 has the N-terminal N–H hydrogen located at about 2.3 Å from the C-terminal C = O oxygen. The corresponding distance is larger in the other energy minima. This observation is qualitatively consistent with the destabilizing effect of β-alanine as seen from comparative IR studies (Aubry and Marraud, 1989; Aubry et al., 1988) on t-Bu-CO-L-Pro-Gly-NHMe and t-Bu-CO-L-Pro-β-Ala-NHMe. The energy-refined models do not favor a βII structure for either of the two compounds studied because the hydrogen bonding interactions needed to create it would lead to excessive (>25 kcal/mole) bond angle strain energies.

The calculated low-energy minima of 6 are consistent with the x-ray crystal structure data of compounds with β-alanine. Most of the conformations of β-alanine in cyclic and linear peptides (Benedetti et al., 1985; Karle et al., 1975; Itoh et al., 1977; Springer et al., 1984) lie within 2 kcal/mole of the global minimum (see Figure 11–7 and Tables 11-7A and 11–7B). Recently reported crystal structures of two cyclic peptides with β-alanine (Di Blasio et al., 1991; Pavone et al., 1990) have conformations ($\phi \sim 170°$ and $\psi \sim 100°$) not found as unique energy minima in our analyses. However, these conformations have an energy of less than 3 kcal/mole relative to the global minimum of 6. The qualitative closeness between the crystallographic data and the results of our calculations is encouraging in light of the fact that our calculations have been done without including crystal packing forces and with a simplistic treatment of electrostatic effects.

Conclusions

Molecular mechanics calculations on six model peptide compounds have been presented. The salient features obtained in our studies are generally consistent with those reported previously. However, our investigations, carried out with an improved force field and by incorporating bond length and bond angle flexibility, show better consistency with the x-ray crystal structures. The effect of steric bulk on the substituent, as in L-$tert$-butyl glycine, is not only to restrict the overall conformational space but to destabilize the left-handed helical conformation more significantly than in either glycine, L-alanine, or Aib. The effect of bond angle widening, as in the ACC-containing model compound, is clearly seen in the stabilization of the γ-turn (2_7) structure as the global minimum, with energetic feasibilities for other standard structures such as α- and 3_{10} helices. The energetically favorable conformations of β-amino-acid-containing compounds clearly exclude β- and γ-turns. The essential features in these model compounds could form the basis of design of peptidomimetics with desired secondary structure characteristics.

Acknowledgements

We thank ImmunoPharmaceutics Inc. and Searle Research and Development (Drug Design) for the computational and graphics facilities.

REFERENCES

Allinger NL (1977): *J Am Chem Soc* 99:8127–8134.

Aubry A, Marraud M (1989): *Biopolymers* 28:109–122.

Aubry A, Boussard G, Cung MT, Marraud M, Bitoux B (1988): *J Chim Phys Phys-Chim Biol* 85:345-359.

Balaji VN (1981): *Int J Quant Chem* 20:347.

Balaji VN, Ramnarayan K (1991): In: *Biologically Active Peptides: Design, Synthesis and Utilization*, Vol. 1, Williams WV, Weiner DB, eds., pp. 35–54. Basel: Technomic Publishing.

Balaji VN, Profeta S, Jr., Dietrich SW (1987): *Biochem Biophy Res Commun* 28:109–122.

Benedetti E, Bavoso A, Di Blasio B, Grimaldi P, Pavone V, Pedone C, Toniolo C, Bonora GM (1985): *Int J Biol Macromol* 7:81–88.

Crisma M, Bonora GM, Toniolo C, Barone V, Benedetti E, Blasio V, Pavone BD, Pedone C, Santini A, Fraternali F, Bavoso A, Lelj F (1989): *Int J Biol Macromol* 11:345-352.

Di Blasio BA, Lomardi A, Yang X, Pedone C, Pavone V (1991): *Biopolymers* 31:1181–1188.

Dutta AS (1989): *Chem Br* 10:159–162.

Fauchere JL (1986): *Adv Drug Res* 15:29–69.

Freidinger RM (1989): *Trends Pharm Sci* 10:270–274.

Itoh H, Yamane T, Ahida T, Kakudo M (1977): *Acta Crystallogr Sect B Struct Crystallogr Cryst Chem* 33:2959-2961.

Jorgensen WL, Gao J (1988): *J Am Chem Soc* 110:4212–4216.

Jorgensen WL, Tirado-Rives J (1988): *J Am Chem Soc* 110:1657–1666.

Karle I, Handa BK, Hassall CH (1975): *Acta Crystallogr Sect B Struct Crystallogr Cryst Chem* 31:555–560.

Karle IL, Kishore R, Raghothama S, Balaram P (1988): *J Am Chem Soc* 110:1958.

Krimm S, Bandekar J (1968): *Adv Protein Chem* 38:181–364.

Meek RD, Lambert DM, Dreyer GB, Carr TJ, Tomaszek A, Moore AL, Strickler JE, Debouck C, Hyland LJ, Matthews TJ, Metcalf BW, Petteway SR (1990): *Nature (London)* 343:90–92.

Milner-White EJ (1989): *Trends Pharm Sci* 10:70–73.

Morgan BA, Gainor JA (1990): *Annu Rep Med Chem* 224:243–252.

Nagarajaram HA, Paul PKC, Ramnarayan K, Soman KV, Ramakrishnan C (1992):

Int J Pept Protein Res 40:383–394.

Pauling L, Corey RB, Branson HR (1951): *Proc Natl Acad Sci USA* 37:205–211.

Pavone V, Lombardi A, Yang X, Pedone C, Di Blasio B (1990): *Biopolymers* 30:189–196.

Ramachandran GN, Sasisekharan V (1968): *Adv Protein Chem* 23:283–437.

Ramakrishnan C, Paul PKC, Ramnarayan K (1985): *Proc Int Symp Biomol Struct Interact Suppl J Biosci* 8:239–251.

Ramnarayan K, Ramakrishnan C (1987): *J Biosci* 12:331–347.

Ravishankar G, Mezei M, Beveridge DL (1986): *J Comp Chem* 7:345–348.

Roberts NA, Martin JA, Kinchington D, Broadhurst AV, Craig JC, Duncan IB, Galpin SA, Handa BK, Kay J, Kroehn A, Lambert RW, Merrett JH, Mills JS, Parkes KEB, Redshaw S, Ritchie AJ, Taylor DL, Thomas GJ, Machin PJ (1990): *Science* 248:358–361.

Ruoslahti E, Pierschbacher MD (1987): *Cell* 44:517–518.

Sasisekharan V, Balaji VN (1979): *Macromolecules* 12:28.

Scheraga HA (1968): *Adv Phys Org Chem* 6:103–184.

Smith GD, Pletnev VZ, Duax WL, Balasubramanian TM, Bosshard HE, Czerwinski EW, Kendrick NE, Mathew FS, Marshall GR (1981): *J Am Chem Soc* 103:1493–1501.

Springer JP, Cole RJ, Dorner JW, Cox RH, Richard JL, Barnes CL, van der Helm D (1984): *J Am Chem Soc* 106:2388–2392.

Valle G, Crisma M, Toniolo C, Holt EM, Tamura M, Bland J, Stammer CH (1989): *Int J Pept Protein Res* 34:56–65.

Varughese KI, Srinivasan AR, Stammer CH (1985): *Int J Pept Protein Res* 26:242–251.

Venkataram Prasad BV, Sasisekharan V (1979): *Curr Sci* 48:517–519.

Weiner SJ, Singh UC, O'Donnell TJ, Kollman PA (1984): *J Am Chem Soc* 106:6243–6245.

III

STUDIES OF PEPTIDE HORMONES

12

THE DESIGN AND SYNTHESIS OF LONG-ACTING OXYTOCIN ANTAGONISTS SUBSTITUTED IN POSITIONS 2, 7, AND 8

Victor J. Hruby, W. Y. Chan, Todd W. Rockway,
Jan Hlavacek, and James Ormberg

Introduction

The design of oxytocin antagonists (for reviews, see Hruby and Mosberg, 1982; Hruby and Smith, 1987; Hruby et al., 1990; Lebl, 1987; Manning and Sawyer, 1989; Sawyer and Manning, 1985) has increasingly involved a search for structural changes that would enhance both in vivo potency and increase duration of action. The discovery of Shulz and du Vigneaud (1966, 1967) and Jost et al. (1961) that substituting more bulky amino acids in either position 1 (penicillamine) or position 2 (O-methyltyrosine) produced oxytocin antagonists has led to numerous further investigations into the structural and conformational requirements important for antagonism at the uterine oxytocin receptor (Hruby, 1985; Hruby et al., 1990; Manning and Sawyer, 1989; Meraldi et al., 1975, 1977). Since these pioneering studies, many important, more potent antagonists have been reported, particularly by the groups of Manning et al., Melin et al., Lebl et al., and Hruby et al. (Hruby and Smith, 1987; Lebl, 1987; Manning and Sawyer, 1985) primarily by incorporating appropriate amino acid substitutions into positions 1, 2, 4, 7, and 8, including linear analogs (Manning et al., 1987). Two new

Peptides: Design, Synthesis, and Biological Activity
Channa Basava and G. M. Anantharamaiah, Editors
©1994 *Birkhäuser Boston*

classes of oxytocin antagonists have been introduced: (1) bicyclic analogs involving bridges between the 1–6 and 4–8 residues (Hill et al., 1988, 1990; Smith et al., 1992); and (2) nonpeptide oxytocin antagonists derived from fermentation broths (Bock et al. 1990; Evans et al., 1992; Williams et al., 1992). Despite all these efforts, there is still much to be done in elucidation of a true pharmacophore for antagonist activity at the oxytocic receptor.

Many of the peptide and nonpeptide analogs exhibited only modest in vivo antagonism. The design of more potent oxytocin antagonists incorporating multiple substitutions, most notably in positions 1 and 2, has produced more efficacious in vivo oxytocin antagonists (Manning et al., 1989). To understand the conformational requirements for potent in vivo oxytocin antagonist activity, Hruby proposed the dynamic model for oxytocin antagonists (Hruby and Mosberg, 1981; Meraldi et al., 1977), which suggests that different peptide conformations are required by receptors for agonists and antagonists (Hruby, 1985, and references therein). Thus, oxytocin antagonists that show restricted rotation of the tyrosine-2 side chain by the neighboring β-methyl groups of penicillamine-1 must adopt a different conformation that prevents the tyrosine-2 side chain from assuming an orientation over the 20-membered disulfide-containing ring, as was proposed for oxytocin agonists in the cooperative model of Walter (1977).

The knowledge obtained from conformational studies of oxytocin antagonists has led to the design of potent oxytocin antagonists incorporating amino acid substitutions in positions 1, 2, and 4; most notably, the highly potent oxytocin antagonist [Pen^1,Phe^2,Thr^4]oxytocin (Hruby et al., 1980). The results obtained from a conformational study of the aforementioned highly potent oxytocin antagonist, [Pen^1,Phe^2,Thr^4]oxytocin (Mosberg et al., 1981), led us to design oxytocin antagonists incorporating amino acid substitutions in positions 2, 7, and 8. We have reported (Chan et al., 1986, 1987) pharmacological studies of oxytocin antagonists substituted in positions 2, 4, 7, and 8 that exhibited similar potency to [Pen^1,Phe^2,Thr^4]oxytocin but showed a marked increase in duration of action. We wish to report here the synthesis and pharmacological studies of these long-acting oxytocin antagonists. The biological results obtained for the analogs described in this chapter have extended our knowledge of the structural and conformational features of oxytocin antagonists required for high potency and extended duration of action.

Results

The protected oxytocin peptide analogs were prepared according to standard solid-phase peptide synthetic methodology, using a semiautomated peptide synthesizer and methods previously reported from this laboratory (Upson and Hruby, 1976). N$^\alpha$-t-Boc-glycine was esterified to chloromethylated Merrifield resin according to the procedure of Gysin (1973), and the growing peptide chain was assembled from the carboxyl terminus using the protocol described later in this chapter. Glutamine and asparagine were coupled as their para-nitrophenyl esters employing the protocol described under **Experimental**. The protected peptides were removed from the solid support by stirring the peptide resin with a saturated ammonia/methanol solution for 4 days at room temperature, followed by extraction of the protected peptide carboxamide from the resin with N,N-dimethylformamide (DMF). The protected peptide carboxamides were deprotected in liquid ammonia with sodium metal and cyclized for 60 min with potassium ferricyanide in 0.1% aqueous acetic acid adjusted to pH 8.3 with 1 N aqueous ammonia. The crude peptides were first purified by partition chromatography on Sephadex G-25 block polymerizate using n-BuOH-HOAc-H$_2$0 (4:1:5, upper phase) followed by gel filtration on Sephadex G-25 with 0.2 N HOAc (and in some cases reversed-phase HPLC). The physicochemical properties and amino acid sequences of each oxytocin antagonist analog described in this work are listed in Table 12–1.

The synthesis of the O-alkylated tyrosine derivatives was performed according to the procedure described by Kolodziejczyk and Manning (1981). The synthesis of the para-alkylated phenylalanine derivatives was accomplished using classic techniques described by Snyder et al. (1945). The N^α-t-Boc-protected para-alkylated phenylalanine derivatives were incorporated into the peptides as racemates. The pure peptide diastereomers were separated from either partition chromatography or reversed-phase HPLC, and

Table 12-1. Amino Acid Sequence and Physichochemical Properties of Oxytocin Antagonist Analogs

Analog	Amino Acid Sequence	Yield (%)	HPLC,κ'^a	$[\alpha]^{23}546$
1	Pen-Tyr(OMe)-Ile-Thr-Asn-Cys-Pro-Orn-Gly-NH$_2$	31	7.5[b]	+95.1
2	Pen-Tyr(OEt)-Ile-Thr-Asn-Cys-Pro-Orn-Gly-NH$_2$	28	5.0[b]	+37.8
3	Pen-Phe(Me)-Ile-Thr-Asn-Cys-Pro-Orn-Gly-NH$_2$	15	5.0[c]	+52.4
4	Pen-D-Phe(Me)-Ile-Thr-Asn-Cys-Pro-Orn-Gly-NH$_2$	15	6.0[c]	-42.5
5	Pen-Phe(Et)-Ile-Thr-Asn-Cys-Pro-Orn-Gly-NH$_2$	14	6.0[c]	+81.9
6	Pen-D-Phe(Et)-Ile-Thr-Asn-Cys-Pro-Orn-Gly-NH$_2$	14	8.5[c]	-60.5
7	Pen-Tyr-Ile-Gln-Asn-Cys-Pro-Orn-Gly-NH$_2$	20	4.8[c]	N.D.[d]
8	Pen-Phe-Ile-Thr-Asn-Cys-$\Delta^{3,4}$Pro-Leu-Gly-NH$_2$	25	12.7[c]	-29.6
9	Pen-Phe-Ile-Thr-Asn-Cys-$\Delta^{3,4}$Pro-Orn-Gly-NH$_2$	20	6.0[c]	N.D.[d]
10	Pen-Tyr-Ile-Gln-Asn-Cys-$\Delta^{3,4}$Pro-Leu-Gly-NH$_2$	25	5.7[c]	-36.0
11	Pen-Tyr-Ile-Thr-Asn-Cys-$\Delta^{3,4}$Pro-Leu-Gly-NH$_2$	25	7.2[c]	-70.1
12	Pen-D-Tyr(OEt)-Ile-Thr-Asn-Cys-Pro-Orn-Gly-NH$_2$	14	5.5[c]	+44.2

[a] $\kappa' = \dfrac{retention\ time - solvent\ front\ time}{solvent\ front\ time}$.

[b] 0.05 M Triethyl ammonium acetate, pH 4; acetonitrile, isocratic; Flow: 2 ml/min.

[c] 0.1% TFA/acetonitrile; linear gradient, 30 min; 20% B → 35% B==20%B; Flow: 2 ml/min.

[d] N.D., Not determined.

the stereochemical integrity of each peptide diastereomer was confirmed by enzymatic digestion of the final peptide product. The preparation of dehydroproline ($\Delta^{3,4}$ Pro) was accomplished utilizing a procedure described by Robertson and Witkop (1962).

The in vitro antagonist potencies and duration of action for analogs **1** to **12** are shown in Table 12-2. The six analogs, **1–6** in Table 12-2, which contain either *O*-alkyl-tyrosine or *p*-alkyl-phenylalanine, exhibit good in vitro anti-oxytocin activity. One of the striking features of these analogs is the effect of alkyl group size on the observed oxytocin antagonism. Notice that either methyl group substitution on the tyrosine hydroxyl or its substitution on the para position of phenylalanine provides antagonist analogs with high potency. Alternatively, increasing the size of the alkyl group for either amino acid to *O*-ethyl or to ethyl provides analogs with an approximately 100-fold decrease in antagonist potency.

The importance of stereochemistry of the *O*-ethyl-tyrosine and *p*-alkyl-phenylalanine derivatives in position **2** was investigated. Here again, both D-*p*-methylphenylalanine, **3**, and L-*p*-methylphenylalanine, **4**, showed high in vitro antagonism. The *p*-ethylphenylalanine peptide diastereoisomers, **5** and **6**, however, showed large differences in their pA$_2$ values with the D-*p*-ethylphenylalanine peptide analog, **6**, exhibiting an approximately 70-fold increase in anti-oxytocin potency over the corresponding L-*p*-ethylphenylalanine peptide diastereomer, **5**. Similar results were observed for the L-*O*-ethyltyrosine, **2**, and the D-*O*-ethyltyrosine, **12**. Analog **12**, the D-*O*-ethyltyrosine peptide diastereomer, again showed a 100-fold increase in anti-oxytocin potency over the corresponding L-*O*-ethyltyrosine diastereoisomer.

Table 12-2. Antioxytotic Potency and Duration of Action of Oxytocin Antagonists

Peptide Analog	In vitro, pA$_2$	Dose range for 50–80% inhibition of OT response, μg	Recovery, t$_{1/2}$ min
1	7.30	3.5–5.0	130 ± 16
2	5.32	6.0–8.0	55 ± 12
3	7.30	3.0–4.0	160 ± 14
4	7.5	2.5	148 ± 11
5	5.80	40–50	110 ± 9
6	7.50	3.5–5.0	155 ± 22
7	6.75	10–20	50 ± 4
8	7.46	5–10	20
9	7.45	5–10	93 ± 2
10	7.12	10–50	20
11	7.21	10–50	20
12	7.36	4.0	45 ± 2

The incorporation of ornithine for leucine in position 8 into analogs 1–7 and 12 provides compounds with an increased duration of action with no loss in antagonist potency. The results of studies addressing prolongation are shown in Table 12–2. Analog 7, [Pen^1,Orn^8]oxytocin, shows a slight (2.5-fold) increase in duration of action over [Pen^1]oxytocin ($t_{1/2}$, ~20 min; Chan et al., 1987) as do analogs 8, 10, and 11, which do not contain an ornithine-8 substitution. Analogs containing multiple amino acid substitutions in position 2, 4, or 7, including ornithine-8 analogs (1–7, 9, 12), all showed much more extended duration of action relative to [Pen^1]oxytocin or its analogs 8, 10, and 11. The analogs exhibiting the most prolonged duration of action contain either O-alkyl-tyrosine or p-alkyl-phenylalanine in position 2. These amino acid substitutions not only enhance anti-oxytocin potency but also prolong the action of the hormone. Comparison of the peptide diastereomers containing substitution in position 2 shows no clear trend as to whether D-amino acid residues or L-amino acid residues enhance the duration of action of the peptide. All the analogs showed increased duration of action relative to [Pen^1]oxytocin. The size of the alkyl group on the Tyr^2 hydroxyl, however, does appear to affect the observed duration of action. O-Methyltyrosine substitution provides an analog, 1, with $t_{1/2}$ = 130 min; however, increasing the size to O-ethyltyrosine decreases duration of action by two- to threefold.

Replacement of proline-7 with dehydroproline ($\Delta^{3,4}$-Pro) provided peptide analogs 8, 9, 10, and 11 with high anti-oxytocin potency approximately equal to [Pen^1,Thr^4]oxytocin (pA$_2$ = 7.5; Hruby et al., 1980). The replacement of proline-7 with $\Delta^{3,4}$proline in oxytocin (Moore et al., 1972) provided an analog with oxytocin potency approximately 1.5 fold greater than oxytocin. Table 12–2 shows that the antagonist potency of analog 10, containing $\Delta^{3,4}$-proline, mirrors this trend. However, when $\Delta^{3,4}$-proline is combined with threonine-4, there is no enhancement in anti-oxytocin potency as would be predicted from the observed antagonist potencies of analogs each containing a single amino acid substitution. In addition, the substitution of $\Delta^{3,4}$-proline has no effect on the observed duration of action. As stated earlier, ornithine-8 incorporation appears to have a significant effect on the observed duration of action; analog 9, which contains orthinine-8, does show increased duration of action.

Discussion

The antagonist analogs described in this chapter all show high anti-oxytocin potency. The data presented suggest that incorporating amino acid residues containing hydrophobic side chains into positions 2, 4, and 7 provides analogs with high anti-oxytocin activity. These results are consistent with the work reported by Manning et al. (1987) and others (Melin et al., 1981,

1986) showing high antagonist potencies in peptide analogs containing combined valine-4 and O-alkyltyrosine-2 substitutions. In addition, we have shown that multiple substitutions in positions 2, 4, and 7 in oxytocin antagonists do not show increased antagonist potency over analogs that have single or double amino acid substitutions. The results obtained for analogs 7, 8, 10, and 11, which have multiple substitutions in these positions, suggest that these positions may be involved in hormone–receptor interactions for the antagonist state.

Substituting leucine-8 with ornithine provides oxytocin antagonists with enhanced duration of action as illustrated, for example, by comparing analogs 8 and 9. The substitution of leucine-8 with ornithine suggests that metabolic breakdown of the peptide by enzymes, probably post-proline-cleaving enzyme, may be retarded. Apparently oxytocin receptor specificity for antagonists is enhanced by ornithine incorporation, although it clearly is diminished for agonists (Hruby and Smith, 1987). Walter (1977) had suggested that leucine-8 was required for receptor interaction or recognition by oxytocin agonists. However, the results presented in this work would appear to substantiate the dynamic model of Hruby, that is, that agonists and antagonists adopt different receptor requirements for observed biological activity (Hruby, 1981, 1985, 1987; Meraldi et al., 1977).

Increasing the size of the para-alkyl substituent in position 2 in conjunction with other substitutions in positions 4 and 8 shows no necessary enhancement of antagonist potency, but generally shows marked increases in observed duration of action. Thus, combining para-alkyl substituted aromatic residues in position 2 and ornithine or other basic unnatural amino acids in position 8 provides highly potent and long-acting oxytocin antagonists. These results suggest that more bulky amino acids in position 2, most notably those containing para-methyl-substituted (or methoxy-substituted) aromatic rings, increases the duration of receptor interaction in the antagonist state, and provides analogs with a prolonged duration of anti-oxytocic activity. These results indicate that, in any series of antagonists for the oxytocic uterine receptor, increased lipophilicity of an aromatic moiety in conjunction with a positive change properly placed topographically is an important feature to consider in the design of potent long-acting oxytocic antagonists.

The analogs presented from this research show that highly potent, long-acting oxytocin antagonists are now available. The most significant finding is the prolonged duration of anti-oxytocin activity possessed by many of these analogs. Combining bulky amino acids in position 2 with ornithine in position 8 has provided peptide analogs that may be useful as clinical agents. Although the apparent specificity for uterine oxytocin receptors has not been unequivocally demonstrated, these analogs could be useful as agents to inhibit preterm labor. In addition, these analogs may provide further impetus to design more specific and longer lasting peptide analogs incorporating further modifications of the peptide or of peptide mimetics.

Experimental

General Methods

Melting points were determined on a Thomas Hoover melting point apparatus and are uncorrected. Nuclear magnetic resonance (NMR) spectra were obtained on a Brucker WM 250 or an AM 250 instrument operating at 250 MHz for ^{1}H. Elemental analyses were performed by Desert Analytics (Tucson, Arizona). Amino acid analyses were performed on a Beckman 120C Amino Acid Analyzer after acid hydrolysis in sealed tubes with 4 N methanesulfonic acid at 100°C for 24–48 h. Standard solid-phase peptide synthesis methodology (Hruby et al., 1977; Stewart and Young, 1984) was used to make the peptides reported. Chloromethylated polystyrene resin, 1%, cross-linked with divinylbenzene (chloride content, 1.02 mequiv/g resin), was used for the syntheses. The C-terminal amino acid (Boc-glycine) was attached to the resin by the methods of Gysin (1973). Either the carbodiimide method of activation by using a 2.5-fold excess of amino acid and dicyclohexylcarbodiimide (DCC), or, for N^α-Boc-Asn and N^α-Boc-Gln, a 3-M excess of the hydroxybenzotriazole active ester were used for the coupling reactions. Completion of reactions was monitored by the ninhydrin test (Kaiser et al., 1970). Purity of the final products was assessed by amino acid analysis, optical rotation, and HPLC (Tables 12–1 and 12–3). Cystine and penicillamine were not determined.

Cleavage of Protected Peptide from the Solid Support

The protected nonapeptides were cleaved from the resin by addition of the dried resin to a 250-ml round-bottom flask containing 150 ml methanol [freshly distilled from Mg(OMe)$_2$] and anhydrous ammonia (freshly distilled from Na) at –5°C. The volume of the flask increased slightly (~20 ml) with the addition of ammonia to methanol. After addition of the resin, the flask was wired shut and stirred in a desiccator containing KOH pellets for 4 days at 25°C. The solvent was removed by aspiration and rotary evaporation in vacuo leaving dry resin material. The cleaved peptide was extracted from the resin by adding 125 ml DMF and heating the resulting slurry at 62°C for 8 h. The mixture was cooled and filtered; 125 ml fresh DMF was added to the resin, which was then heated at 85°C for 2 h. The resin mixture was cooled and filtered, and the resulting DMF extracts were combined and concentrated to approximately 15 ml in vacuo. Deionized water (125 ml) was added dropwise to the DMF concentrate with swirling, resulting in a white precipitate. The solution containing the solvent was cooled in an ice bath for 2 h to induce further solid precipitation from the solution. The precipitate was collected by suction filtration, washed with water

Table 12-3. Amino Acid Analysis of Oxytocin Antagonist Analogs

Analog	Gly	Ile	Pro $\Delta^{3,4}$Pro[c]	X-Phe[a] X-Tyr[b]	Thr Gln[c]	Asx	Orn Leu[d]
			Amino Acid Analysis (theory)				
1	1.06 (1.0)	0.84 (1.0)	1.03 (1.0)	0.96 (1.0)[b]	0.95 (1.0)	1.04 (1.0)	0.94 (1.0)
2	1.14 (1.0)	0.84 (1.0)	1.13 (1.0)	0.94 (1.0)[b]	0.91 (1.0)	1.04 (1.0)	0.93 (1.0)
3	0.99 (1.0)	1.04 (1.0)	1.06 (1.0)	0.61 (1.0)[a]	0.96 (1.0)	1.01 (1.0)	1.01 (1.0)
4	1.00 (1.0)	1.01 (1.0)	1.06 (1.0)	0.61 (1.0)[a]	0.95 (1.0)	1.05 (1.0)	1.07 (1.0)
5	1.03 (1.0)	1.00 (1.0)	1.01 (1.0)	0.97 (1.0)[b]	0.95 (1.0)	0.99 (1.0)	0.97 (1.0)
6	1.02 (1.0)	0.96 (1.0)	1.02 (1.0)	1.08 (1.0)[a]	0.95 (1.0)	1.03 (1.0)	0.92 (1.0)
7	1.00 (1.0)	0.92 (1.0)	1.10 (1.0)	0.90 (1.0)[b]	0.92 (1.0)[c]	1.04 (1.0)	0.95 (1.0)
8	1.07 (1.0)	0.99 (1.0)	1.03 (1.0)[c]	0.98 (1.0)[a]	0.89 (1.0)	1.02 (1.0)	1.03 (1.0)[d]
9	1.06 (1.0)	0.97 (1.0)	0.95 (1.0)[c]	0.92 (1.0)[a]	1.02 (1.0)	1.01 (1.0)	1.03 (1.0)
10	0.95 (1.0)	0.98 (1.0)	1.01 (1.0)[c]	0.90 (1.0)[b]	0.98 (1.0)[c]	1.00 (1.0)	1.07 (1.0)[d]
11	1.00 (1.0)	0.88 (1.0)	1.00 (1.0)[c]	1.00 (1.0)[b]	0.85 (1.0)	0.99 (1.0)	1.06 (1.0)[d]
12	1.00 (1.0)	1.02 (1.0)	1.00 (1.0)	0.97 (1.0)[b]	0.98 (1.0)	1.00 (1.0)	0.98 (1.0)

(2 × 20 ml) and ether (2 × 20 ml), and dried for 1 h at room temperature and then in vacuo, leaving a white powder. A second crop of protected nonapeptide was obtained by lyophilization of the mother liquor. The resulting lyophilizate was analyzed for purity by comparison of melting point and by amino acid analysis with the solid material obtained by trituration with water.

Deprotection and Disulfide Formation of Oxytocin Analogs

A typical reaction included the following general procedure: A sample of 250 mg of protected nonapeptide was dissolved in 200 ml anhydrous ammonia (freshly distilled from Na). The solution was warmed to the boiling point and treated with a sodium stick until a blue color persisted for 60 sec. If the blue color persisted for longer than 60 sec, addition of a few milligrams of NH_4Cl crystals rapidly dissipated the color and prevented cleavage of the proline residue. The ammonia was evaporated under the N_2 stream and the last 20 ml was removed by lyophilization. The white powder resulting from lyophilization was dissolved in 650 ml deaerated 0.1% HOAc under an N_2 atmosphere. The pH of the peptide solution was adjusted to 8.5 with 3 M NH_4OH and then oxidized with addition of excess 0.01 N $K_3Fe(CN)_6$. The resultant dark-yellow solution was stirred for 30 min while maintaining the pH at 8.5. The excess ferro- and ferricyanide ions were removed from the solution by first adjusting the solution to pH with 20% HOAc and then adding 5 ml (wet volume) anion exchange resin (Rexyn 203 (Cl⁻ cycle) Fisher Chemical Company, Pittsburgh, Pennsylvania) or BioRad 3-X4A (BioRad Laboratories, Richmond, California). After the peptide solution was stirred for 20 min, the resin was removed by filtration and washed with 20% HOAc (3 × 20 ml) to ensure complete exchange of the peptide material from the resin. Approximately 75 ml of butanol (to reduce bumping) was added to the aqueous peptide solution, which was concentrated in vacuo at 20°–30°C to about 100 ml and lyophilized. The resulting product was then purified by partition chromatography followed by gel filtration.

Partition Chromatography and Gel Filtration

The lyophilized product was initially purified by partition chromatography on Sephadex G-25 block polymerizate (Pharmacia Fine Chemicals, Piscataway, New Jersey) using the organic phase of biphasic butanol:water (containing 3.5% acetic acid and 1.5% pyridine) (1:1), butanol:acetic acid:water (4:1:5), or butanol:ethanol:H_2O (containing 3.5% acetic acid, 1.5% pyridine) (4:1:5) systems. Fractions of 4 ml each were collected and analyzed for peptide material using either UV measurement at 280 nm or Folin–Lowry analysis. The fractions corresponding to the product were pooled, rinsed with 20% HOAc and 0.2 M HOAc, then lyophilized. The resulting white power was further purified by gel filtration on Sephadex G-25 (240–270 mesh) using either aqueous 0.2 M HOAc or 20% HOAc as the eluent solvent. The fractions corresponding to the major peak were pooled and lyophilized, yielding a white powder of the purified peptide material.

Acknowledgments

This work was supported by grants from the U.S. Public Health Service (DK 17420) and from the National Science Foundation.

REFERENCES

Bock MG, DiPardo RM, Williams PD, Pettibone DJ, Clineschmidt BV, Ball RG, Veber DF, Freidinger RM (1990): *J Med Chem* 33:2321–2323.
Chan WY, Rockway TW, Hruby VJ (1987): *Proc Soc Exp Biol Med* 185:187–192.
Chan WY, Hruby VJ, Rockway TW, Hlavacek J (1986): *J Pharmacol Exp Ther* 239:84–87.
Evans BE, Leighton JL, Rittle KE, Gilbert KF, Lundell GF, Gould NP, Hobbs DW, DiPardo RM, Veber DF, Pettibone DJ, Bluneschmidt BV, Anderson PS, Freidinger RM (1992): *J Med Chem* 35:3919–3927.
Gysin BF (1973): *Helv Chim Acta* 56:1476–1482.
Hill PA, Slaninova J, Hruby VJ (1988): In: *Peptides: Structure and Function*, Marshall G, ed., pp. 468–470. Leiden: ESCOM.
Hill PS, Smith DD, Slaninova J, Hruby VJ (1990): *J Am Chem Soc* 112:3110–3113.
Hruby VJ (1981): In: *Topics in Molecular Pharmacology*, Vol. 1, Burgen ASV, Roberts

GCK, eds., pp. 99–126. Amsterdam: Elsevier/North-Holland Biomedical.

Hruby VJ (1985): In: *Oxytocin: Clinical and Laboratory Studies*, Amico JA, Robinson AG, eds., pp. 405–414. New York: Elsevier/North Holland.

Hruby VJ (1987): *Trends Pharmacol Sci* 8:336–339.

Hruby VJ, Mosberg HI (1981): In: *Neurohypophyseal Peptide Hormones and Other Biologically Active Peptides*, Schlesinger DH, ed., pp. 227–237. New York: Elsevier/North-Holland.

Hruby VJ, Mosberg HI (1982): In: *Hormone Antagonists*, Agarwal MK, ed., pp. 433–474. Berlin: Walter de Gruyter.

Hruby VJ, Smith CW (1987): In: *The Peptides: Analysis, Synthesis, Biology, Vol. 8., Chemistry, Biology and Medicine of Neurohypophyseal Hormones and Their Analogues*, Smith CW, ed., pp. 77–207. New York: Academic Press.

Hruby VJ, Chow M-S, Smith DD (1990): *Annu Rev Pharmacol Toxicol* 30:501–534.

Hruby VJ, Upson DA, Agarwal NS (1977): *J Org Chem* 42:3552–3557.

Hruby VJ, Mosberg HI, Hadley ME, Chan WY, Powell AM (1980): *Int J Pept Protein Res* 16:372–381.

Jost K, Sorm F, Rudinger J (1961): *Collect Czech Chem Commun* 26:2673–2684.

Kaiser E, Colescott RL, Bossinger CD, Cook PI (1970): *Anal Biochem* 34:595–548.

Kolodziejczyk AM, Manning M (1981): *J Org Chem* 46:1944–1946.

Lebl M (1987): In: *Handbook of Neurohypophyseal Hormone Analogs*, Vol. 2, Part 1, Jost K, Lebl M, Brtnik F, eds., pp. 17–74. Boca Raton: CRC Press.

Manning M, Sawyer WH (1989): *J Lab Clin Med* 114:617–632.

Manning M, Przybylski JP, Olma A, Klis WA, Kruszynski M, Wo NC, Pelton GH, Sawyer WH (1987): *Nature (London)* 329:839–840.

Manning M, Kruszynski M, Bankowski K, Olma A, Lammek B, Cheng LL, Klis WA, Seto J, Holder J, Sawyer WH (1989): *J Med Chem* 32:382–391.

Meraldi J-P, Hruby VJ, Brewster AI, Brewster R (1977): *Proc Natl Acad Sci USA* 74:1373–1377.

Meraldi J-P, Yamamoto D, Hruby VJ, Brester AIR (1975): In: *Peptides: Chemistry, Structure and Biology*, Walter R, Meienhofer J, eds., pp. 803–814. Ann Arbor: Ann Arbor Science.

Mosberg HI, Hruby VJ, Meraldi J-P (1981): *Biochemistry* 20:2822–2828.

Robertson AV, Witkop B (1962): *J Am Chem Soc* 84:1697–1701.

Sawyer WH, Manning M (1985): In: *Oxytocin: Clinical and Laboratory Studies*, Amico JA, Robinson AG, eds., pp. 423–432. Amsterdam: Elsevier.

Schulz H, du Vigneaud V (1966): *J Med Chem* 9:647–650.

Schulz H, du Vigneaud V (1967): *J Med Chem* 10:1037–1039.

Smith DD, Slaninova J, Hruby VJ (1992): *J Med Chem* 35:1558–1563.

Snyder HR, Shekleton JF, Lewis CD (1945): *J Am Chem Soc* 67:310–311.

Stewart JM, Young JD (1984): *Solid Phase Peptide Synthesis*, 2d Ed. Rockford: Pierce Chemical Company.

Walter R (1977): *Fed Proc* 36:1872–1878.

Williams PD, Boch MG, Tung RD, Garsky VM, Perlow DS, Erb JM, Lindell GF, Gould NP, Whitter WL, Hoffmann JB, Kaufman MJ, Clineschmidt BV, Pettibone DJ, Freidinger RM, Veber DF (1992): *J Med Chem* 35:3905–3918.

13

CALCITONIN: A MINIREVIEW

Channa Basava

Introduction

Calcitonin (CT) is a 32-amino-acid, single-chain polypeptide hormone that plays important roles in calcium homeostasis and bone remodeling. Endogenous calcitonin is secreted primarily by the parafollicular cells referred to as the "C" cells. These cells are scattered throughout the thyroid in mammals but constitute a distinct organ, the ultimobranchial body, in submammalian species. The major biological function of calcitonin is to inhibit osteoclast-induced mineral resorption from bone. It regulates serum calcium concentrations by opposing the bone and renal effects of parathyroid hormone and by inhibiting bone resorption, resulting in hypocalcemia, hypophosphatemia, and decreased urinary calcium concentrations.

Another beneficial property of this hormone is an analgesic effect induced by the central nervous system (CNS). The combination of hypocalcemic and analgesic properties of calcitonin make it an agent of choice for the treatment of disorders associated with hypercalcemia, excessive bone resorption, and bone pain. Salmon, human, and porcine calcitonins, and

Peptides: Design, Synthesis, and Biological Activity
Channa Basava and G. M. Anantharamaiah, Editors
©1994 *Birkhäuser Boston*

an analog of eel hormone (Elcatonin), are in clinical use for the treatment of Paget's disease, certain kinds of osteoporosis, and the hypercalcemia of malignancy. Calcitonin is one of the most successful peptide drugs, with a long history of safe and effective therapeutic uses in the treatment of bone and mineral disorders.

Even though the discovery of calcitonin dates back almost 30 years and although this hormone has been in clinical use for more than two decades, a number of laboratories still continue to pursue research in this field with a great deal of interest, evidenced by such developments as the recent characterization of calcitonins from dogfish, stingray, rabbit, and dog, the discovery of new, superpotent human calcitonin analogs and calcitonin antagonists, and characterization of the human calcitonin receptor. Earlier studies of the discovery, isolation, characterization, and biosynthesis of calcitonin and structure–activity studies of numerous synthetic analogs have been reviewed extensively (Azria, 1989; Copp, 1992a, 1992b; Guttmann, 1981; MacIntyre et al., 1987; Potts, 1976, 1992; Potts et al., 1971; Rosenfeld et al., 1992; Zaidi et al., 1990, 1991, 1993). The objective of this chapter is to summarize some recent developments in calcitonin field with particular emphasis on its current and future therapeutic applications.

Isolation and Structure

The hypocalcemic action of calcitonin was first recognized by Copp (Copp et al., 1962). MacIntyre and co-workers demonstrated the origin of calcitonin to be the thyroid gland (Foster and MacIntyre, 1964), specifically the parafollicular "C" cells. Following this discovery, amino acid sequences of porcine (Potts et al., 1968), human (Neher et al., 1968), bovine (Brewer and Ronan, 1969), and salmon (Niall et al., 1969) calcitonin were determined. Amino acid sequences of calcitonins given in Figure 13–1 include the peptides from stingray (Takei et al., 1991) and dogfish (Sasayama et al., 1993).

Common structural features of calcitonins from various species include an N-terminal 1–7 cystine disulfide bridge and a C-terminal proline amide residue. Amino acid residues at seven positions—1 (Cys), 4 (Leu), 5 (Ser), 6 (Thr), 7 (Cys), 28 (Gly), and 32 (Pro-NH_2)—are invariant among species, and residues at position 9 (Leu) and 16 (Leu) are common to 11 of 12 known sequences. On the basis of sequence similarities, Guttmann (1981) subdivided the calcitonins into three broad subgroups: hormones from human lineage (human, rat), pig lineage (porcine, bovine, ovine), and salmon lineage (salmon, eel). Sasayama et al. (1992) included chicken and goldfish hormones in the subgroup of salmon lineage. This classification could be further broadened to include rabbit calcitonin in the human lineage hormones, stingray calcitonin in the salmon lineage hormones, and canine calcitonin in the pig lineage hormones (Fig. 13–2).

Species																																	Reference
															Calcitonin sequence																		
	1	2	3	4	5	6	7	8	9	10	11	12	13	14	15	16	17	18	19	20	21	22	23	24	25	26	27	28	29	30	31	32	
Human	C	G	N	L	S	T	C	M	L	G	T	Y	T	Q	D	F	N	K	F	H	T	F	P	Q	T	A	I	G	V	G	A	P	Neher et al., 1968
Rat	C	G	N	L	S	T	C	M	L	G	T	Y	T	Q	D	L	N	K	F	H	T	F	P	Q	T	S	I	G	V	G	A	P	Raulais et al., 1976
Rabbit	C	G	N	L	S	T	C	M	L	G	T	Y	T	Q	D	L	N	K	F	H	T	F	P	Q	T	A	I	G	V	V	A	P	Martial et al., 1990
Dog	C	S	N	L	S	T	C	V	L	G	T	Y	S	K	K	L	N	N	F	H	T	F	S	G	I	G	F	G	A	E	T	P	Mol et al., 1991
Sheep	C	S	N	L	S	T	C	V	L	G	A	Y	W	D	K	L	N	N	Y	H	R	Y	S	G	M	G	F	G	P	E	T	P	Potts et al., 1972
Cattle	C	S	N	L	S	T	C	V	L	G	A	Y	W	D	K	L	N	N	Y	H	R	Y	S	G	M	G	F	G	P	E	T	P	Brewer and Ronan 1969
Pig	C	S	N	L	S	T	C	V	L	G	K	Y	W	R	N	L	N	N	F	H	R	F	S	G	M	G	F	G	P	E	T	P	Potts et al., 1968
Salmon	C	S	N	L	S	T	C	V	L	G	K	L	S	Q	E	L	H	K	L	Q	T	Y	P	R	T	N	T	G	S	G	T	P	Niall et al., 1969
Eel	C	S	N	L	S	T	C	V	L	G	K	L	S	Q	E	L	H	K	L	Q	T	Y	P	R	T	D	V	G	A	G	T	P	Otani et al., 1976
Chicken	C	A	S	L	S	T	C	V	L	G	K	L	S	Q	E	L	H	K	L	Q	T	Y	P	R	T	D	V	G	A	G	T	P	Homma et al., 1986
Goldfish	C	S	S	L	S	T	C	V	L	G	K	L	S	Q	E	L	H	K	L	Q	T	Y	P	R	T	N	V	G	A	G	T	P	Sasayama et al., 1993
Stingray	C	T	S	L	S	T	C	V	V	G	K	L	S	Q	Q	L	H	K	L	Q	N	I	Q	R	T	D	V	G	A	A	T	P	Takei et al., 1991

Figure 13–1. Amino acid sequences of calcitonins from various species.

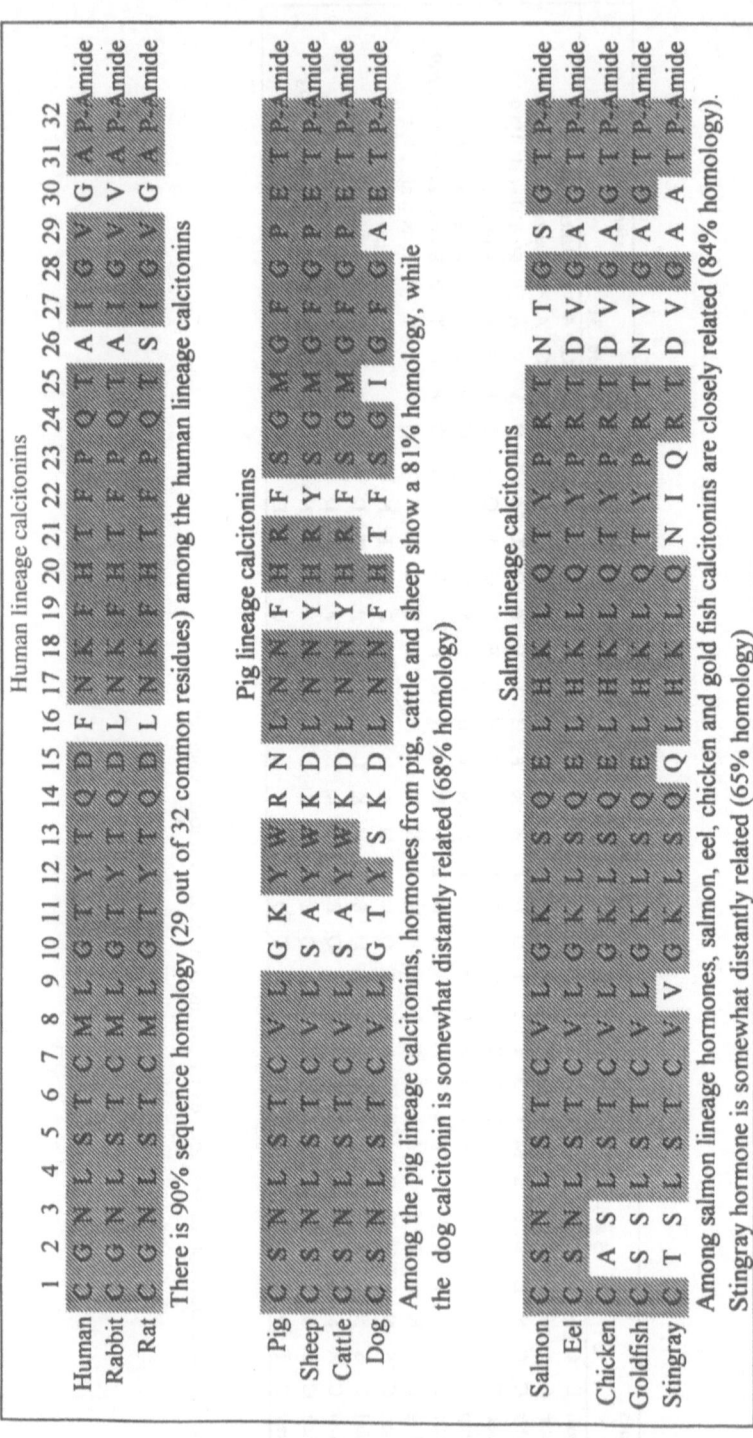

Figure 13–2. Sequence homologies among calcitonins.

Human lineage (human, rat, and rabbit) calcitonins have more than 90% sequence homology (29 of 32 residues in common), the only variations occurring at positions 16, 26, and 30. Among the pig lineage hormones, porcine, bovine, and ovine calcitonins have a sequence homology greater than 81% as a group (26 of 32 common residues). They also show somewhat distant similarity of 68% with the canine hormone (22 of 32 common residues). Among the salmon lineage calcitonins, salmon, eel, chicken, and goldfish hormones show a sequence homology of 87% (28 of 32 common residues). Stingray calcitonin is somewhat distantly related to this group, having a homology of 68% (22 of 32 common residues). Sequences of human and salmon calcitonins differ in 16 of the 32 positions.

Molecular Biology and Biosynthesis

The calcitonin gene complex consists of a small family of peptides: calcitonin, calcitonin gene-related peptide (CGRP) encoded in chromosome 11, and a newly discovered member, amylin, which is encoded in chromosome 12. It is suggested that chromosomes 11 and 12 arose from a common ancestral chromosome, which may explain structural and functional similarities among these peptides. All three hormones show varying degrees of osteoclast-inhibiting action and vasodialatory action; calcitonin is the most potent inhibitor of osteoclastic activity. The major biological effect of CGRP is vasodialation, while amylin exhibits an antiinsulin action in carbohydrate metabolism. Tissue-specific splicing of the calcitonin gene results primarily in two distinct gene products. Calcitonin is the primary product of translation in C cells, whereas CGRP is the major processed product in the neurons (Bennett and Amara, 1992; Deftos and Roos, 1989; MacIntyre, 1992; Rosenfeld et al., 1983, 1992; Zaidi et al., 1991).

Biological Activities and Bioassays

Calcitonin potencies are measured by the standardized hypocalcemic bioassay in immature male rats (Kumar et al., 1965; Sturtridge and Kumar, 1968). Calcitonin hypocalcemic potency is reported in international units per milligram (IU/mg); the quantity of peptide required to bring about a 10% drop in the serum calcium in immature male rats 60 min after subcutaneous administration represents 10 IU. International standards for salmon calcitonin, eel calcitonin, and Elcatonin have been established by the World Health Organization (WHO), each with an assigned potency in IU (available from the National Institute for Biological Standards and Control, Potters Bar, Hertfordshire EN6 3QG, United Kingdom) (Zanelli et al., 1990).

Radioimmunoassay is useful for measuring calcitonin levels in biological samples and could be used to diagnose hypercalcitoninemia associated

Table 13-1. Hypocalcemic Potencies of Calcitonins from Various Species

Species	Potency (IU/mg)	Remarks
Human	100–200	Guttman, 1981
Rat	400	Guttman, 1981
Ovine	100–200	Guttman, 1981
Bovine	100–200	Guttman, 1981
Porcine	100–200	Guttman, 1981
Salmon	4000–6000	Guttman, 1981
Eel	4300	Morikawa et al., 1976
Goldfish (*Carassius auratus*)	3470	Sasayama et al., 1993
Chicken	4500	Homma et al., 1986
Stingray (*Dasyatis akajei*)	1500–3800	Sasayama et al., 1992

with medullary thyroid carcinoma (Azria, 1989). Calcitonin RIA kits are available commercially.

A high-performance liquid chromatographic (HPLC) method is described for the assay of salmon calcitonin. The results obtained by this method are reported to correlate with the results obtained by the biological assay method (Buck and Maxl, 1990).

As a group, mammalian hormones, having ahypocalcemic potency of 100–400 IU/mg, are considerably less active than calcitonins of ultimobranchial origin, which have a potency of 2000–6000 IU/mg. The higher potency of ultimobranchial calcitonins is attributed to their increased affinity toward calcitonin receptors and resistance to degradation (Potts, 1992). Two recently isolated calcitonins from the ultimobranchial glands of goldfish (*Carassius auratus*) and stingray (*Dsyatis akajei*) show hypocalcemic potencies similar to that of nonmammalian hormones (Table 13-1).

Structure–Activity Relationships

Because of the therapeutic importance of calcitonins, much research has been directed toward understanding the structural basis for calcitonin activity. C-Terminal prolinamide and the 1–7 disulfide bridge are considered essential for biological activity. An analog of eel calcitonin in which the disulfide is replaced by an ethylene bridge, [Asu^{1-7}]-eCT (Elcatonin), exhibits full biological activity (Morikawa et al., 1976) and is currently in clinical use. An asymmetric disulfide analog of salmon calcitonin in which the peptide bond between residues Cys^1 and Ser^2 is eliminated (i.e., a free cysteine is bridged to Cys^7 by a disulfide bond) is reported to have potency similar to the native hormone (Cardinaux et al., 1988). Branched chain analogs of eel calcitonin containing two peptide chains linked to the two amino groups of lysine at position 7 (in place of Cys^7) also show high biological activity (Basava and Hostetler, 1992b). Orlowski et al. (1987) reported

Table 13-2. Hypocalcemic Potencies of Some Nondisulfide Calcitonin Analogs

Analog	Potency (IU/mg)	Relative Potency sCT-1	Reference
[N$^\alpha$-Propionyl Di-Ala^{1,7}, des-Leu^{19}]-sCT	7435	1.53	Yates et al., 1990
[(N$^\alpha$-Isocaproyl-Ser)^5, Ala^7]-sCT (5-32)		1.37	Cardinaux et al., 1988
[(Adamentanacetyl-Ser)^5, Ala^7]-sCT (5-32)		1.20	Cardinaux et al., 1988
[(Cyclohexylpropionyl-Ser)^5, Ala^7]-sCT (5-32)		1.23	Cardinaux et al., 1988
[(Ser-Asn-Leu-Ser-Thr-NH-CH-CO-)Val^8]-sCT (8-32) | CH$_2$-S-S-CH$_2$-CH(NH$_2$)-COOH		Similar to sCT	Cardinaux et al., 1988
[(Ser-Asn-Leu-Ser-Thr-NH-CH-CO-)Val^8]-sCT (8-32) | CH$_2$-S-S-CH$_2$-COOH		Similar to sCT	Cardinaux et al., 1988
[Ala^{1,7}]-sCT	5500		Orlowski et al., 1987
[Cys(Acm)^{1,7}]-sCT	4250		Orlowski et al., 1987
[(Cyclohexylpropionyl-Ser-Thr)$_2$-Lys^7]-eCT (7-32)	5000		Basava and Hostetler, 1992b
[CO-Ser-Asn-Leu-Ser-Thr-NH-CH-CO-Leu^8]-eCT (8-32) | | CH$_2$-CH$_2$-CH$_2$-CH$_2$-CH$_2$————— [Elcatonin]	3400		Morikawa et al., 1976
[CO-Ser-Asn-Leu-Ser-Thr-NH-CH-CO-Leu^8]-CT (8-32) | | CH$_2$CH$_2$CO-NHCH$_2$CH$_2$CH$_2$CH$_2$	4000		Basava and Hostetler, 1992a

that compounds lacking the disulfide bridge, [Ala^{1,7}]-sCT and [Cys(Acm)^{1,7}]-sCT, show hypocalcemic potency equal to salmon calcitonin (Table 13-2). Other investigators also have reported linear calcitonin analogs showing significant hypocalcemic potency (Yates et al., 1990). Epand et al. (1988) have reported a series of deletion analogs of salmon calcitonin that retain the essential biological and conformational features of the intact molecule. A model peptide designed to mimic the amphipathic structure of salmon calcitonin showed potent calcitonin-like biological activity (Moe and Kaiser, 1985). Replacement of Val^8 by a leucine residue and extending the N terminal by an additional leucine led to salmon and eel calcitonin analogs with enhanced hypocalcemic potencies (Basava and Hostetler, 1992b). Feyen et al. (1992) described the preparation of N-terminal truncated sequences of salmon calcitonin that act as calcitonin antagonists (Table 13-3).

Salmon calcitonin and Elcatonin are used widely as clinical agents compared to human calcitonin becaue of their superior potency. Salmon calcitonin, differing from the human hormone in 16 of the 32 positions, is reported to produce antibodies (Grauer et al., 1990; Levy et al., 1988; Muff et al., 1991), which may result in the development of clinical resistance. Other reports indicate that human calcitonin may be effective in treating patients who have developed clinical resistance to salmon calcitonin (Muff et al., 1990; Singer et al., 1980). The design of minimally substituted human calcitonin analogs with high potency, therefore, has been an objective of a number of investigators. Earlier studies by Maier and co-workers (Maier, 1976; Maier et al., 1974, 1975, 1976, 1977) led to a series of compounds in which certain amino acid residues in the human sequence were systematically replaced by those in salmon hormone. A number of compounds with potencies higher than human calcitonin were reported, the most potent of

Table 13-3. Hypocalcemic Potencies of Some Potent Calcitonin Analogs

Analog	Potency (IU/mg)	Relative Potency sCT=1	Reference
[des-Leu[19]]-sCT	8000	1.78	Epand et al., 1988
[des-Leu[19],Gln[20],Thr[21],Tyr[22]]-sCT	6300	1.40	Epand et al., 1988
[Leu[8]]-sCT	5000	1.25	Basava and Hostetler, 1992b
[Leu[0,8]]-sCT	6000	1.50	Basava and Hostetler, 1992b
[Leu[8]]-eCT	5000	1.25	Basava and Hostetler, 1992b
[Leu[0,8]]-eCT	6000	1.50	Basava and Hostetler, 1992b
[Leu[12,16,19]]-hCT		0.2	Guttman, 1981
[Leu[12,16,19],Tyr[22]]-hCT		0.3–0.4	Guttman, 1981
[Leu[8,12]]-hCT	2000	0.5	Basava and Hostetler, 1992a
[Leu[0,8,12]]-hCT	4000	1	Basava and Hostetler, 1992a
[His[17],Leu[19],Gln[20],Tyr[22],Arg[24],Asn[26],Thr[27,31], Ser[29]]-hCT		Similar to sCT	Kozono et al., 1992

these being [Leu[12,16,19], Tyr[22]]-hCT. However, this analog was reported to be less than half as potent as salmon calcitonin (Guttmann, 1981).

Kozono et al. (1992) have reported a chimeric molecule that combines the N-terminal half of human sequence with the C-terminal part of salmon calcitonin. This chimeric molecule is reported to exhibit potency similar to that of salmon calcitonin but with reduced side effects. The sequence of this molecule still differs from the native human peptide in nine positions. The optimal combination of greatest potency with minimal modification to the human sequence has been attained in a series of leucine-substituted human calcitonin analogs. For example, [Leu[8,12]]-hCT exhibits a hypocalcemic potency of 2000 IU/mg, and this activity is doubled by extending the N terminal by an additional leucine. The tri-leucine-substituted compound [Leu[0,8,12]]-hCT, showing a hypocalcemic potency of 4000 IU/mg, is equipotent with salmon calcitonin but differs from human sequence in only three positions (Basava and Hostetler, 1992a, 1992b).

Physiological Functions

Calcitonin, together with parathyroid hormone, participates in the regulation of mineral metabolism and homeostatic regulation of calcium levels in the blood. The primary physiological function of calcitonin is the maintenance of skeletal integrity during periods of calcium stress such as growth, pregnancy, and lactation. Normal bone remodeling consists of osteoclast-induced bone resorption and bone formation that is influenced by osteoblasts. Calcitonin binds to specific receptors on osteoclasts and thus reduces mineral resorption by reducing osteoclast volume and activity. Parathyroid hormone acts as a physiological antagonist of calcitonin by stimulating osteoclastic activity. Calcitonin and parathyroid hormone may exert opposing effects on the transport of calcium between intracellular, extracellular, and mitochondrial compartments. Calcitonin regulates the renal function and calcium homeostasis by acting on the receptors present in the proximal tubules and other parts of the kidney and plays a role in the regulation of intestinal absorption of calcium.

Calcitonin also is reported to act as a neurotransmitter and brings about receptor-mediated analgesia, possibly through the release of β-endorphin in the brain (Gennari et al., 1991). Various interactions between osteoclasts, calcitonin and other agents, and their effects on bone resorption have been reviewed by Zaidi et al. (1993). Calcitonin is reported to inhibit bone resorption by inducing both quiescence (Q effect) and retraction (R effect) in osteoclasts, and this action is mediated by intracellular calcium. Two structurally related members of the calcitonin gene peptide family, calcitonin gene-related peptide (CGRP) and amylin, inhibit osteoclastic bone resorption selectively via the Q effect (Alam et al., 1993). Calcitonin receptors from a porcine kidney epithelial cell line and human ovarian small cell carcinoma line have been cloned and characterized. The calcitonin receptor is homologous to the parathyroid hormone–parathyroid hormone-related peptide receptor, indicating that the receptors for these hormones, which regulate calcium homeostasis, represent a new family of G protein-coupled receptors (Gorn et al., 1992; Lin et al., 1991).

Therapeutic Applications

Calcitonin has been successfully used during the past 25 years for the treatment of Paget's disease, a metabolic bone disorder characterized by excessive resorption of the bone accompanied by imbalanced formation of new bone. Calcitonin therapy effectively reduces bone resorption, as indicated by the lowered levels of alkaline phosphatase and hydroxyproline, serum markers for this disease. Also, the analgesic actions of calcitonin provide relief from the pain and tenderness associated with Paget's disease. Calcitonin is effective in the treatment of hypercalcemia associated with carcinoma, bone metastasis, hyperthyroidism, and vitamin D intoxication. Calcitonin therapy also is useful in the treatment of osteoporosis, which is marked by progressive loss of bone density leading to fractures. Calcitonin therapy appears to increase bone density and reduces bone pain.

Some of the side effects of calcitonin therapy are the appearance of neutralizing antibodies leading to clinical resistance (associated with nonhuman calcitonins), gastrointestinal discomfort, and facial flushing. These side effects notwithstanding, however, calcitonin therapy has been accepted as safe and effective for a variety of bone disorders. Alternative calcitonin formulations for nasal or oral delivery, which would improve patient acceptance, are under development. New generations of calcitonin molecules, especially those with reduced side effects, are expected to further enhance the usefulness of calcitonin therapy.

Therapeutic uses of calcitonin have been reviewed extensively (Chestnut, 1992; Milhaud, 1992; Singer, 1991; Wimalawansa, 1993; Wisneski, 1992). Calcitonin is a valuable therapeutic agent in the treatment of Paget's disease, particularly in patients with osteolytic lesions. Synthetic salmon calcitonin administered as a nasal spray in Pagetic patients decreased serum alkaline phosphatase and the urinary hydroxyproline/creatinine ratio; intranasal calcitonin can counteract early postmenopausal bone loss (Reginster et al., 1987, 1988a, 1988b). In healthy subjects, 200 IU of intranasal salmon calcitonin caused a fall in serum calcium, a fall in serum phosphorus, and a transient rise in parathyroid hormone levels similar to that observed after the intramuscular (im) injection of 80 IU of the hormone (Reginster et al., 1987). In osteoporosis, calcitonin exerts an analgesic effect that is unrelated to its effect on bone. Although the precise mechanism has yet to be clarified, there is some evidence that the analgesic effect of calcitonin may be mediated through the endogenous opioid system. The intranasal administration of calcitonin seems to be more effective than parenteral administration in producing analgesia (Gennari et al., 1991).

Treatment with calcitonin is reported to produce significant, dose-dependent, analgesic effects (Ljunghall et al., 1991), and the analgesic effect of calcitonin might be mediated by increased β-endorphin release (Laurian et al., 1986). Calcitonin exerts a beneficial effect on back pain following a vertebral crush fracture caused by postmenopausal osteoporosis (Lyritis et al., 1991). In women with high-turnover osteoporosis, therapy using intranasal salmon calcitonin results in a net gain of bone in both the peripheral and axial skeleton (Overgaard et al., 1990). A retrospective, population-based, case control survey of a large number of postmenopausal women taking drugs affecting bone metabolism indicates that therapy with calcitonin, calcium, or estrogen decreased the risk of hip fracture (Kanis et al., 1992). With long-term treatment with salmon calcitonin, a significant number of patients developed antibodies, and human calcitonin may be effective in treating patients who have developed clinical resistance (Levy et al., 1988; Singer et al., 1980). Other studies have indicated that intranasal administration of salmon calcitonin does not give rise to side effects even in patients known to be intolerant to intramuscularly administered salmon calcitonin (Reginster and Franchimont, 1985).

Conclusion

In clinical use, calcitonin has been found to be a safe and beneficial treatment for a number of bone disorders. It has been used as a treatment for Paget's disease, postmenopausal bone loss, high-turnover osteoporosis, and hypercalcemia caused by malignancy, and is a drug of choice for osteolytic bone lesions. Second-generation analogs having high potency, increased nasal bioavailabilities, and the availability of new dosage forms (nasal and, potentially, oral) are expected to make calcitonin therapy much more widely accepted and useful.

Acknowledgments

I sincerely thank Professor Sivanandaiah for introducing me to the exciting field of peptide chemistry and biology, and for the kind guidance he has provided throughout my association with him. The calcitonin work presented here was carried out during my tenure at Vical Inc., San Diego, California. I thank all my collegues at Vical for their contributions to this project.

REFERENCES

Alam AS, Bax CM, Shankar VS, Bax BE, Bevis PJ, Huang CL, Moonga BS, Pazianas M, Zaidi M (1993): *J Endocrinol* 136(1):7–15.

Azria M (1989): In: *Progress in Clinical Biochemistry and Medicine*, Vol. 9, pp. 3–34. Berlin: Springer-Verlag.

Basava C, Hostetler KY (1992a): In: *Peptides: Chemistry and Biology*, Proceedinga of the 12th American Peptide Symposium, Smith JA, Rivier JE, eds., pp. 20–22. Leiden: ESCOM.

Basava C, Hostetler KY (1992b): United States Patent: 5,175,146.

Bennett MM, Amara SG (1992): *Ann NY Acad Sci* 657:36–49.

Brewer HB, Jr., Ronan R (1969): *Proc Natl Acad Sci USA* 63(3):940–947.

Buck RH, Maxl F (1990): *J Pharm Biomed Anal* 8(8-12):761–769.

Byfield PG, McLoughlin JL, Matthews EW, MacIntyre I (1976): *FEBS Lett* 65(2):242–245.

Cardinaux F, Pless J, Buck RH (1988): United States Patent: 4,758,550.

Chestnut CH, III (1992): *Bone Miner* 16(3):211–212.

Copp DH (1992a): *Endocrinology* 131(3):1007–1008.

Copp DH (1992b): *Bone Miner* 16(3):157–159.

Copp DH, Cameron EC, Cheney BA, Davidson AGF, Heneze KG (1962): *Endocrinology* 70:638–639.

Deftos LJ, Roos B (1989): In: *Bone and Mineral Research*, Peck WA, ed., pp. 267–316. Amsterdam: Excerpta Medica.

Epand RM, Epand RF, Stafford AR, Orlowski RC (1988): *J Med Chem* 31(8):1595–1598.

Feyen JH, Cardinaux F, Gamse R, Bruns C, Azria M, Trechsel U (1992): *Biochem Biophys Res Commun* 187(1):8–13.

Foster GV, Baghdiantz A, Kumar MA, Slack E, Soliman HA, MacIntyre I (1964): *Nature (London)* 202:1303–1305.

Gennari C, Agnusdei D, Camporeale A (1991): *Calcif Tissue Int* 49(Suppl. 2):S9–S13.

Gorn AH, Lin HY, Yamin M, Auron PE, Flannery MR, Tapp DR, Manning CA, Lodish HF, Krane SM, Goldring SR (1992): *J Clin Invest* 90(5):1726–1735.

Grauer A, Raue F, Schneider HG, Frank-Raue K, Ziegler R (1990): *J Bone Miner Res*

5(4):387–391.

Guttman S (1981): In: *Calcitonin 1980*, Proceedings of the International Symposium, Pecile A, ed., pp. 11–24. Amsterdam: Excerpta Medica.

Homma T, Watanabe M, Hirose S, Kanai A, Kangawa K, Matsuo H (1986): *J Biochem (Tokyo)* 100(2):459–467.

Kanis JA, Johnell O, Gullberg B, Allander E, Dillsen G, Gennari C, Lopes Vaz AA, Lyritis GP, Mazzuoli G, Miravet L (1992): *Br Med J* 305(6862):1124–1128.

Kozono T, Hirata M, Endo K, Satoh K, Takanashi H, Miyauchi T, Fukushima N, Kumagai E, Abe S, Matsuda E (1992): *Endocrinology* 131(6):2885–2890.

Kumar MA, Slack E, Edwards A, Soliman HA, Baghdiantz A, Foster GV, MacIntyre I (1965): *J Endocrinol* 33:469–475.

Laurian L, Oberman Z, Graf E, Gilad S, Hoerer E, Simantov R (1986): *Horm Metab Res* 18(4):268–271.

Levy F, Muff R, Dotti-Sigrist S, Dambacher MA, Fischer JA (1988): *J Clin Endocrinol & Metab* 67(3):541–545.

Lin HY, Harris TL, Flannery MS, Aruffo A, Kaji EH, Gorn A, Kolakowski LF, Jr., Lodish HF, Goldring SR (1991): *Science* 254:102–124.

Ljunghall S, Gardsell P, Johnell O, Larsson K, Lindh E, Obrant K, Sernbo I (1991): *Calcif Tissue Int* 49(1):17–19.

Lyritis GP, Tsakalakos N, Magiasis B, Karachalios T, Yiatzides A, Tsekoura M (1991): *Calcif Tissue Int* 49(6):369-3-72.

MacIntyre I (1992): *Bone Miner* 16:160–161.

MacIntyre I, Alevizaki M, Bevis PJ, Zaidi M (1987): *Clin Orthop* (217):45–55.

Maier R (1976): *Calcif Tissue Res* 21(Suppl.):317–2013.

Maier R, Riniker B, Rittel W (1974): *FEBS Lett* 48(1):68–71.

Maier R, Kamber B, Riniker B, Rittel W (1975): *Horm Metab Res* 7(6):511–514.

Maier R, Kamber B, Riniker B, Rittel W (1976): *Clin Endocrinol* 5(Suppl.):327S–332S.

Maier R, Brugger M, Bruckner H, Kamber B, Riniker B, Rittel W (1977): *Acta Endocrinol (Copenhagen)* 85(1):102–108.

Martial K, Minvielle S, Jullienne A, Segond N, Milhaud G, Lasmoles F (1990): *Biochem Biophys Res Commun* 171(3):1111–1114.

Milhaud G (1992): *Bone Miner* 16(3):201–210.

Moe GR, Kaiser ET (1985): *Biochemistry* 24(8):1971–1976.

Mol JA, Kwant MM, Arnold IC, Hazewinkel HA (1991): *Regul Pept* 35(3):189–195.

Morikawa T, Munekata E, Sakakibara S, Noda T, Otani M (1976): *Experientia (Basel)* 32:1104–1106.

Muff R, Dambacher MA, Fischer JA (1991): *Osteoporos Int* 1(2):72–75.

Muff R, Dambacher MA, Perrenoud A, Simon C, Fischer JA (1990): *Am J Med* 89(2):181–184.

Neher R, Riniker B, Rittel W, Zuber H (1968): *Helv Chim Acta* 51(8):1900–1905.

Niall HD, Keutmann HT, Copp DH, Potts JT, Jr. (1969): *Proc Natl Acad Sci USA* 64(2):771–778.

Orlowski RC, Epand RM, Stafford AR (1987): *Eur J Biochem* 162(2):399–402.

Otani M, Yamauchi H, Meguro T, Kitazawa S, Watanabe S, Orimo H (1976): *J Biochem (Tokyo)* 79(2):345–352.

Overgaard K, Hansen MA, Nielsen VA, Riis BJ, Christiansen C (1990): *Am J Med* 89(1):1–6.

Potts JT, Jr. (1976): In: *Peptide Hormones*, Parsons JA, ed., p. 424. Baltimore: University Park Press.

Potts JT, Jr. (1992): *Bone Miner* 16(3):169–173.

Potts JT, Jr., Niall HD, Deftos LJ (1971): *Curr Top Exp Endocrinol* 1:151–173.

Potts JT, Jr., Niall HD, Keutmann HT, Lequin RM (1972): In: *Calcium, Parathyroid Hormone and the Calcitonin*, Talmage RV, Munson P, eds., pp. 121–127. Amsterdam: Excerpta Medica.

Potts JT, Jr., Niall HD, Keutmann HT, Brewer HB, Jr., Deftos LJ (1968): *Proc Natl Acad Sci USA* 59(4):1321–1328.

Raulais D, Hagaman J, Ontjes DA, Lundblad RL, Kingdon HS (1976): *Eur J Biochem* 64(2):607–611.

Reginster JY, Franchimont P (1985): *Clin Exp Rheumatol* 3(2):155–157.

Reginster JY, Denis D, Albert A, Franchimont P (1987): *Bone Miner* 2(2):133–140.

Reginster JY, Jeugmans-Huynen AM, Albert A, Denis D, Franchimont P (1988a): *J Bone Miner Res* 3(3):249–252.

Reginster JY, Denis D, Albert A, Deroisy R, Lecart MP, Fontaine MA, Lambelin P, Franchimont P (1988b): *Lancet* ii(8574):1481–1483.

Rosenfeld MG, Emeson RB, Yeakley JM, Merillat N, Hedjran F, Lenz J, Delsert C (1992): *Ann NY Acad Sci* 657:117.

Rosenfeld MG, Mermod JJ, Amara SG, Swanson LW, Sawchenko PE, Rivier J, Vale WW, Evans RM (1983): *Nature (London)* 304:129–135.

Sasayama Y, Suzuki N, Oguro C, Takei Y, Takahashi A, Watanabe TX, Nakajima K, Sakakibara S (1992): *Gen Comp Endocrinol* 86(2):269–274.

Sasayama Y, Ukawa K, KaiYa H, Oguro C, Takei Y, Watanabe TX, Nakajima K, Sakakibara S (1993): *Gen Comp Endocrinol* 89(2):189–194.

Singer FR (1991): *Calcif Tissue Int* 49(Suppl.)2:S7–S8.

Singer FR, Fredericks RS, Minkin C (1980): *Arthritis Rheum* 23(10):1148–1154.

Sturtridge WC, Kumar MA (1968): *J Endocrinol* 42:501–503.

Takei Y, Takahashi A, Watanabe TX, Nakajima K, Sakakibara S, Sasayama Y, Suzuki N, Oguro C (1991): *Biol Bull* 180:485–488.

Wimalawansa SJ (1993): *Calcif Tissue Int* 52(2):90–93.

Wisneski LA (1992): *Bone Miner* 16(3):213–216.

Yates AJ, Gutierrez GE, Garrett IR, Mencel JJ, Nuss GW, Schreiber AB, Mundy GR (1990): *Endocrinology* 126(6):2845–2849.

Zaidi M, Moonga BS, Bevis PJ, Bascal ZA, Breimer LH (1990): *Crit Rev Clin Lab Sci* 28(2):109–174.

Zaidi M, Moonga BS, Bevis PJ, Alam AS, Legon S, Wimalawansa S, MacIntyre I, Breimer LH (1991): *Vitam Horm* 46:87–164.

Zaidi M, Alam AS, Shankar VS, Bax BE, Bax CM, Moonga BS, Bevis PJ, Stevens C, Blake DR, Pazianas M (1993): *Biol Rev Cambr Philos Soc* 68(2):197–264.

Zanelli JM, Gaines-Das RE, Corran PH (1990): *Bone Miner* 11(1):1–17.

14

IMPORTANCE OF Ca²⁺-HORMONE INTERACTION IN CONFORMATION-ACTIVITY CORRELATIONS

Vettai S. Ananthanarayanan

Introduction

The enormous strides in peptide research made in the past few decades are the result of the pioneering efforts of scientists who foresaw the power of synthetic peptide chemistry in unravelling the structure–function correlations in peptide hormones. In this chapter, I present an overview of recent studies in my laboratory that address the question of the bioactive structures of peptide hormones.

The multifarious roles of Ca^{2+} in the living cell are often mediated by proteins that exhibit specific binding to this cation. This has led to a plethora of studies on Ca^{2+}-binding proteins and model peptides (Strynadka and James, 1989). Most of these studies concern aqueous systems, and thus our understanding of Ca^{2+} binding in a nonpolar milieu such as the lipid bilayer is meager. In the past few years, we have attempted to delineate the minimal conformational requirement for Ca^{2+} binding in nonpolar media through the use of short linear synthetic peptides (Ananthanarayanan et al., 1985, in press; Michel et al., 1992; Rehse, 1985). The results obtained formed the basis for our subsequent studies on the interaction of peptide hormones with Ca^{2+} and other divalent cations. These studies (Ananthanarayanan and Orlicky, 1992; Brimble and Ananthanarayanan,

Peptides: Design, Synthesis, and Biological Activity
Channa Basava and G. M. Anantharamaiah, Editors
©1994 *Birkhäuser Boston*

1992, 1993) brought out some very interesting aspects of hormone structures and hormone–receptor interactions (Ananthanarayanan, 1991) that we believe will be of use in the design of potent hormone analogs and in understanding the initial events in signal transduction by hormones.

Studies on Synthetic Peptide–Ca^{2+} Interactions

We selected the following proline-containing peptides that would facilitate the formation of a set of consecutive β-turns, a plausible template for Ca^{2+} binding (Vogt et al., 1979): tert-Boc-Pro-Gly-Ala-NHCH$_3$, Gly-Val-Pro-Gly-Val, tert-Boc-Pro-D-Ala-Ala-NHCH$_3$, and tert-Boc-Leu-Pro-Tyr-Ala-NHCH$_3$. Of these, the first two peptides are substrates and the third peptide an inhibitor of collagen prolyl hydroxylase (Atreya and Ananthanarayanan, 1991); the last peptide is a tyrosine kinase substrate (Tinker et al., 1988). As is to be expected, the β-turn conformation in these peptides was not significantly populated in aqueous media because of strong solvent–peptide interactions. This was consistent with the very weak binding of Ca^{2+} by these peptides in water as monitored by circular dichroism (CD) spectral changes (Ananthanarayanan et al., 1985; Rehse, 1985). [In addition to the flexiblity of the peptides, the relatively high degree of hydration of the Ca^{2+} ion (Sussman and Weinstein, 1989) would also prohibit these peptides from binding the cation in aqueous solutions.] However, in less polar solvents such as acetonitrile (ACN) and trifluoroethanol (TFE), all these peptides exhibited stoichiometric binding of Ca^{2+}, which was accompanied by substantial changes in the peptide conformation (Ananthanarayanan et al., 1985; Michel et al., 1992; Rehse, 1985).

Analysis of the binding isotherm indicated the 2:1 peptide–Ca^{2+} complex (known as the ion "sandwich" complex) as the dominant species in all cases. A preliminary study (Ananthanarayanan et al., 1985; Rehse, 1985) of the CD, ^{13}C- and ^{1}H NMR (nuclear magnetic resonance), and IR data on tert-Boc-Pro-Gly-Ala-NHCH$_3$ and tert-Boc-Pro-D-Ala-Ala-NHCH$_3$ indicated that, in each case, the free peptide adopted a consecutive β-turn. Ca^{2+} binding involved the breaking of the intramolecular hydrogen bonds and the reorientation of the peptide carbonyl groups so as to enable their liganding to the cation (Ananthanarayanan et al., 1985). In the resulting conformation the Xxx-Pro bond was all trans, in contrast to a mixture of cis and trans in the free peptide. Thus, Ca^{2+} binding appeared to significantly reduce the conformational freedom of the peptide. A detailed conformational study of the Pro-D-Ala peptide (Michel et al., 1992) using random search, energy minimization, and molecular dynamics procedures, revealed that among the low-energy conformers containing single and consecutive β-turns in the peptide the latter group had the proper orientation of three carbonyl oxygens conducive to the formation of a stable 2:1 Ca^{2+}–peptide sandwich

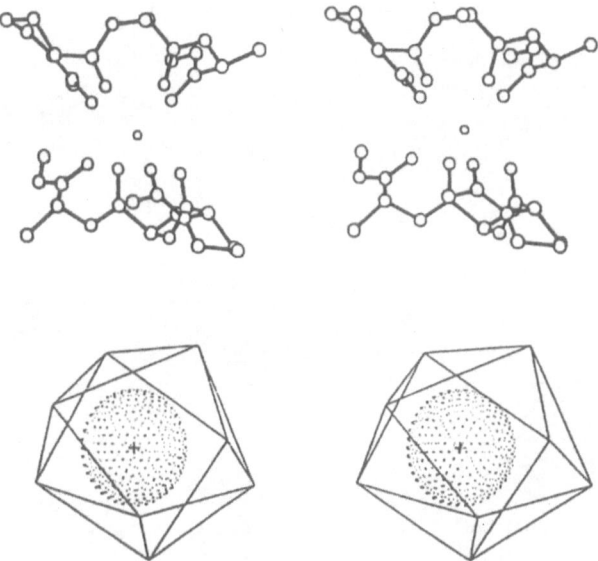

Figure 14-1. Stereoviews of sandwich complex between *N*-acetyl-L-Pro-D-Ala-L-Ala-NHCH₃ and Ca²⁺. Upper part: peptide geometry; lower part: slightly distorted octahedral geometry of Ca²⁺ coordination. Oxygen atoms occupy corners of octahedron. (Reprinted with permission of Adenine Press from Michel et al., 1992.)

complex. The dynamics of the complex formation resulted in a conformational rearrangement leading to an 8-coordinated dodecahedral Ca²⁺ complex (Figure 14–1). The energetically facile interconvertibility among the different β-turn conformers in the free peptide was found to shift the equilibrium in favor of the consecutive β-turn during the cation-complexing process.

Detailed ¹H NMR studies have since been carried out on *tert*-Boc-Pro-D-Ala-Ala-NHCH₃ (Saint-Jean et al., 1992, and unpublished data) and on *tert*-Boc-Leu-Pro-Tyr-Ala-NHCH₃ (Ananthanarayanan et al., in press) using two-dimensional NOESY and ROESY methods to obtain *inter*proton distances and an energy minimization program that utilized the NOESY-derived distance constraints. The results confirmed our earlier suggestion (Ananthanarayanan et al., 1985) and recent calculations (Michel et al., 1992) that the optimum conformation is one in which Ca²⁺ is sandwiched between two peptide molecules (Figure 14–2). Such sandwich complexes have so far been characterized only in the case of cyclic peptides such as cyclo(Pro-Gly)₃ in water (Kartha et al., 1982) and cyclo(Ala-Leu-Pro-Gly)₂ in acetonitrile (Jois et al., 1992).

In the sandwich complex, the cation is held in the polar interior of the complex, whose exterior surface is largely composed of the nonpolar side

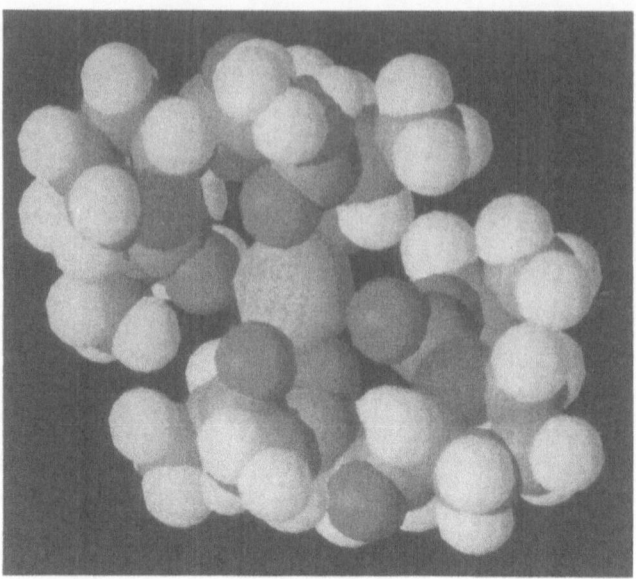

Figure 14-2. Space-filled model of "sandwich" Ca^{2+} complex of *tert*-Boc-Leu-Pro-Tyr-Ala-NHCH$_3$ obtained by Monte Carlo method of random structure generation followed by energy minimization.

chain groups. This prompted us to investigate the suitability of such a molecule as a carrier of Ca^{2+} across synthetic bilayer vesicles. Large unilamellar vesicles (LUV) of dimyristoylphosphatidylcholine (DMPC), containing the Ca^{2+}-sensitive dye Arsenazo III trapped within them, were employed for this purpose (Sokolove and Kester, 1989). The results obtained with the foregoing synthetic peptides demonstrated that all acted as Ca^{2+} ionophores, albeit to different extents (Ananthanarayanan and Porter, 1988, also, unpublished data; Shastri et al., 1986). Their efficacy as ionophores was, however, much less when compared to that of well-known Ca^{2+} ionophores such as A23187.

Studies on Hormone–Ca^{2+} Interactions

Our studies on synthetic peptides illustrated that Ca^{2+} binding by linear peptides is a thermodynamically favorable process in low dielectric media such as nonpolar solvents (used in the binding studies) and lipids (used in the transport studies), and that the conformational prerequisite for binding is a flexible structure such as [but not necessarily (Michel et al., 1992)] the β-turn. Anticipating peptide hormones as the possible biological counterparts of the synthetic peptides, we initiated the study of their interaction with Ca^{2+}. It is well known that in general, peptide hormones adopt structures in aqueous solvents that represent an ensemble of many different conformations rather than a unique structure (Rose et al., 1985). One of these conformations has been suggested to be the β-turn (Rose et al., 1985). Transfer to nonpolar media such as detergent micelles and lipids often stabilizes the β-turn or α-helix-like (including 3_{10} helical) conformations in these hormones (Wooley and Deber, 1987). These latter structures are considered to be more relevant to the bioactive conformations of the hormones than the structures prevalent in water.

Using TFE or TFE-ACN mixtures as a mimic of the lipid environment (Gronenborn et al., 1987) (see following), we measured the CD and fluorescence spectral changes in several peptide hormones caused by their interaction with Ca^{2+}. The hormones were ACTH(1–10), bombesin, bradykinin, Leu-enkephalin, Met-enkephalin, D-Met²-Pro⁵-enkephalin, glucagon, gonadotropin-releasing hormone (GnRH), insulin, kentsin, oxytocin, and substance P. The data showed that although hormones like kentsin and oxytocin formed a 2:1 peptide:Ca^{2+} sandwich complex (as observed in the case of the synthetic peptides described earlier), others formed 1:1 [e.g., ACTH(1–10), bombesin] or 1:2 (e.g., substance P, GnRH) peptide-Ca^{2+} complexes. The estimated binding constants for Ca^{2+} binding lay in the 10^4 M^{-1} range.

Ca²⁺-Binding Domains in Hormones

Details of the Ca^{2+}-binding and ionophoretic characteristics of substance P, glucagon, insulin, bombesin, and GnRH have been examined in our recent studies; these are summarized here. Substance P showed negligible cation binding in water. However, in an 80:20 (vol/vol) mixture of ACN and TFE, the hormone underwent dramatic CD (Figure 14–3) and fluorescence spectral changes (Ananthanarayanan and Orlicky, 1992), indicating a significant conformational change. Mg^{2+} binding was also observed but was relatively weaker. A biphasic binding curve for Ca^{2+} was observed that suggested two independent Ca^{2+}-binding domains in the hormone molecule. Using synthesized fragments of the hormone, one of these domains was identified to be the C-terminal region spanning residues 7 to 11. This fragment and the intact hormone elicited the influx of Ca^{2+} into DMPC vesicles while an N-terminal fragment 1–6 did not (Ananthanarayanan and Orlicky, 1992). With the 7–11 peptide, a large part of the Ca^{2+} influx occurred from membrane leak and fusion. The intact hormone thus seems to attenuate the membrane-disrupting effect of the C-terminal domain while still retaining the ability for ion transport. Interestingly, much of the biological activity of substance P seems to reside in the C-terminal 7–11 fragment

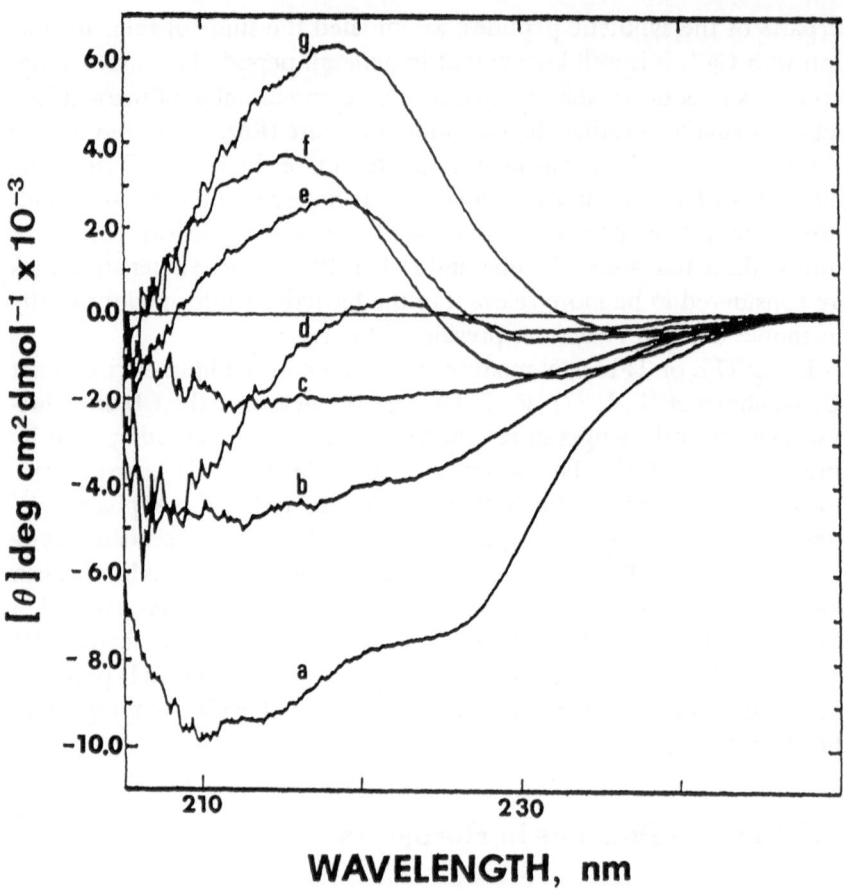

Figure 14-3. CD spectra of substance P (0.45–0.65 mM) at 25°±0.1°C in (a) 80:20 (vol/vol) ACN:TFE; (b) TFE with 2 M excess $Mg(ClO_4)_2$; (c) 100% TFE; (d) water; (d) 80:20 (vol/vol) ACN:TFE with 2 M excess $Ca(ClO_4)_2$; (f) TFE with 2 M excess $Mg(ClO_4)_2$ followed by 2 M excess $Ca(ClO_4)_2$; (g) TFE with 2 M excess $Ca(ClO_4)_2$. (Reprinted with permission of John Wiley & Sons, Inc. from Ananthanarayanan and Orlicky, 1992.)

(Stavropoulos et al., 1991). Such a *regiospecific localization* of Ca^{2+} binding and bioactivity was also observed in the case of glucagon and insulin.

In glucagon, the C-terminal 19–29 region, which exhibits some of the hormone activities in vivo (Blache et al., 1990), contained both the two Ca^{2+}-binding sites that we observed in the parent hormone in a 98% TFE:water mixture (Brimble and Ananthanarayanan, 1993). Ca^{2+} binding altered the helix content and tertiary structure of the hormone and the 19–29 fragment as monitored by CD and fluorescence, respectively (Figure 14-4). It is interesting to note that Tb^{3+}, a Ca^{2+} mimic with higher binding affinity, caused a CD change in glucagon in TFE similar to that of Ca^{2+} and

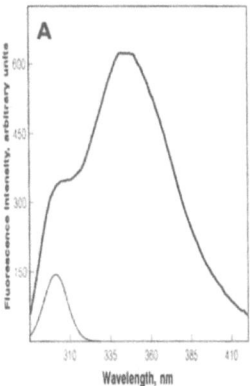
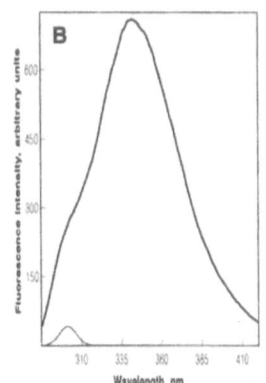
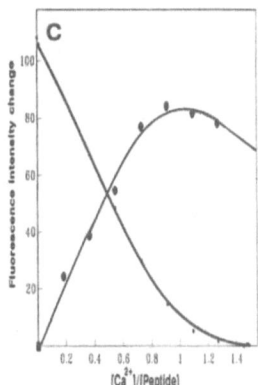

Figure 14–4. Fluorescence emission spectra and analysis at 22±1°C of glucagon (44 μM) in 98% TFE (excitation: 270 nm): (**A**) (heavy line), emission spectra of free peptide; (single line), contribution from tyrosine residue; (**B**) (heavy line), emission spectra of the peptide with equimolar CaCl₂; (single line), contribution from tyrosine; (**C**) Ca²⁺-binding isotherms obtained by using individual tryptophan (–·–) and tyrosine (–●–) contributions to observed emission spectra. (Reprinted with permission from Brimble and Ananthanarayanan, 1993. Copyright 1993, American Chemical Society.)

a much more enhanced CD change in water than did Ca²⁺ (Brimble and Ananthanarayanan, unpublished data). Both peptides translocated Ca²⁺ in the synthetic liposome system (Figure 14–5). Molecular modeling of the 19–29 glucagon fragment in the free and Ca²⁺-bound forms was carried out using a Monte Carlo generation of random conformations and subsequent energy minimization (Figure 14–6).

In the case of insulin, the B-chain has been shown to have a Ca²⁺-binding site (Hill et al., 1991). It also exhibits independent bioactivity and has been identified as the signal transducing region of insulin (Mirmira et al., 1991). We found that the B-chain and the intact hormone, but not the A-chain, caused Ca²⁺ transport in DMPC and egg lecithin vesicles (Brimble and Ananthanarayanan, 1992); the latter contained Fura-2 as the Ca²⁺-influx monitoring dye (Figure 14–7).

Our current studies on bombesin (Saint-Jean and Ananthanarayanan, 1993) augment this trait of the "domain structure" in hormones. While this hormone exhibited a nearly random coil structure in water, it showed a tranferred NOE ¹H NMR spectrum in the presence of large unilamellar vesicles of DMPC. Comparison with the NOESY data obtained in TFE showed that the hormone adopts a predominantly α-helical structure in this solvent and when it is bound to the lipid bilayer. This justified the use of TFE as a membrane mimetic in our detailed spectral studies on this and other hormones. Ca²⁺ binding appears to be confined to the C-terminal

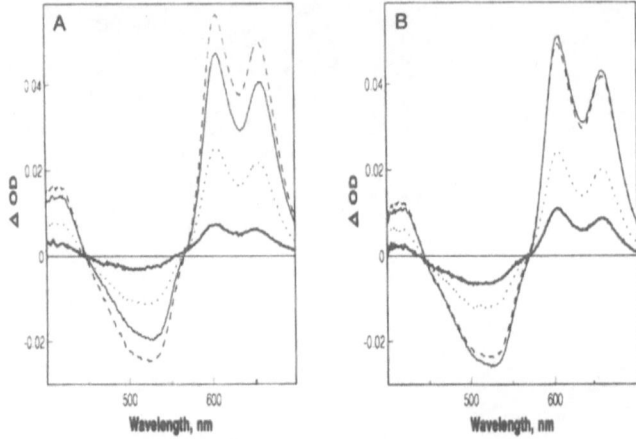

Figure 14–5. Ca^{2+} influx into DMPC LUV (3.5 µmol) measured using the Arsenazo III technique at 37°±1°C. Sample cuvette contained LUV containing 3.6 mM Arsenazo III incubated with 3.5 mM external CaCl$_2$ and 30 µM (24 nmol in 0.8 ml) of either (**A**) glucagon or (**B**) glucagon 19–29 fragment at pH 7.2; reference cuvette contained all components except peptide. Difference spectra were recorded at (heavy line), 2 min; (dotted line), 5 min; (dashed line), 12 min; and (single line), after addition of EDTA (final concentration, 5.0 mM), 13 min. (Reprinted with permission from Brimble and Ananthanarayanan, 1993. Copyright 1993, American Chemical Society)

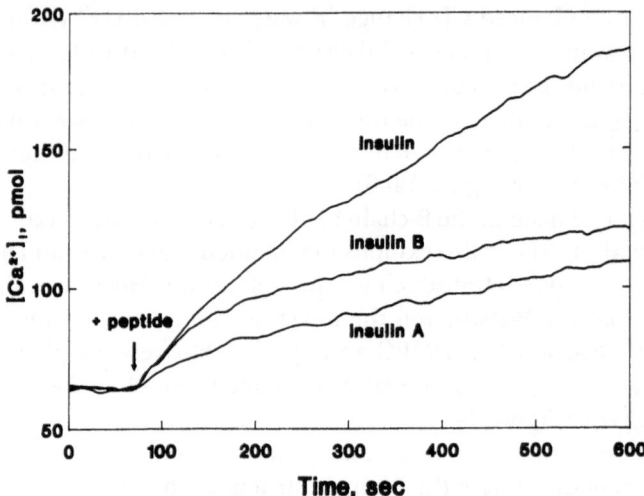

Figure 14–6. Insulin-mediated Ca^{2+} transport monitored by the fura-2 method using egg PC MLV at 20°C containing 100 µM fura-2 in 10 mM Hepes (pH 7.2) and 145 mM KCl. External Ca^{2+}, 2.0 mM); fluorescence emission wavelength, 510 nm. Excitation spectra shown correspond to (a) 30 µM insulin, 10 min; (b) 10 nM A23187, 10 min; (c) 30 µM insulin + EGTA (final concentration, 5 mM), 10 min; (d) 10 nM A23187 + EGTA, 10 min; (e) Ca^{2+}-free fura-2, (f) Ca^{2+}-bound fura-2. (Reprinted with permission of Elsevier Science Publishers BV from Brimble and Ananthanarayanan, 1992.)

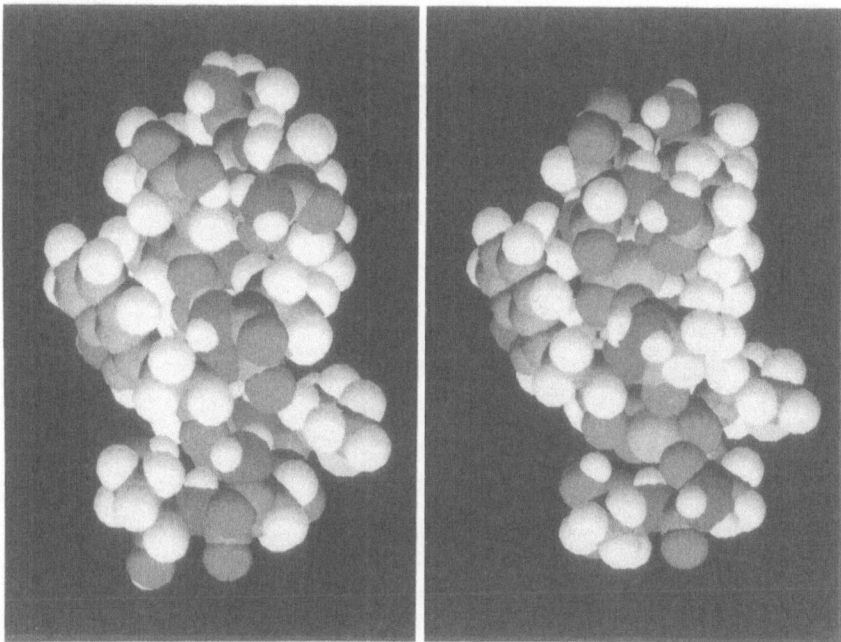

Figure 14-7. Molecular models of 19–29 peptide fragment of glucagon (left) and its Ca²⁺ complex (right) obtained by energy minimization. A BioGraf program (Molecular Simulations, Inc., Massachusetts) was used.

part of this hormone (Broccardo et al., 1975). Interestingly, this region shows amino acid composition identity to the C-terminal parts of glucagon, substance P, and a few other hormones. These hormones presumably, share a common Ca²⁺-binding motif.

Structure–Activity Correlation in Peptide Hormones

The results just described revealed a hitherto unrecognized common property among peptide hormones, namely, their interaction with Ca²⁺ in the lipid milieu. This shared characteristic led us to propose that the bioactive conformation of a peptide hormone would be its Ca²⁺-bound form (Ananthanarayanan, 1991). The latter would specify a unique conformation of the hormone that is recognized by its membrane-bound receptor (in contrast to an ensemble of flexible conformations prevailing in the free hormone). In this context, the Ca²⁺ ionophoretic character of the hormones may be viewed as indicating their ability to interact with their receptors (often inside the membrane interior regions) with the bound Ca²⁺ ion.

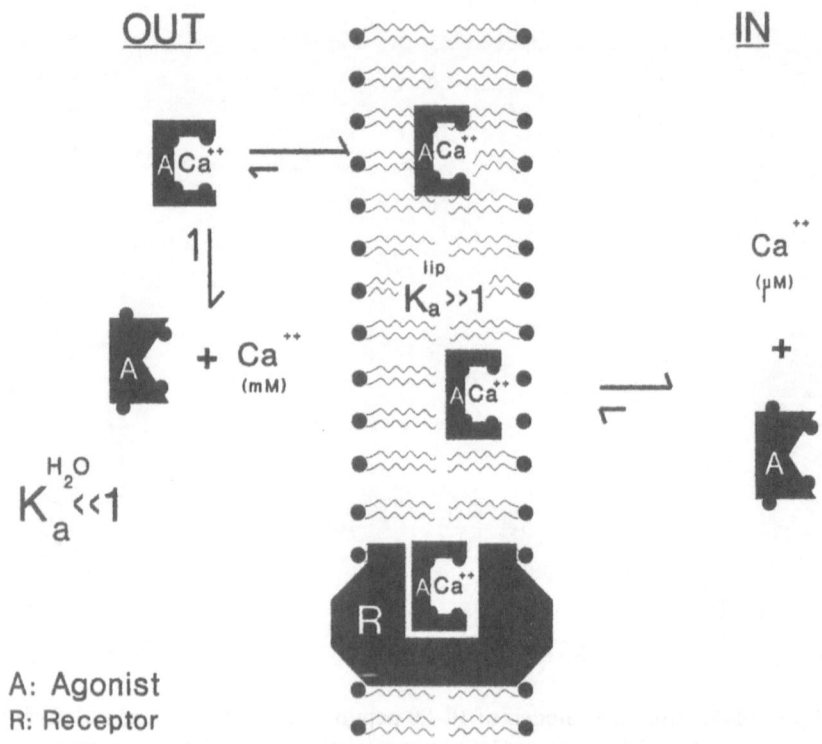

Figure 14–8. Scheme for agonist-mediated transport of polar Ca^{2+} ion through the nonpolar cell membrane. The agonist is shown as undergoing a conformational change on calcium binding; this is shown as involving enhancement of agonist amphiphilicity. Dark circles on agonist surface represent polar liganding groups; K_a refers to association constant. Variations of this scheme (for example, partitioning of the agonist into the lipid before cation binding) are possible. In the presence of a receptor (not shown), Ca^{2+} translocation by the agonist will be intercepted by the receptor. (Reprinted with permission of National Research Council of Canada from Ananthanarayanan, 1991.)

We have further proposed (Ananthanarayanan, 1991) and obtained some evidence (Ananthanarayanan and Horne, 1990) that the receptors, on their part, would also interact with Ca^{2+} such that the ion becomes an essential cofactor in the receptor–hormone interaction. We suggest a generalized model for a Ca^{2+}-mediated interaction of agonists with receptors whereby the "delivery" of Ca^{2+} by the hormone to the receptor would cause a conformational change in the latter that would be the first step in signal transduction. Figure 14–8 shows a schematic representation of our proposal. The generality of this model is indicated by our results on other agonists such as chemotactic peptides (B. Pathinathan and V. S. Ananthanarayanan, unpublished data) and drug molecules (Ananthanarayanan et al., 1993b; Tetreault and Ananthanarayanan, 1993) that bind and translocate Ca^{2+} in our model systems.

Current and future studies in our laboratory are designed to examine, in detail: (a) the correlation of observed bioactivities in a series of hormone analogs with their respective Ca^{2+}-binding abilities, and (b) the role of Ca^{2+} in the in vitro and in vivo interaction of the ligand-binding regions of specific receptors with the respective hormones. With regard to the first objective, it is gratifying to note that, in a series of GnRH agonists, interaction with Ca^{2+} parallels their bioactivities; in contrast, antagonists of the hormone do not bind Ca^{2+} appreciably (Ananthanarayanan and Salehian, 1993). Such a structure-based distinction of GnRH analogs has not been possible by other means (Karten and Rivier, 1986). With respect to the second goal, we have obtained evidence for the requirement of extracellular Ca^{2+} for the interaction of insulin with its receptor in a frog oocyte in vivo system (Vassilakos et al., in manuscript).

Acknowledgments

It is a pleasure to recall my association with Dr. Sivanandiah and his colleagues during the past many years. (I still distinctly remember traveling in the early years from the Indian Institute of Science to Dr. Sivandaiah's laboratory at Central College on a "scooter" to carry out peptide syntheses that required the nasty phosgene gas.) I thank my colleagues in my laboratory who have contributed to the experimental studies referred to in this chapter. The studies presented here were supported by the Medical Research Council of Canada.

REFERENCES

Ananthanarayanan VS (1991): *Biochem Cell Biol* 69:93–95.
Ananthanarayanan VS, Horne C (1990): In: *Peptides. Chemistry, Structure and Biology*, Rivier JE, Marshall GR, eds., pp. 527–532. Leiden: Escom.
Ananthanarayanan VS, Orlicky S (1992): *Biopolymers* 32:1765–1773.
Ananthanarayanan VS, Porter R (1988): In: *Advances in Gene Technology, Protein Engineering and Production*, Vol. 8, ICSU Short Reports, Brew K et al., eds., pp. 216–217. New York: IRL Press.
Ananthanarayanan VS, Saint-Jean A, Cheesman B, Hughes DW, Bain A: *J Biomol Struct Dyn* (in press).
Ananthanarayanan VS, Salehian O (1993a): Poster presentation at the 13th American Peptide Symposium, Edmonton, Canada.
Ananthanarayanan VS, Tetreault S, Saint-Jean A (1993b): *J Med Chem* 36:1324–1332.
Ananthanarayanan VS, Attah-Poku SK, Mukkamala PL, Rehse PH (1985): *J Biosci Suppl* 8:209–221.

Atreya PL, Ananthanarayanan VS (1991): *J Biol Chem* 266:2852–2858.

Blache P, Kervran A, Dufour M, Martinez J, Le-Nguyen D, Lotersztajn S, Pavoine C, Pecker F, Bataille D (1990): *J Biol Chem* 265:21514–21519.

Brimble KS, Ananthanarayanan VS (1992): *Biochim Biophys Acta* 1105:319–327.

Brimble KS, Ananthanarayanan VS (1993): *Biochemistry* 32:1632–1640.

Broccardo M, Falconieri GE, Melchiorri P, Negri L, De Castiglione R (1975): *Br J Pharmacol* 55:221–227.

Gronenborn AM, Bovermann G, Marius CG (1987): *FEBS Lett* 215:88–94.

Hill CP, Dauter Z, Dodson EJ, Dodson GG, Dunn MF (1991): *Biochemistry* 30:917–924.

Jois DSS, Easwaran KRK, Bednarek M, Blout ER (1992): *Biopolymers* 32:993–1001.

Karten M, Rivier J (1986): *Endocr Rev* 7:44–66.

Kartha G, Varughese KL, Aimoto S (1982): *Proc Natl Acad Sci USA* 79:4519–4522.

Michel A, Jeandenans C, Ananthanarayanan VS (1992): *J Biomol Struct & Dyn* 10:281–293.

Mirmira RG, Nakagawa SH, Tager HS (1991): *J Biol Chem* 266:1428–1436.

Rehse PH (1985): *Synthesis and Conformational Studies on Proline-Containing Peptides: Ion Binding by Linear Tetrapeptides.* Master's thesis, Memorial University of Newfoundland, St. John's, Newfoundland, Canada.

Rose GD, Gierasch LM, Smith JA (1985): *Adv Protein Chem* 37:1–109.

Saint-Jean A, Cheesman B, Ananthanarayanan VS (1992): In: *Peptides: Chemistry and Biology*, Smith JA, Rivier JE, eds. Leiden: Escom.

Saint-Jean A, Ananthanarayanan VS (1993): Poster presentation at the 13th American Peptide Symposium, Edmonton, Canada.

Shastri BP, Rehse PH, Attah-Poku SK, Ananthanarayanan VS (1986): *FEBS Lett* 200:58–62.

Sokolove PM, Kester MB (1989): *Anal Biochem* 177:402–406.

Stavropoulos G, Karagiannis K, Cordopatis P, Hall D, Gilon C, Bar-Akiva G, Selinger Z, Chorev M (1991): *Int J Pept Protein Res* 37:180–184.

Strynadka NCJ, James MNG (1989): *Annu Rev Biochem* 58:951–998.

Sussman F, Weinstein H (1989): *Proc Natl Acad Sci USA* 86:7880–7884.

Tetreault S, Ananthanarayanan VS (1993): *J Med Chem* 36:1017–1023.

Tinker DA, Krebs EG, Feltham IC, Attah-Poku SK, Ananthanarayanan VS (1988): *J Biol Chem* 263:5024–5026.

Vogt H-P, Strassburger W, Wollmer A, Fleischhauer J, Bullard B, Mercola D (1979): *J Theor Biol* 76:297–310.

Wooley GA, Deber CM (1987): *Biopolymers* 26:S109–S121.

IV

OTHER BIOLOGICALLY ACTIVE PEPTIDES

VI

Other Biologically
Active Peptides

15

THE BINDING OF PEPTIDES AND PROTEINS TO MEMBRANES CONTAINING ANIONIC LIPID

Marian Mosior and Richard M. Epand

Introduction

The interaction of proteins with lipids is one of the central problems of membrane biophysics. Of particular interest is that some proteins require a distinct category of lipids for their function. For example, several functionally related groups of proteins that interact preferentially with acidic lipids were discovered in recent years. They include vitamin K-dependent blood coagulation proteins (Jackson and Nemerson, 1980), annexins (Geisow et al., 1987), calpactins (Glenney, 1986), synexins (Creutz et al., 1983), the protein kinase C family (Nishizuka, 1989), and actin-severing or actin-capping proteins (Stossel, 1989). Many other proteins, particularly enzymes, also require acidic lipids for activation (Cornell, 1991; Enyedi et al., 1987; Moritz et al., 1992). There are excellent reviews available on many of the particular groups of proteins that interact with acidic lipids (Geisow et al., 1987; Glenney, 1986; Jackson and Nemerson, 1980; Stossel, 1989). Therefore, we decided to focus this chapter on the roles played by acidic lipids in lipid–protein interactions. For the sake of clarity, we used a limited number of examples to describe the four distinct functions performed by acidic lipids. We also review recent models of the mechanism of acidic lipid–protein interaction.

Peptides: Design, Synthesis, and Biological Activity
Channa Basava and G. M. Anantharamaiah, Editors
©1994 *Birkhäuser Boston*

Apparent Increase of Protein Affinity for Membrane

Association of positively charged molecules with the membrane can be significantly increased by the nonspecific accumulation of these molecules at the membrane–solution interface by the electrostatic potential of the membrane produced by acidic lipids. The Gouy–Chapman theory provides an accurate description of the electrostatic properties of a membrane containing monovalent acidic lipids (reviewed by McLaughlin, 1989). This theory has been confirmed by a variety of experimental techniques (Cafiso et al., 1989), and its essential features have remained unaltered with the appearance of more sophisticated theories (Carnie et al., 1984; Langner et al., 1990). The magnitude of the electrostatic potential of the membrane depends on the surface charge density as well as on the valency and concentration of ions in solution (McLaughlin, 1977, 1989). At physiological concentrations of KCl and at the mole percent of acidic lipids in the cytoplasmic side of the plasma membrane, the surface potential of the model membrane is approximately equal to -30 mV (McLaughlin, 1989). As predicted by the Gouy–Chapman theory, the electrostatic potential decays approximately exponentially with the distance from the membrane (Langner et al., 1990; McLaughlin, 1989). This decay is characterized by the Debye length, the distance at which the potential decreases e-fold, where e is the base of the natural logarithm. The Debye length is equal to about 1 nm when the concentration of monovalent salts is 0.1 M. The concentration of ions at any given distance from the membrane is linked to the electrostatic potential via the Boltzmann distribution. Hence, for a surface potential of -30 mV, the concentration of divalent cations at the interface is 10 fold higher than that in the bulk solution (McLaughlin, 1977). Tetravalent cations such as gentamicin or spermine are concentrated 100 fold by the same potential (Chung et al., 1985).

Not only do inorganic cations accumulate at the membrane interface, but there is also a nonspecific accumulation by the electrostatic potential of peptides including model peptides (Kim et al., 1991; Mosior and McLaughlin, 1992a), toxins (Beschiaschvili and Seelig, 1990), neuropeptides (Seelig and Macdonald, 1989), and peptide sequences derived from proteins (Mosior and McLaughlin, 1991; Rebecchi et al., 1992). One of the most thoroughly studied examples is melittin, the main component of bee venom. Melittin is a cationic peptide that adopts the conformation of an amphipathic helix in the presence of lipid. This peptide binds to the phospholipid membrane by orienting its hydrophobic face toward the hydrocarbon core of the membrane (Stanislawski and Ruterjans, 1987). When melittin binds to a membrane composed of zwitterionic lipids, its positive charges produce an electrostatic potential that repels other molecules of the peptide from the membrane (Kuchinka and Seelig, 1989). In contrast, when anionic lipids are included in the membrane, the initial affinity of melittin toward the membrane increases significantly (Beschiaschvili and Seelig, 1990). In both cases, however, the binding of the peptide to the membrane could be characterized by a single partitioning constant, if the concentration of melittin at the interface were calculated by means of the Gouy–Chapman theory and the Boltzmann distribution (Beschiaschvili and Seelig, 1990; Kuchinka and Seelig, 1989).

Substance P, a neuropeptide abundant in the nervous system, binds very weakly to membranes composed of zwitterionic lipids, with an association constant of 1 M^{-1}. Under physiological conditions, its binding to membranes containing anionic lipids increases by three orders of magnitude. The combination of the Gouy–Chapman theory with the Boltzmann distribution accounted, with a good accuracy, for the binding isotherms of this peptide to the phospholipid bilayer (Seelig and Macdonald, 1989). In light of the very weak association of substance P with electrically neutral membranes, the nonspecific accumulation of this neuropeptide in the layer immediately adjacent to anionic membrane surfaces indicates the critical role of the electrostatic potential in determining the partitioning of this peptide into the membrane. Such an interaction may have a physiological role, because the association of substance P with the lipid portion of the postsynaptic membrane has been postulated to be a prerequisite for its subsequent interaction with its specific receptor (Schwyzer, 1987).

Most proteins bear a net negative charge at physiological pH, so they would be repelled rather than attracted to the membrane by the electrostatic potential produced by acidic lipids. However, the linear dimensions of a 100-kDa protein are an order of magnitude larger than the Debye length. It is likely, then, that even protein with an overall negative charge could orient itself as a dipole and a positively charged domain could be attracted by the negative potential of the membrane. The evidence supporting this speculation has yet to be found. The studies on the proteins like myristoylated alanine-rich-kinase C substrate (MARCKS), neuromodulin, and neurogranin, all of which contain a large, well-defined, positively charged domain, can elucidate the role of electrostatic potential in protein–lipid interactions (Mosior and McLaughlin, 1992a).

The electrostatic potential produced by acidic lipids can exert a less direct effect on protein–membrane interactions through the nonspecific accumulation of Ca^{2+} or other biologically relevant cations in the layer immediately adjacent to the interface. Bazzi and Nelsestuen (1991a, 1991b) presented evidence that annexins and protein kinase C constitute a new family of Ca^{2+}-binding proteins. The high stoichiometry binding of Ca^{2+} to these proteins occurred only in membrane–protein complexes. They concluded that the binding of Ca^{2+} occurs only at the lipid–protein interface. The binding of PKC to the membrane indeed depends on the interfacial concentration of Ca^{2+} (Mosior and Epand, unpublished observations).

Reduction of Dimensionality

The rate of collisions between molecules is a primary factor determining the kinetics of chemical reactions. The low concentrations of the molecules involved in the chemical reactions occurring in living matter require special devices to assure fast rates of reaction. Adam and Delbrück (1968) developed the concept of the reduction of dimensionality in the diffusion-regulated processes occurring at various levels of organization in living matter. They proposed that the diffusion of molecules to membrane-bound receptors can occur in two stages. First, a molecule diffuses freely over a short distance in three-dimensional space in solution and then adsorbs to a surface containing another kind of molecule participating in the reaction. In the second stage, the adsorbed molecule diffuses on the surface of the membrane, colliding freely with the molecules embedded therein. As one of the examples, Adam and Delbrück (1968) considered an enzymatic reaction occurring on the membrane surface. They showed that the mean diffusion time required for the substrate to meet its target enzyme was much shorter if the substrate diffusion was divided into two stages, that is, a three-dimensional stage and a two-dimensional stage, than if diffusion occurred only in three dimensions. This particular mechanism of diffusion, termed reduction of dimensionality, was suggested for a number of molecules binding to specific receptors in membranes. Substance P, discussed in the previous paragraph, may serve as an example. The binding of this neuropeptide to the lipid component of the postsynaptic membrane is likely to be a prerequisite for its subsequent binding to a specific receptor (Schwyzer, 1987).

Anionic lipids can function for membrane-binding proteins in a manner analogous to the way membrane receptors act toward their specific ligands. The binding of proteins to acidic lipids can also reduce the dimensionality of subsequent protein–protein interactions. The proteins of the blood coagulation cascade appear to constitute a good example of this phenomenon. Binding of the blood coagulation proteins to anionic lipids, chiefly phosphatidylserine (PS), initiates the formation of a fibrin clot. The enzymatic conversion of prothrombin to the active serine protease, thrombin, is a key event in this process (Jackson and Nemerson, 1980; Mann et al., 1990). Thrombin production can occur at slow rates in solution; however, the translocation to the membrane surface of all proteins required for this process speeds the enzymatic reactions by orders of magnitude (Mann et al., 1990) and allows for rapid cascade amplification. Prothrombin and several other proteins involved in the fibrin clot formation, such as factors V, VIII, IX, and X, bind to acidic lipids in the presence of Ca^{2+} (Jackson and Nemerson, 1980). All these proteins enclose a highly homologous domain containing 9–12 γ-carboxyglutamic acid (Gla) residues (Furie and Furie, 1988; Tulinsky et al., 1988). These domains have been shown to bind to model membranes composed of a mixture of anionic and zwitterionic lipids with characteristics similar to those of the proteins from which they were obtained (Dombrose et al., 1979; Pearce et al., 1992).

The binding of these proteins to acidic lipids occurs presumably through the Ca^{2+}-mediated interaction of Gla residues with the headgroups of acidic lipids (Dombrose et al., 1979; Lim et al., 1977). Lentz and co-workers (Jones and Lentz, 1986) have shown that the binding of prothrombin and factor X to the phospholipid bilayer does not cause any extensive aggregation of acidic lipid in the membrane. They concluded that there are only a few binding sites specific for acidic lipids on each of these proteins. The fit of their theoretical model to the experimental data was consistent with three or four binding sites for acidic lipids on prothrombin and factor X (Cutsforth et al., 1989). Prothrombin has a few specific high-affinity binding sites for Ca^{2+} and some additional lower affinity sites that have less specificity toward divalent cations (Bloom and Mann, 1978; Wei et al., 1982). The binding of divalent cations to prothrombin was postulated as a mechanism of activation through the change of conformation of this proenzyme (Borowski et al., 1986). Rosing et al. (1988) reported that the binding of divalent cations to prothrombin is not a necessary condition for its activation. They showed that prothrombin can bind to membranes containing positively charged lipids like stearylamine in the absence of divalent cations. Such membranes also activated prothrombin in the presence of the factor Xa–Va complex. Prothrombin derivatives lacking the Gla domain neither bound to these membranes nor were converted into thrombin. These results strongly suggested that the reduction of dimensionality is a primary factor in the activation of the blood coagulation cascade.

Protein kinase C (PKC) is an important regulatory enzyme that has been implicated in the control of differentiation, mitogenesis, tumorigenesis, and many other cellular processes (for reviews, see Lester and Epand, 1992; Nishizuka, 1989). In cells, PKC is activated by two second messengers, Ca^{2+} and diacylglycerol; the latter can be substituted by a phorbol ester (Ashendel, 1985). Association of PKC substrates with membranes was found to be a prerequisite of the effective phosphorylation by the enzyme (Bazzi and Nelsestuen, 1987). At least a few of the in vivo substrates of PKC, such as MARCKS (Thelen et al., 1991), neuromodulin, neurogranin (Houbre et al., 1991), and myosin I (Swanljung-Collins and Collins, 1991), are membrane bound before the phosphorylation. In vitro studies have shown that acidic lipids are a necessary cofactor in the activation of PKC by membranes (Lester and Epand, 1992; Nishizuka, 1989). Further, the activation of PKC by acidic lipids exhibits a threshold with respect to their mole percent in the membrane, having highly sigmoidal characteristics (Newton and Koshland, 1989). PKC binding to acidic lipids alone is too weak to cause translocation of the enzyme to the membrane in the absence of other activating components (Mosior and Epand, 1993). However, anionic lipids are necessary for PKC–membrane association, at least at the physiological Ca^{2+}

level (Bazzi and Nelsestuen, 1992; Mosior and Epand, 1993). The binding of PKC to acidic lipids plays an important role in the reduction of the dimensionality. Although the activation of PKC coincides with the binding of the enzyme to the membrane (Mosior and Epand, 1993), the rate of phosphorylation catalyzed by the enzyme depends also on many other factors, as discussed next.

Regulation of Physiological Processes

Transient binding of proteins to acidic lipids in the membrane activates or inhibits several physiologically relevant processes. The best known example is activation of the cascade of blood coagulation proteins by the translocation of the acidic lipid phosphatidylserine from the inner to the outer leaflet of the plasma membrane of stimulated platelets (Jackson and Nemerson, 1980). We discussed the plausible binding mechanism of prothrombin and other vitamin K-dependent proteins to membranes in the previous section. Prothrombin and other proteins containing the Gla domain exhibit a sigmoidal dependence of the binding to the membrane on the mole percent acidic lipid (Cutsforth et al., 1989). Hence, the physiologically relevant translocation of these proteins to the membrane and the subsequent formation of a fibrin clot can occur only when the mole percent PS in the outer leaflet of the membrane increases above a certain threshold level. We discuss a possible mechanism of this phenomenon in the next section.

Polyphosphoinositides constitute a class of phospholipids implicated in the regulation of a variety of cellular processes through the second messenger system (Berridge and Irvine, 1984). In this chapter we examine another case in which the direct binding of proteins to phosphoinositides regulates the polymerization state of actin. A number of actin-severing or actin-capping proteins have been identified, including profilin (Lassing and Lindberg, 1985), cofilin (Nishida et al., 1984), gelsolin (Yin and Stossel, 1979), villin (Bretscher and Weber, 1979), severin (Brown et al., 1982), fragmin (Hasegawa et al., 1980), adseverin/scinderin (Del Castillo et al., 1990; Maekawa et al., 1989), and gCap39 (Yu et al., 1990). These proteins are functionally regulated by Ca^{2+} and phosphoinositides. In vitro studies showed that profilin (Goldschmidt-Clermont et al., 1990), gelsolin (Janmey et al., 1992), and severin (Eichinger and Schleicher, 1992) bind to phosphatidylinositol bisphosphate (PIP_2) in the membrane or micelle. Binding of these proteins to PIP_2 induces dissociation of their complexes with actin and hence promotes the polymerization of actin filaments. An increase of intracellular Ca^{2+} activates PIP_2-specific phospholipase C, PLC (Berridge and Irvine, 1984), which can be subsequently phosphorylated by the epidermal growth factor (EGF) receptor tyrosine kinase. This phosphorylated form of PLC is able to hydrolyze PIP_2 and release the proteins bound to this lipid

(Goldschmidt-Clermont et al., 1991). Subsequently, these proteins bind to and sever actin filaments. A decrease of Ca^{2+} concentration (Yin, 1979) and the synthesis of polyphosphoinositides (Janmey and Stossel, 1987) induce once again the dissociation of actin complexes with the actin-severing or actin-capping proteins.

This straightforward picture of the regulation of actin polymerization by polyphosphoinositides requires, however, further clarification. For example, severin also binds in vitro to membranes containing PS as the only acidic lipid (Eichinger and Schleicher, 1992). PS is significantly more abundant in the plasmalemma than are phosphatidylinositols. Many other functionally related proteins that demonstrate a preference for PIP_2 over other acidic lipids have not been studied in experiments with appropriate controls.

Both profilin (Goldschmidt-Clermont et al., 1990, 1991) and cofilin (Yonezawa et al., 1991) inhibited the hydrolysis of PIP_2 by several isoforms of PLC. These proteins may be involved in the regulation of the inositol triphosphate second messenger system (Goldschmidt-Clermont et al., 1990; Yonezawa et al., 1991). Cofilin seems to bind to phosphatidylinositol regardless of its phosphorylation state, although this protein displays high specificity toward PI over other acidic lipids (Yonezawa et al., 1991). Yonezawa et al. (1991) identified a short sequence in cofilin that appears to be responsible for the binding of this protein to phosphatidylinositol (PI). The dodecapeptide mimicking this sequence displayed lipid-binding specificity identical to that of the intact protein. Identification of a PIP_2-binding domain on gelsolin and villin was also reported. The peptides mimicking these putative PIP_2-binding sites competed with gelsolin for PIP_2 at an efficiency a few orders higher than that of the basic peptides derived from either of the other domains on gelsolin and villin or unrelated proteins (Janmey et al., 1992). However, the PIP_2 specificity of these peptides has not been demonstrated. Charge density is likely to be the primary factor determining the association of severin with membranes containing anionic lipids (Eichinger and Schleicher, 1992). This protein bound equally well to membranes containing PS or PIP_2 when the charge density on the membrane was identical (PS was threefold PIP_2). Both the lipid-specific and non-lipid-specific binding to acidic lipids, as well as the interaction with the electrostatic potential of the membrane, may contribute to the overall free energy change in the association of the actin-severing/actin-capping proteins with the membrane. Untangling the relative contributions of these interactions may prove to be a challenging task.

Acidic lipids have been also implicated in the regulation of calmodulin (CaM) interaction with several CaM-binding substrates of PKC such as MARCKS (Mosior and McLaughlin, 1992a), neuromodulin (Houbre et al., 1991), neurogranin (Houbre et al., 1991), and myosin I (Swanljung-Collins and Collins, 1992). At the intracellular Ca^{2+} levels encountered in a quiescent cell, CaM remains tightly bound to these proteins. A transient rise of the Ca^{2+} concentration results in the dissociation of CaM from these proteins, which can be subsequently phosphorylated by PKC. The phosphorylated proteins exhibit little affinity toward CaM (Alexander et al., 1987; Graff et al., 1989; Swanljung-Collins and Collins, 1992). Because the phosphorylation of PKC substrates requires their association with membranes, Houbre et al. (1991) postulated that the highly basic sequences on neuromodulin and neurogranin, containing both the CaM-binding and phosphorylation sites, are also involved in the binding of these proteins to acidic lipids in the membrane. They showed that the phosphorylation of neuromodulin and neurogranin decreases their affinity toward membranes composed of acidic lipids. Swanljung-Collins and Collins (1992) demonstrated that the binding of myosin I to membranes containing PS occurs simultaneously with the dissociation of CaM from myosin. The CaM-binding sites on myosin I display sequence homology to the respective binding sites on neuromodulin and neurogranin, particularly with regard to the number and location of basic residues. Binding of these basic sequences to acidic lipids facilitates the phosphorylation of the CaM binding sites by PKC. The phosphorylation of neuromodulin and neurogranin extends the duration of an otherwise very transient release of CaM, and thus was postulated to constitute a "molecular switch" for this messenger protein (Alexander et al., 1987; Mosior and McLaughlin, 1992a).

Protein Translocation and Topology on the Membrane

Acidic lipids have been implicated in the translocation of proteins to appropriate cellular compartments as well as the determination of the orientation of integral membrane proteins. A strong indication for the general involvement of acidic lipids in these events came from the statistical analysis of the primary structure of transmembrane proteins and signal peptides. The transmembrane proteins from both prokaryotes and eukaryotes display a striking correlation of transmembrane orientation with the distribution of charged residues in the polar domains connecting the transmembrane segments of the proteins. The domains containing more positively charged residues were usually found on the cytoplasmic side of the membrane (von Heijne, 1986). The topology of transmembrane proteins on the rough endoplasmic reticulum seemed to be determined by the net charge difference between amino- and carboxyl termini (Hartmann et al., 1989). Signal peptides typically contain a positively charged amino terminus composed of 1–5 residues (von Heinje, 1990). Experimental studies on genetically engineered variants of the protein leader peptidase from the inner membrane of E. coli showed that the addition of basic residues to the N terminus of the protein resulted in the reversal of its orientation with respect to the membrane (Nilsson and von Heijne, 1990). The positively charged residues were found to be the sole determinant of the protein orientation (Andersson et al., 1992). Binding of positively charged residues to acidic lipids in the cytoplasmic membrane was suggested as one of the possible mechanisms determining the orientation of transmembrane proteins (Nilsson and von Heijne, 1990).

There is experimental evidence that anionic lipids are essential for the efficient translocation of proteins in E. coli (De Vrije et al., 1988; Kusters et al., 1991). The synthetic analog of the signal peptide of the E. coli outer membrane protein, PhoE, interacts preferentially with membranes containing acidic lipids (Demel et al., 1990). An acidic lipid-specific insertion of signal peptides was demonstrated also for the synthetic analogs of other signal peptides (Demel et al., 1990). Apocytochrome C, a representative of another class of proteins that are synthesized in the cytoplasm and later translocated to the target mitochondrial membranes, lacks a signal sequence; nevertheless, in in vitro studies it showed a preference for membranes containing acidic lipids. Negatively charged lipids are also present at the outside of the outer mitochondrial membrane, to which apocytochrome C binds in vivo (Nicholson et al., 1989). The binding of this protein to model membranes is followed by spontaneous partial translocation of the N terminus of the protein across the lipid bilayer. This spontaneous translocation across the membrane is, however, specific for apocytochrome C. Other mitochondrial proteins require specific receptors or mitochondrial enzymes to be efficiently translocated across the membrane (Jordi et al., 1992). An initial association with acidic lipids may, however, be crucial for the subsequent interaction with the specific receptor (see pp. 240–242).

Both the statistical and experimental studies indicate that the asymmetric distribution of acidic lipid in the opposite leaflets of cellular membranes plays an important role in protein translocation and the determination of protein orientation in the membrane. However, many more experimental studies are required to elucidate the mechanism of this particular acidic lipid–protein interaction.

Models of Protein Binding to Acidic Lipids

The binding of proteins to acidic lipids in the membrane was a crucial event for the functioning of proteins discussed in the preceding sections. The putative binding sites on proteins for acidic lipids are usually composed of short sequences rich in basic amino acid residues (Janmey et al., 1992; Houbre et al., 1991; Mosior and McLaughlin, 1991; Swanljung-Collins and Collins, 1992). The interaction of polycationic peptides with acidic lipids in membranes has been investigated for the past two decades (Kim et al., 1991, and references therein). Only recently, however, partly because of technical advances in biophysical methods, has a consistent picture of this interaction begun to emerge. We discussed earlier in this chapter the role of the electrostatic potential in the binding of cationic amphipathic helices to the membrane. The electrostatic potential produced by anionic lipids plays a similar role in the membrane binding of other cationic peptides, such as pentalysine, that do not penetrate the membrane interior (Kim et al., 1991; Roux et al., 1988) and display little affinity toward membranes composed solely of zwitterionic lipids. The association of polylysines (Kim et al., 1991) and other basic peptides (Mosior and McLaughlin, 1991, 1992a; Rebecchi et al., 1992) can be described by a combination of the Gouy–Chapman theory of electrostatic potential, the Boltzmann distribution of charged molecules in the electrostatic field, and the sequential mass action model.   McLaughlin and co-workers showed that each basic residue on the peptide, either lysine or arginine, can bind to an acidic lipid molecule with a free energy change of about 1 kcal/mole. There was little specificity with respect to either the acidic lipid or basic residue. The affinity of the model basic peptides toward acidic lipid decreased only slightly when the basic residues were separated by one or two alanine residues (Kim et al., 1991; Mosior and McLaughlin, 1992a). One of the most interesting findings was the apparent cooperativity with respect to acidic lipids, exhibited by basic peptides binding to the membrane (Mosior and McLaughlin, 1991, 1992a, 1992b). McLaughlin and co-workers identified two mechanisms involved in this apparent cooperativity (Mosior and McLaughlin, 1992b). First, the basic peptides are concentrated at the membrane surface by the electrostatic potential produced by acidic lipid. The concentration of charged molecules at the interface depends approximately exponentially on the surface charge of the membrane and thus also on the mole percent of acidic lipid. Second, the binding of the first basic residue to the acidic lipid molecule is concurrent with an increase of the local concentration of acidic lipid for other basic residues on the peptide. The increase of the local concentration of anionic lipid is mathematically equivalent to the increase of affinity toward anionic lipids by subsequent binding sites on the peptide (Mosior and McLaughlin, 1992b). Such a phenomenon is not unique for peptides binding to acidic lipids. It was theoretically considered for the binding of other multivalent ligands to membrane receptors (Reynolds, 1979). This particular binding model of basic peptides to acidic lipids was successfully applied to the basic peptides derived from PKC (Mosior and McLaughlin, 1991) and PLC (Rebecchi et al., 1992).

Binding of proteins to membranes is usually described as an association of the protein with the membrane binding sites composed of N lipid molecules (Epand and Epand, 1992), and a suitable mass action equation is used. Lentz and co-workers (Cutsforth et al., 1989) showed that for prothrombin and factor X, the dissociation constants and the size of protein binding site, N, calculated from the fit of this model to the experimental data, differ by an order of magnitude for membranes containing various fractions of acidic lipids. In particular, an eightfold increase in the mole percent of PS resulted in a 100-fold increase of the affinity of prothrombin toward the membrane. The binding of prothrombin and factor X to membranes was, however, accurately described by a sequential mass action model assuming that these proteins have three or four discrete binding sites for acidic lipids. The experimental data presented there display the apparent cooperativity with respect to acidic lipids in the binding of these proteins to membranes.

A similar effect was observed when these proteins bound to membranes containing positively charged stearylamine instead of acidic lipids (Rosing et al., 1988). A few other acidic lipid-dependent proteins display similar sigmoidal characteristics of either the function or membrane binding with respect to the acidic lipid content of the membrane. Examples include protein kinase C (Hannun et al., 1985; Mosior and Epand, 1993; Newton and Koshland, 1989), phosphocholine cytidyltransferase (Cornell, 1991), and phosphatidylinositol-4-phosphate kinase (Moritz et al., 1992). Cooperative sequestering of PS molecules in the membrane was proposed to explain the sigmoidal dependence of the enzyme activation on the mole percent of PS (Newton and Koshland, 1989). A recent study on PKC binding to the membrane demonstrated, however, that the mechanism of this apparent cooperativity is at least in part similar to that invoked in the binding of basic peptides to acidic lipids in the membrane (Mosior and Epand, 1993).

Conclusions

The scope of this chapter has been limited to large classes of proteins sharing common features in their interaction with acidic lipids. We identified four of the functions served by the interactions of proteins with acidic lipids. A particular protein–acidic lipid interaction usually performs more than one task. For example, the change in the distribution of acidic lipids across the membrane of platelets initiates the formation of the fibrin clot through the reduction of dimensionality in enzymatic reactions catalyzed by a cascade of proteases.

The mechanism(s) of the protein–acidic lipids interaction have only recently begun to be revealed. A study on the binding of basic peptides to acidic lipids in the membrane has allowed the formulation of an elementary model of this interaction. Its application to the protein–acidic lipids interaction is currently under extensive investigation. Protein domains involved in the interaction of proteins with acidic lipids were identified in several cases. A combination of structural and functional studies on artificial protein constructs is the next step in the elucidation of the details of the interaction between protein and acidic lipids.

REFERENCES

Adam G, Delbrück M (1968): In: *Structural Biochemistry and Molecular Biology*, Rich A, Davidson N, eds., pp. 198–215. San Francisco: Freeman.

Alexander KA, Cimler B, Meier K, Storm DR (1987): *J Biol Chem* 262:6108–6113.

Andersson H, Bakker E, von Heijne G (1992): *J Biol Chem* 267:1491–1495.

Ashendel CL (1985): *Biochim Biophys Acta* 882:219–242.

Bazzi MD, Nelsestuen GL (1987): *Biochemistry* 26:5002–5008.

Bazzi MD, Nelsestuen GL (1991a): *Biochemistry* 30:7961–7969.

Bazzi MD, Nelsestuen GL (1991b): *Biochemistry* 30:7969–7977.

Bazzi MD, Nelsestuen GL (1992): *Biochemistry* 31:1125–1134.

Berridge MJ, Irvine RF (1984): *Nature (London)* 341:197–205.

Beschiaschvili G, Seelig J (1990): *Biochemistry* 29:52–58.

Bloom JW, Mann KG (1978): *Biochemistry* 17:4430–4438.

Borowski M, Furie BC, Bauminger S, Furie B (1986): *J Biol Chem* 261:14969–14975.

Bretscher A, Weber K (1979): *Proc Natl Acad Sci USA* 76:2321–2325.

Brown SS, Yamaoto K, Spudich JA (1982): *J Cell Biol* 93:205–210.

Cafiso D, McLaughlin A, McLaughlin S, Winiski A (1989): *Methods Enzymol* 171:342–364.

Carnie SL,Torrie GM (1984): *Adv Chem Phys* 56:141–253.

Chung L, Kaloyanides R, McDaniel R, McLaughlin A, McLaughlin S (1985): *Biochemistry* 24:442–452.

Cornell RB (1991): *Biochemistry* 30:5873–5880.

Creutz CE, Dowling LG, Sando JJ, Villar-Palasi C, Whipple JH, Zaks WJ (1983): *J Biol Chem* 258:14664–14674.

Cutsforth GA, Whitaker RN, Hermans J, Lentz BR (1989): *Biochemistry* 28:7453–7461.

Del Castillo AR, Lemaire S, Tchakarov L, Jeyapragasan M, Doucet J-P, Vitale L, Trifaro J-M (1990): *EMBO J* 9:43–52.

Demel RA, Goormagtigh E, de Kruijff B (1990): *Biochim Biophys Acta* 1027:155–162.

De Vrije T, de Swart RL, Dowhan W, Tommassen J, de Kruijff B (1988): *Nature (London)* 334:173–175.

Dombrose FA, Gitel SN, Zawalich K, Jackson CM (1979): *J Biol Chem* 254:5027–5040.

Eichinger L, Schleicher M (1992): *Biochemistry* 31:4779–4787.

Enyedi A, Flura M, Sarkadi B, Gardos G, Crafoli E (1987): *J Biol Chem* 262:6425–6430.

Epand RM, Epand RF (1992): In: *The Structure of Biological Membranes*, Yeagle P, ed., pp. 573–601. Boca Raton: CRC Press.

Furie B, Furie BC (1988): *Cell* 53:505–518.

Geisow MJ, Walker JH, Boustead C, Taylor W (1987): *Biosci Rep* 7:291–298.

Glenney JR (1986): *J Biol Chem* 261:7247–7252.

Goldschmidt-Clermont PJ, Machesky LM, Baldassare JJ, Pollard TD (1990): *Science* 247:1575–1578.

Goldschmidt-Clermont PJ, Kim JW, Machesky LM, Rhee SG, Pollard TD (1991): *Science* 251:1231–1233.

Graff JM, Young TM, Johnson JD, Blackshear PJ (1989): *J Biol Chem* 264:21818–21823.

Hannun YA, Loomis CR, Bell RM (1985): *J Biol Chem* 260:10039–10043.

Hartmann E, Rapoport TA, Lodish HF (1989): *Proc Natl Acad Sci USA* 86:5786–5780.

Hasegawa T, Takashi S, Hayashi H, Hatano S (1980): *Biochemistry* 19:2677–2683.

Houbre D, Duportail G, Deloulme JC, Baudier J (1991): *J Biol Chem* 266:7121–7131.

Jackson CM, Nemerson Y (1980): *Annu Rev Biochem* 49:765–811.

Janmey PA, Stossel TP (1987): *Nature (London)* 325:362–364.
Janmey PA, Lamb J, Allen PG, Matsudaira PT (1992): *J Biol Chem* 267:11818–11823.
Jones ME, Lentz BR (1986): *Biochemistry* 25:567–574.
Jordi W, Hergersberg C, de Kruijff B (1992): *Eur J Biochem* 204:841–846.
Kim J, Mosior M, Chung L, Wu H, McLaughlin S (1991): *Biophys J* 60:135–148.
Kuchinka E, Seelig J (1989): *Biochemistry* 28:4216–4221.
Kusters R, Dowhan W, de Kruijff B (1991): *J Biol Chem* 266:8659–8705.
Langner M, Cafiso D, Marcelja S, McLaughlin S (1990): *Biophys J* 57:335–349.
Lassing I, Lindberg U (1985): *Nature (London)* 314:472–475.
Lester D, Epand RM (1992): *Protein Kinase C: Current Concepts and Future Perspectives*. Chichester, England: Ellis Horwood.
Lim TK, Bloomfield VA, Nelsestuen GL (1977): *Biochemistry* 16:4177–4181.
Maekawa S, Toriyama M, Hisanaga S-I, Yonezawa N, Endo S, Hirokawa N, Sakai H (1989): *J Biol Chem* 264:7458–7465.
Mann KG, Nesheim ME, Church WR, Haley P, Krishnaswamy S (1990): *Blood* 76:1–16.
McLaughlin S (1977): *Curr Top Membr Transp* 7:71–144.
McLaughlin S (1989): *Annu Rev Biophys Biophys Chem* 18:113–136.
Moritz A, De Graan PNE, Gispen WH, Wirtz KWA (1992): *J Biol Chem* 267:7207–7210.
Mosior M, Epand RM (1993): *Biochemistry* 32:66–75.
Mosior M, McLaughlin S (1991): *Biophys J* 60:149–159.
Mosior M, McLaughlin S (1992a): *Biochemistry* 31:1768–1773.
Mosior M, McLaughlin S (1992b): *Biochim Biophys Acta* 1105:185–187.
Newton AC, Koshland DE, Jr. (1989): *J Biol Chem* 264:14909–14915.
Nicholson DW, Hergersberg C, Neupert W (1989): *J Biol Chem* 263:19034–19042.
Nilsson I, von Heijne G (1990): *Cell* 62:1135–1141.
Nishida E, Maekawa S, Sakai H (1984): *Biochemistry* 23:5307–5313.
Nishizuka Y (1989): *Nature (London)* 334:6661–6666.
Pearce KG, Hiskey RG, Thompson NL (1992): *Biochemistry* 31:5983–5985.
Rebecchi MJ, Peterson AA, McLaughlin S (1992): *Biochemistry* 31:12742–12747.
Reynolds JA (1979): *Biochemistry* 18:264–269.
Rosing J, Tans G, Speijer H, Zwaal RFA (1988): *Biochemistry* 27:9048–9055.
Roux M, Neumann J-M, Bloom M, Devaux PF (1988): *Eur Biophys J* 16:267–273.
Schwyzer R (1987): *EMBO J* 6:2255–2259.
Seelig A, Macdonald PM (1989): *Biochemistry* 28:4216–4221.
Stanislawski B, Ruterjans H (1987): *Eur Biophys J* 15:1–12.
Stossel TP (1989): *J Biol Chem* 264:18261–18264.
Swanljung-Collins H, Collins JH (1992): *J Biol Chem* 267:3445–3454.
Thelen M, Rosen A, Nairn AC, Aderem A (1991): *Nature (London)* 351:320–322.
Tulinsky A, Park CH, Skrzypczak-Jankun E (1988): *J Mol Biol* 203:885–901.
von Heijne G (1986): *EMBO J* 5:3021–3027.
von Heinje G (1990): *J Membr Biol* 115:195–201.
Wei GJ, Bloomfield VA, Resnick RM, Nelsestuen GL (1982): *Biochemistry* 21:1949–1959.
Yin H (1979): *Nature (London)* 281:583–586.
Yin HL, Stossel TP (1979): *Nature (London)* 281:581–583.
Yonezawa N, Homma Y, Yahara I, Sakai H, Nishida E (1991): *J Biol Chem* 266:17218–17221.
Yu F-X, Johnston PA, Sudhof TC, Yin HL (1990): *Science* 250:1413–1415.

16

SYNTHETIC PEPTIDES MIMIC THE ACTIVE SITES OF FIBRONECTIN RECEPTORS FROM GRAM-POSITIVE BACTERIA

Sivashankarappa Gurusiddappa and Magnus Höök

Introduction

Fibronectin is a large (~440 kDa) dimeric glycoprotein found in body fluids and the extracellular matrix of higher animals. This protein has been shown to affect numerous biological processes. Most of the biological functions of fibronectin appear to be related to its ability to serve as a substrate for the adhesion of eukaryotic cells (for review, see Hynes, 1985; Yamada, 1983). The cellular receptors that mediate cell adhesion to fibronectin are of the integrin type, a family of heterodimeric receptors consisting of an α-chain and a β-chain. Several integrins recognize structures in the fibronectin molecule. Thus, $\alpha_5\beta_1$ and $\alpha_v\beta_3$ recognize and bind to a Arg-Gly-Asp (RGD) sequence located in the central part of fibronectin (Hynes, 1992).

During the past decade it has become apparent that some microorganisms that require colonizing the host tissue have developed surface structures which serve as receptors for adhesive extracellular matrix components of the host. The best characterized group of bacterial receptors for matrix molecules are the fibronectin-binding receptors present on gram-positive bacteria. A generic model of a member of this class of bacterial receptor proteins is shown in Figure 16–1. The primary ligand binding domain of these receptors has been localized to a segment composed of a 35- to 40-

Peptides: Design, Synthesis, and Biological Activity
Channa Basava and G. M. Anantharamaiah, Editors
©1994 *Birkhäuser Boston*

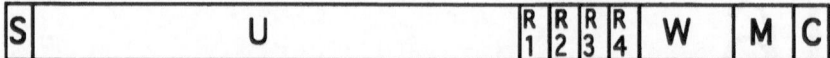

Figure 16-1. Generic model of fibronectin receptor from gram-positive bacteria. Abbreviations: S, signal sequence; U, unique sequence; R, repeat motif containing fibronectin-binding sites; W, cell wall-spanning domain; M, membrane-spanning domain; C, cytoplasmic domain.

amino-acid unit (called R) that is repeated three to five times (Lindgren et al., 1993; Signäs et al., 1989; Talay et al., 1992). Recombinant fusion proteins that contain the segment of R repeats of the bacterial receptors have fibronectin-binding activity and appear to specifically recognize the N-terminal domain of fibronectin (Mosher and Proctor, 1980; Speziale et al., 1984). This fibronectin domain is composed of five so-called type I motifs. Studies in which one or more of the type I motifs in the N-terminal fibronectin domain was deleted through site-directed mutagenesis indicate that all five type I motifs must be intact for the domain to be recognized by the bacterial receptors (Sottile et al., 1991).

Synthetic Repeat Motifs Bind Fibronectin

The fibronectin receptors from gram-positive bacteria that have been examined so far include two receptors each from *Staphylococcus aureus* and *Streptococcus dysgalactiae* (Flock et al., 1987; Jönsson et al., 1991; Lindgren et al., 1992). The overall structures of these receptors are similar, and the primary sequences of the receptors from *Staphylococcus aureus* are analogs and almost identical in the repeat motifs. On the other hand, the two fibronectin receptors from *Streptococcus dysgalactiae* have dramatically different primary sequences throughout the entire protein including the repeat motifs (Lindgren et al., 1992); none of the *Streptococcus dysgalactiae* proteins are very similar to the *Staphylococcus aureus* receptors. The sequences of the repeated units in the four characterized receptors and the terminology used to identify them are shown in Figure 16-2.

Peptides mimicking the repeat units from the different receptors were synthesized and tested for their ability to inhibit binding of fibronectin to bacterial cells. Most of the synthetic repeat units were found to recognize fibronectin, as indicated by their ability to inhibit fibronectin binding to bacteria (Figure 16-3). Somewhat surprisingly, we found that the different peptides showed the same relative inhibitory activity regardless of whether *Staphylococcus aureus* or *Streptococcus dysgalactiae* was used as target cells (McGavin et al., 1993). This observation indicates that the A, B, and D motifs form a common structure that is recognized by fibronectin despite the apparent lack of sequence identity between them. This issue is discussed further here.

FnBPA

```
D1   QNSGN QSFEE DTEED KPKYE QGGNI VDIDF DSVPQ IHG
     || ||  |||||  ||| |  |||||  ||||  |||| ||||  |||
D2   QNKGN QSFEE DTEKD KPKYE HGGNI IDIDF DSVPH IHG
     ||           || || || || || ||      || ||
D3   FNKHT EIIEE DTNKD KPSYQ FGGHN S-VDF EEDTL PKV
```

FnBPB

```
D1   QNSGN QSFEE DTEED KPKYE QGGNI VDIDF DSVPQ IHG
     || ||  |||||  ||| |  |||||  |||||  |||| |||
D'2  QNNGN QSFEE DTEKD KPKYE QGGNI IDIDF DSVPH IHG
     |         || || || || ||  ||         ||
D'3  FNKHT EIIEE DTNKD KPNYQ FGGHN S-VDF E-DTL PQV
```

FnBA

```
A1   EDTQT SQEDI V.LGG PGQVI DFTED SQPGM SGNNS HTIT
     ||      ||||  |  || ||||  |||||  | ||  || ||  ||
A2   EDSKP SQEDE VIIGG QGQVI DFTED TQSGM SGDNS HTDGT VLE
     ||||| ||||| ||||| ||||| ||||| || || ||
A3   EDSKP SQEDE VIIGG QGQVI DFTED TQTGM SGAGQ VESP
```

FnBB

```
B1   EETLP TEQGQ SGSTT EVEDT KGPEV IIGGQ GEIVD I
     || ||  |||||  |||||  |||||  |||||  |||||  || || |
B2   EENLP TEQGQ SGSTT EVEDT KGPEV IIGGQ GEVVD I
     || ||  |||||  ||||| ||||  |          |
B3   EESLP TEQGQ SGSTT EVEDS KPKLS IHFDN EWPKE D
```

Figure 16–2. Synthetic peptides mimicking individual repeats from FnBPA and FnBPB of *Staphylococcus aureus* (Flock et al., 1987; Jönsson et al., 1991) and FnBA and FnBB of *Streptococcus dysgalactiae* S2 (Lindgren et al., 1992). Vertical line indicates identical amino acids. Residues in FnBPB motifs that are not conserved with respect to FnBPA motifs are shown in bold print.

Chemical Modification of Active Peptides

To identify amino acid residues in active synthetic peptides that may participate in the binding to fibronectin or may be required for an active structure, peptides designated A2, B3, and D3 were chosen and subjected to

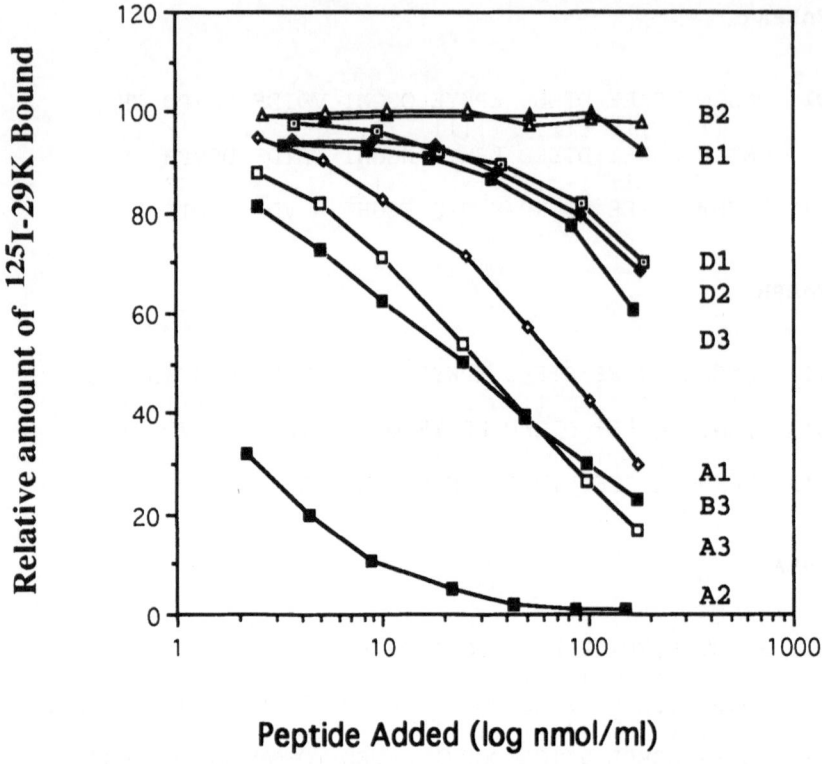

Peptide Added (log nmol/ml)

Figure 16-3. Inhibition of the N-terminal ^{125}I-29kDa fibronectin fragment binding to *Staphylococcus aureus* by synthetic peptides corresponding to repetitive D motifs of FnBPA, A motifs of FnBA, and B motifs of FnBB.

chemical modification of selected residues. The procedures used included reductive dihydroxypropylation of the amino side chain of lysine residues (Acharya et al., 1984), modification of the carboxylic side chains of glutamic and aspartic residues through 1-ethyl-3-(3-dimethyl-aminopropyl) carbodiimide (EDC)-mediated condensation of glycine methyl ester (Lundblad and Noyes, 1984a), and tetranitromethane-mediated oxidation of the phenyl side chains of tyrosine residues (Lundblad and Noyes, 1984b). The efficiency of the chemical modification reaction was monitored by analyses of the amino acid composition of the various peptides before and after the attempted modification.

Modified peptides were tested for their ability to inhibit the binding of fibronectin to bacterial cells (McGavin et al., 1991, 1993). These experiments showed that modification of the carboxyl groups of A2, B3, or D3 yielded inactive peptides; however, when the amino groups of lysine residues were blocked, the inhibitory activity of the modified peptide was only slightly reduced. Oxidation of the phenyl group of tyrosine, which was only tried for the D3 peptide, resulted in a compound with only marginally reduced activity. These data suggested that an acidic amino acid residue is either directly involved in fibronectin binding or is required for an active conformation of the peptide.

Active Fragments of the Repeat Units

To further define the amino acid residues required for fibronectin binding, the active synthetic repeat units A2, B3, and D3 were subjected to enzymatic or chemical cleavage; the generated fragments were purified by HPLC and tested for their ability to inhibit the binding of fibronectin to bacterial cells (Figure 16-4). After digestion of D3 with endoprotease, Glu-C fragments corresponding to amino acid residues 1-6, 11-30, and 31-37 were isolated and shown to be inactive. Also, fragments covering residues 1-21 and 22-37 obtained by chymotrypsin digestion were shown to be essentially inactive. A fragment covering residues 15-36 and isolated after trypsin digestion was shown to be almost as active as intact D3. These results locate the active site to the C-terminal half of the D3 peptide. Analyses of synthetic peptides covering various segments of this domain confirmed these results and also suggested that further truncations at the C terminal or N terminal resulted in reduction of activity. Thus, peptides covering residues 17-33 or 20-36 and 21-36 were about 10 fold and 100 fold, respectively, less active than a peptide corresponding to residues 16-36.

When the peptide A2 was cleaved with chymotrypsin, two fragments covering residues 1-22 and 23-43 were generated and found to be inactive. On the other hand, after treatment of A2 with cyanogen bromide, an active fragment corresponding to residues 1-30 could be isolated. The cyanogen bromide-generated fragment is about six fold less active than the intact A2 based on the concentration of peptide required for 50% inhibition of ^{125}I-fibronectin binding to cells of *Streptococcus dysgalactiae*.

Fragmentation studies were also conducted with peptide B3. Chymotrypsin digestion resulted in cleavage at F_{28} and yielded a highly active fragment, C1-C28, and an inactive fragment, C29-C36. Trypsin cleavage produced fragments covering residues 1-23 and 24-36, both of which were inactive.

The A and D Motifs Contain Conserved Residues, Some of Which Are Required for Activity

A close examination of the amino acid sequences of the repeated units of the A and D motifs reveals some identical or similar residues at conserved

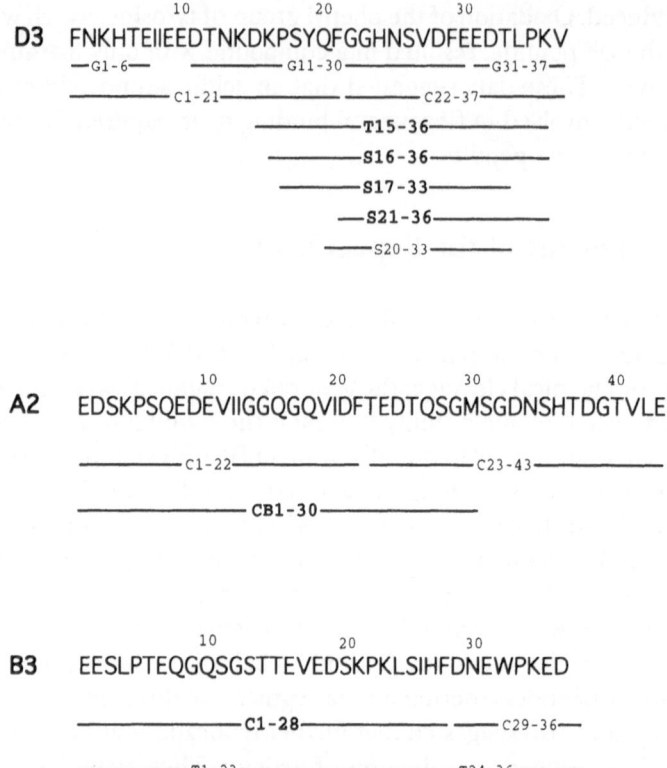

Figure 16–4. Amino acid sequences of D3, A2, and B3 peptides. Illustrated are the sequences of several proteolytic cleavage products, chemical cleavage products, and synthetic peptides used in our studies. Peptides are identified by a two-number code preceded by one or two letters. Numbers are position of amino acid residues of each peptide within the sequences of D3, A2, and B3. Letters G, T, C, and CB indicate cleavage products isolated from endoprotease Glu-C, trypsin, chymotrypsin digestion, or cyanogen bromide treatment, respectively. S designates peptides generated by chemical synthesis. Active peptide fragments are shown in bold.

```
D1    FEEDTEEDKP-KYEQGGNIVDIDFDSVPQIHG
D2    FEEDTEKDKP-KYEHGGNIIDIDFDSVPHIHG
D3    IEEDTNKDKP-SYQFGGHN-SVDFEEDTLPKV
A1    VVEDTQTSQED-IVLGGPGQVIDFTEDSQPGM
A2    ITEDSKPSQEDEVIIGGQGQVIDFTEDTQSGM
A3    LEEDSKPSQEDEVIIGGQGQVIDFTEDTQSGM
```

Figure 16–5. Conserved residues within structural motifs from *Staphylococcus aureus* FnBPA (D1, D2, D3) and *Streptococcus dysgalactiae* FnBA (A1, A2, A3). Residues that are identical or conserved substitutions in all motifs are shown in shaded boxes with bold print.

positions (Figure 16-5). Of these, the EDT sequence is located outside the part of intact peptides identified as important for fibronectin binding in the fragmentation studies (see earlier), whereas the other residues are within the active core segments of the A2 and D3 peptides, respectively.

Focusing on the A2 peptide, we have made a series of analogs in which conserved residues are individually substituted. The results of these experiments showed that some of the conserved residues are essential for activity although conserved substitutions may be acceptable in other cases. These ongoing studies also aim at determining the three-dimensional structure of active peptides.

Acknowledgments

Research reviewed here was supported by grant AI 20624 from the National Institutes of Health. We thank Alice Morales for typing the manuscript.

REFERENCES

Acharya AS, Sussman LG, Manjula BN (1984): *J Chromatogr* 297:37–40.
Flock JI, Fröman G, Jönsson K, Guss B, Signäs C, Nilsson B, Raucci G, Höök M, Wadström T, Lindberg M (1987): *EMBO J* 6:2351–2357.
Hynes RO (1985): *Annu Rev Cell Biol* 1:67–90.
Hynes RO (1992): *Cell* 69:11–25.
Jönsson K, Signäs C, Müller HP, Lindberg M (1991): *Eur J Biochem* 202:1041–1048.
Lindgren PE, McGavin MJ, Signäs C, Guss B, Gurusiddappa S, Höök M, Lindberg M (1993): *Eur J Biochem* 214:819–827.
Lindgren PE, Speziale P, McGavin MJ, Monstein HJ, Höök M, Visai L, Kostiainen T, Bozzini S, Lindberg M (1992): *J Biol Chem* 267:1924–1931.
Lundblad RL, Noyes CM (1984a): In: *Chemical Reagents for Protein Modification, Vol II*, Lundblad RL, Noyes CM, eds. Boca Raton, Florida: CRC Press, Inc.
Lundblad RL, Noyes CM (1984b): In: *Chemical Reagents for Protein Modification, Vol II*, Lundblad RL, Noyes CM, eds. Boca Raton, Florida: CRC Press, Inc.
McGavin MJ, Gurusiddappa S, Lindgren PE, Lindberg M, Raucci G, Höök M (1993): *J Biol Chem* 268:23946–23953.
McGavin MJ, Raucci G, Gurusiddappa S, Höök M (1991): *J Biol Chem* 266:8343–8347.
Mosher DF, Proctor RA (1980): *Science* 209:927–929.
Signäs C, Raucci G, Jönsson K, Lindgren PE, Anantharamaiah GM, Höök M, Lindberg M (1989): *Proc Natl Acad Sci* 86:699–703.
Speziale P, Höök M, Switalski LM, Wadstrom T (1984): *J Bacteriol* 157:420–427.
Sottile J, Schwarzbauer J, Selegue J, Mosher DF (1991): *J Biol Chem* 266:12840–12843.
Talay SR, Valentin-Weigand P, Jerlstrom PG, Timmis KN, Chhatwal GS (1992): *Infect Immun* 60(9):3837–3844.
Yamada KM (1983): *Annu Rev Biochem* 52:761–799.

17

ANALYSES OF VARIOUS FOLDING PATTERNS OF THE HIV-1 LOOP

Goutam Gupta and Gerald Myers

Introduction

The surface of the human immunodeficiency virus (HIV-1), which causes the immunodeficiency syndrome (AIDS), is studded with several copies of the surface glycoprotein, gp120 (Allan et al., 1985; Robey et al., 1985; Veronese et al., 1985). As shown in Figure 17–1, the glycoprotein gp120 consists of multiple (S–S)-bridged loops (Leonard et al., 1990). The amino acid sequences of the loops vary across different HIV-1 isolates. Of particular importance is the third variable or the V3 loop (see Figure 17–1). Antibodies elicited by the V3 loop or the parent gp120 block virus infectivity, thus neutralizing the virus (Goudsmit et al., 1988; Javaherian et al., 1988; Putney et al., 1986). Neutralizing antibodies can also block viral infection by inhibiting fusion of HIV-infected cells with CD4-positive uninfected cells (Rusche et al., 1988). It has also been shown that the changes in sequence inside the V3 loop affect the pattern of cell fusion (Freed and Risser, 1991; Robey and Axel, 1990). The V3 loop has been implicated as a determinant in HIV-1 tropism (Wertervelt et al., 1989). Neutralizing determinants are also able to serve as epitopes for both cytotoxic T cells (Takahashi et al., 1989) and helper T cells (Webster et al., 1982). The role of the V3 loop in

Peptides: Design, Synthesis, and Biological Activity
Channa Basava and G. M. Anantharamaiah, Editors
©1994 *Birkhäuser Boston*

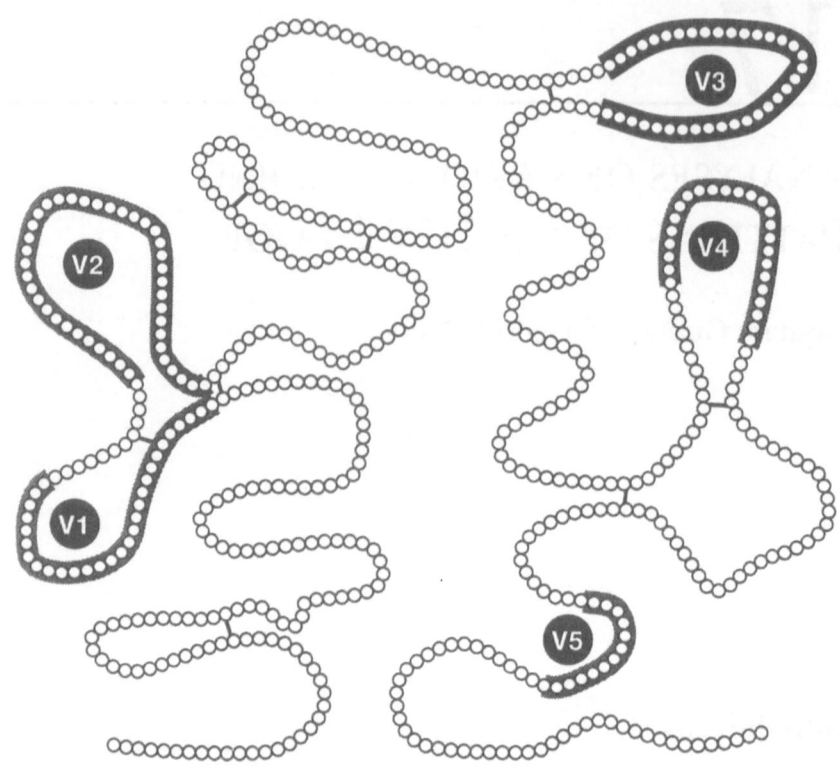

Figure 17–1. Schematic representation of the glycoprotein, gp120, that studs the surface of the AIDS-causing HIV-1. This surface glycoprotein contains several variable domains (shaded and labeled V1 through V5). Each open circle in this diagram represents an amino acid. Disulfide (S–S) bridges are shown as solid bars connecting two cystines. Primary attachment point of the gp120 molecule on the T4 receptor, CD4 (also a glycoprotein), lies between V4 and V5. However, because of its involvement in neutralization, cell tropism, and cell fusion, the (S–S)-bridged V3 loop has been the subject of the most intense research investigation. The V3 loop is also the most variable region of gp120.

virus neutralization, in cell fusion, and in determining cell tropism has made it a primary focus of vaccine development against HIV-1 infection.

Successful vaccine development, however, has been impeded by the amino acid sequence variability found among different isolates of HIV-1, particularly within the V3 loop sequence. It is probable that HIV-1, like the influenza virus, undergoes changes in the V3 loop to escape selective pressure imposed by neutralizing antibodies in vivo (Hart et al., 1990): neutralizing antibodies elicited by the V3 loop from one HIV-1 isolate may not neutralize HIV-1 isolates with V3 loops with different amino acid sequences (LaRosa et al., 1990). It is therefore important to analyze three-dimensional structures of V3 loop sequences from a large number of HIV-1 isolates to develop a broadly reactive vaccine.

Antibody–V3 Loop Interactions

There is little information about the specific interactions that determine the structure and stability of the antibody–V3 loop complex. However, single crystal studies reveal that protein and polypeptide antigens undergo little conformational change upon binding to specific antibodies (a "lock-and-key" mechanism) (Davies et al., 1990). Assuming such a mechanism, the degree of contact of complementary accessible surfaces of the V3 loop and its antibody (approaching each other as rigid bodies) should determine the specificity of the complex; that is to say, it is important to study the V3 loop structure in the free state because the latter will have a direct bearing on the several thermodynamic factors that determine the contact specificity of the V3 loop–antibody complex. Some of these factors are (i) the loss of entropy in the complex, resulting from the freezing of the mobile backbone segments and the side chains in the V3 loop, which in turn is directly related to the equilibrium tertiary folding and the fluctuations of the secondary structural elements in the fold; (ii) the gain in entropy from the loss of water layers, which is related to the pattern of water relaxation at or near atoms or groups in the V3 loop structure in the free state; and (iii) enthalpic contributions from van der Waals' interactions, H-bonding, and salt bridges, which are related to the surface properties (that is, to orientations of the aliphatic, aromatic, and charge groups with respect to the surface of the V3 loop in the free state).

Surface complementarity between the V3 loop and the antibody might also be achieved, however, via an "induced fit" mechanism in which the V3 loop, the antibody, or both undergo conformational changes to obtain greater surface complementarity. A particularly important situation emerges when two conformationally distinct V3 loop sequences bind the same antibody with similar affinity by exploiting the flexibility of the single binding site in the antibody. Because such a flexibility can potentially expand the antibody repertoire by allowing a single combining site to recognize a range of conformationally distinct V3 loop epitopes, this situation would therefore have a special significance in vaccine development. Whether the "lock-and-key" or the "induced fit" mechanism is operative, knowledge of the structural properties of V3 loops in the free state is essential for explaining the roles of the tertiary fold and the amino acid sequence at the contact region and for determining the structure and specificity of V3 loop–antibody complexes.

Two Assumptions

As just explained, the first step in analyzing the V3 loop–antibody interaction is the structural study of the V3 loop. These structural analyses are relevant because of two important facts: (i) an antibody recognizes a specific three-dimensional structure of the antigen (Davies et al., 1990), and (ii) the (S–S)-bridged V3 loop is the smallest part of gp120 that is likely to present the antigenic-determinant site to the antibody in a manner similar to the entire envelope protein. Therefore, it is essential to analyze the various V3 loop sequences in terms of *the conformational flexure* of their three-dimensional structures. This knowledge will, in turn, help identify the critical residues that determine the stereospecificity of antibody–V3 loop interactions.

Conformational Flexure of the V3 Loop

Analyses of amino acid sequences of the V3 loops from various HIV-1 isolates show that the variability in amino acid sequence occurs only in specified regions of the V3 loop, leaving three regions that remain fairly conserved in the amino acid sequence (Gupta and Myers, 1990). The relatively conserved regions are (1) a site of glycosylation [NN*NT, where N* is the site of sugar attachment and N*XT or N*XS (X being any amino acid) is the sequence requirement for glycosylation], (2) the GPG crest, and (3) the C-terminal helix GDIRQAHC. Our modeling studies on 20 different V3 loop sequences suggest that these invariant amino acid segments have very interesting structural properties (Gupta and Myers, 1990).

NN*NT: A Type I β-Turn

The presence of NN*NT leads to a type I β-turn (Rose et al., 1985; Wilmot and Thornton, 1988) where N* is exposed to the environment, thereby making it accessible for glycosylation. From the analysis of various glycoproteins, accessibility of N*, usually as a member of a β-turn, is viewed as an obligatory stereochemical requirement for glycosylation (Bush, 1982).

GPG Crest: A Type II β-Turn

The residue occurring most frequently in the sequence after GPG is R/Q, followed in frequency by K. Based on simulated annealing studies (Kirkpatrick et al., 1983), a type II β-turn appears to be energetically the most favored structure for the GPGR/Q/K crest. The presence of the GPGR/Q-like sequence (henceforth referred to as the GPG crest) induces a chain folding, which in turn facilitates the S–S bridge between two invariant cystines in the V3 loop.

GDIRQAHC: A Stretch of Helix

A helix is predicted for the (DIRQAHC) segment. D and Q are the most variable sites in this stretch: D is most often replaced by N (D and N show a preference for similar secondary structures), and Q is replaced by R or K (Q, R, and K are all helix formers). Computer modeling studies, by fully accounting for the variability of D and Q (Gupta and Myers, 1990) show that the DIRQAHC segment in the V3 loop tends to adopt a helical conformation. The presence of the fairly conserved G before the helical segment perhaps helps to retain the integrity of the helix and yet allows an appropriate orientation of the helix by utilizing the flexibility at the preceding G such that an (S–S) bridge can be formed between the two invariant cystines.

Thus it is clear that variability in the V3 loop sequence of HIV-1 is somewhat limited if the virus is to remain functionally active but escape the pressure imposed by neutralizing antibodies in vivo. Our computer modeling studies reveal that the amino acid sequence variability of the V3 loop is largely confined to the two sides of the highly conserved GPGR/Q crest (Gupta and Myers, 1990).

The most effective neutralizing antibodies map at or near the GPGR/Q crest (Gorny et al., 1991; Javaherian et al., 1989; Ohno et al., 1991), making direct contact to five to seven amino acids. The two regions flanking the GPG crest, being hypervariable, are the sites for potential antigenic drift (gradual accumulation of point mutations), so that changes in the amino acid sequence in these regions can either alter the structure and stability of the GPG-crest or induce a structural change in the flanking regions, or both. Such changes in the amino acid sequence in the regions flanking the GPG crest drastically reduce the binding affinity of the antibody produced by the host in response to the virus, and the virus thus escapes a neutralizing effect.

Assuming that the "conserved" (less variable) regions of the V3 loop are also conserved in their secondary structures (i.e., the site of glycosylation, the GPG crest, and the C-terminal helix in Figure 17-2), analyses of sequence variability and structures of the V3 loops can focus on the effect of the two hypervariable regions flanking the GPG crest on the structure and stability of the V3 loop, to which we now turn.

Classification of Tertiary Folding Patterns

Figure 17-2 schematically describes the flowchart of the method of analyzing the three-dimensional structures of the V3 loops belonging to different folding motifs. The technical details of the methodology are described in the Appendix. Following this methodology, we can construct a

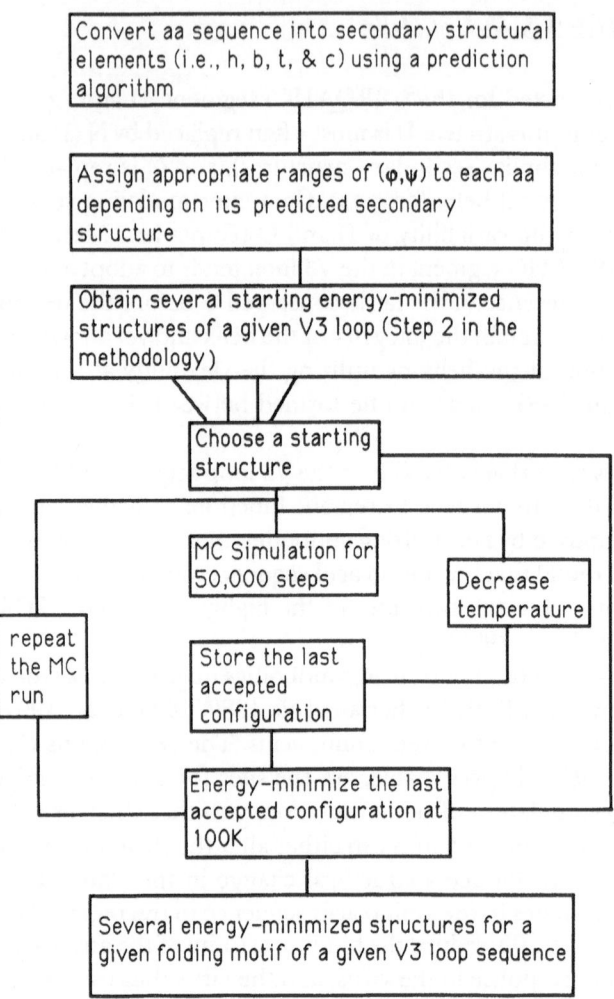

Figure 17-2. Flowchart of the methodology that combines secondary structure prediction, Monte Carlo simulated annealing, and energy minimization. Several starting structures are obtained after step 2 of our methodology. From this set, about 20 such structures with lower energies are chosen as starting structures for simulated annealing. The first MC run (with 50,000 steps) is performed at 1000 K. Temperatures of subsequent MC runs are gradually lowered in 50 temperature cycles to final temperature of 100 K. The 500,000-step MC run for 50 temperature cycles is repeated 20 times for the same starting structure using different random number generators such that the variables are chosen and varied in different ways in different MC runs. This is likely to guarantee conformationally different energy-minimized structures at the end of the calculation. Structures obtained at the end of simulated annealing and energy-minimization are again used as starting structures. Finally, we select 100 low-energy structures for each folding motif for a given V3 loop.

SEQUENCE

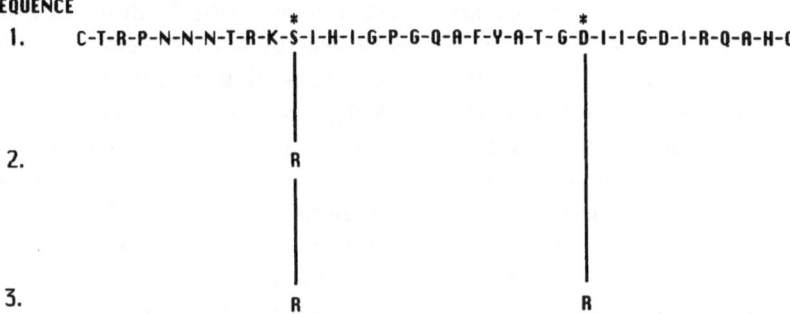

1.   C-T-R-P-N-N-N-T-R-K-S-I-H-I-G-P-G-Q-A-F-Y-A-T-G-D-I-I-G-D-I-R-Q-A-H-C

2.   R

3.   R   R

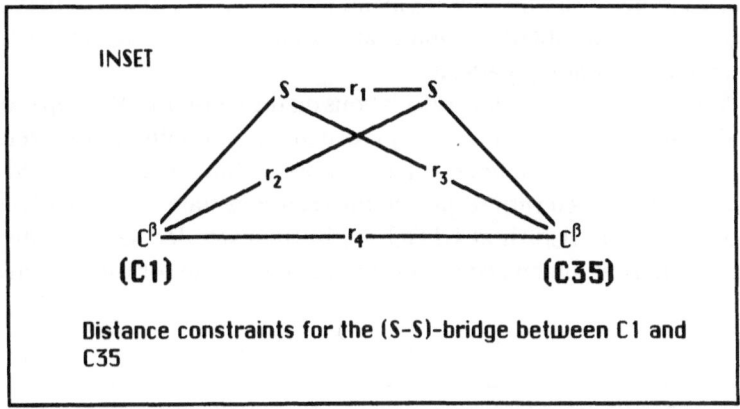

INSET

$$S \!-\! r_1 \!-\! S$$

r_2 r_3

C^β ———————— r_4 ———————— C^β

(C1)   (C35)

Distance constraints for the (S–S)-bridge between C1 and
C35

Figure 17-3. Three sequences used in our calculations: sequence 1, consensus
(Fletcher, 1984); sequence 2, single site mutation, S11R; sequence 3, from double
mutations, S11R and D25R. The invariant cystines, C1 and C35, are involved in the
(S–S) bridge formation. Inset: Four distance constraints for (S–S) bridge between
C1 and C35.

Table 17-1. A List of Representative Folding Patterns Expected
for V3 Loop Sequences

Pattern				NNNT		GPGR/Q	DIRQAHC	
1.	hh	$H_3^+ \, N^- C$	turn	helix	turn	helix	helix	$C\text{-}COO^-$
2.	hb	C	turn	helix	turn	beta	helix	C
3.	bh	C	turn	beta	turn	helix	helix	C
4.	bb	C	turn	beta	turn	beta	helix	C
5.	cb	C	turn	coil	turn	beta	helix	C
6.	ch	C	turn	coil	turn	helix	helix	C
7.	bc	C	turn	beta	turn	coil	helix	C
8.	hc	C	turn	helix	turn	coil	helix	C
9.	cc	C	turn	coil	turn	coil	helix	C

set of V3 loop sequences that are expected to be drastically different from one another in terms of their secondary structures. Each member in this set should represent a given type of tertiary folding pattern. Basing our classification purely on phenomenological grounds (i.e., step 1 of our methodology), assuming a type I turn for the site of glycosylation, a type II turn for the GPGR crest, and a helical stretch for DIRQAHC, and by fully accounting for the variability in the two regions flanking the GPG crest by assigning all possible secondary structural states, we can classify the folding patterns into the categories shown in Table 17-1.

Variable secondary structural elements flanking the conserved GPGR/ Q turn span four to five amino acids immediately preceding or following the GPGR turn. Classification of the V3 loops in terms of their tertiary folding patterns immediately provides us with an opportunity to use fewer trial V3 loops in vaccine development. Before vaccine trials can begin, however, we need to obtain complete and accurate knowledge about each of these V3 loop folding patterns.

We carried out modeling calculations on the consensus V3 loop sequence shown in Figure 17-3. Low-energy structures belonging to different folding catagories were obtained. The relative stabilities of the folded structures are calibrated with respect to the reference state in which all residues except the type II turn at GPGQ are in the extended state. Figure 17-4 shows different folded states and the reference state for the consensus V3

Figure 17-4. Seven folding motifs of consensus V3 loop (sequence 1 in Figure 17-3) and reference extended form. In the refrence form, all residues except putative GPGQ-turn are in extended form. As discussed for Figure 17-2, seven folded forms shown here are the average of several structures in same family. Top, left to right: reference state; 'bb'; 'hb'; 'cb1'. Bottom, left to right): 'bh'; 'hc'; 'cc'; 'cb2'. Secondary structural elements are color coded: helix, red; β/extended, green; turn/ coil, blue. C-terminal helix is present in all folded forms. Cb atoms of C1 and C35, white; S atoms of C1 and C35, magenta. Although folding motifs 'cb1' and 'cb2' belong to same family, the degeneracies of the coil state allow obtaining two variants with similar energies belonging to the same 'cb' motif. The two forms, 'cb1' and 'cb2', are shown to illustrate that there could be significant conformational variation even within the same folding family. Relative energy of stabilization of the folded states is computed as $(ETOT)_{folded} - (ETOT)_{ref}$. ETOTs for each folded form and for reference form are averages of several sampled minima (structures) in same family. Relative energies (kcal/mole) are −32 ('bb'); −45 ('hb'); −17('bh); −35 ('cb1' and 'cb2'); +10 ('cc'); −10('hc'). In starting structures, for a stretch of residues in the coil state no two neighboring residues belong to the same (φ, ψ) region. However, after simulated annealing and energy minimization of starting structures belonging to the 'cb' family, two or more neighboring residues adopted the β or extended conformation. This may be why they show similar stability. However, the 'bb' motif is richer than the 'cb' in secondary structure content.

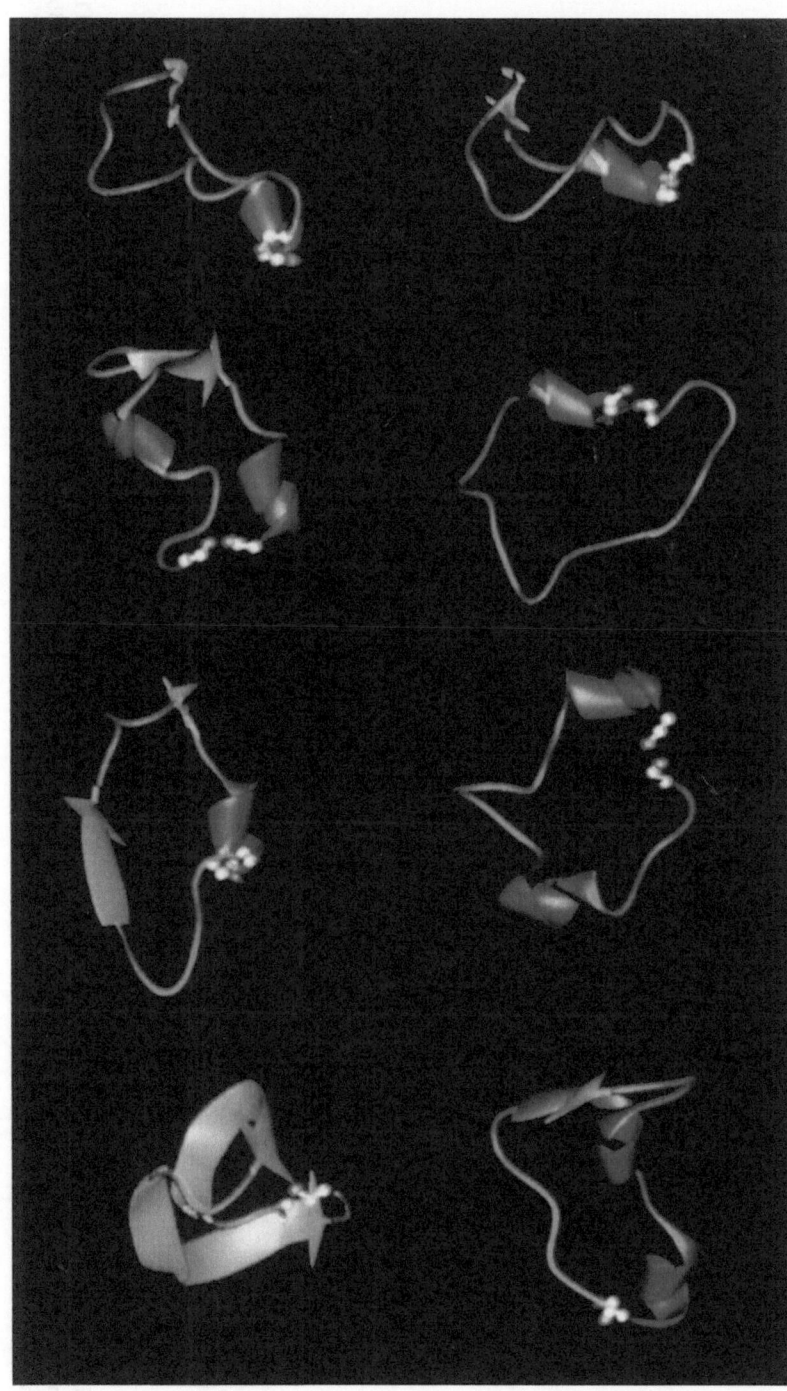

Figure 17-4. See figure legend on previous page.

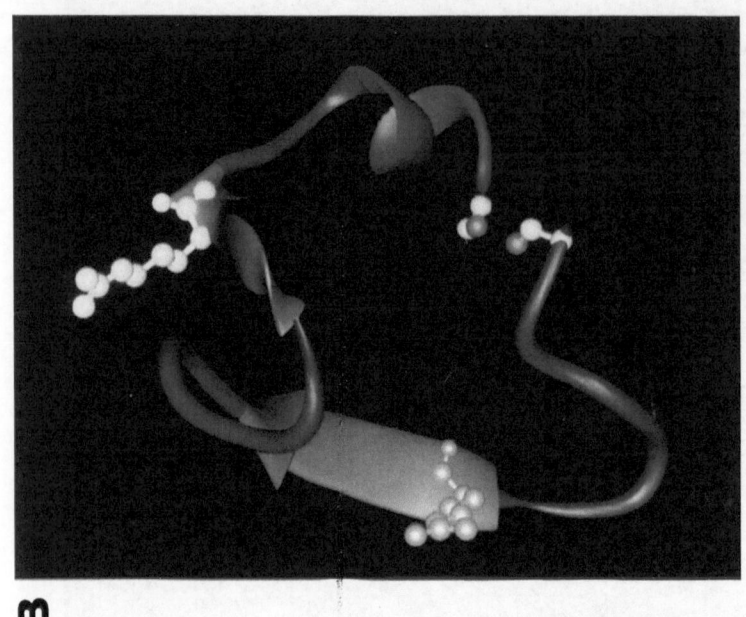

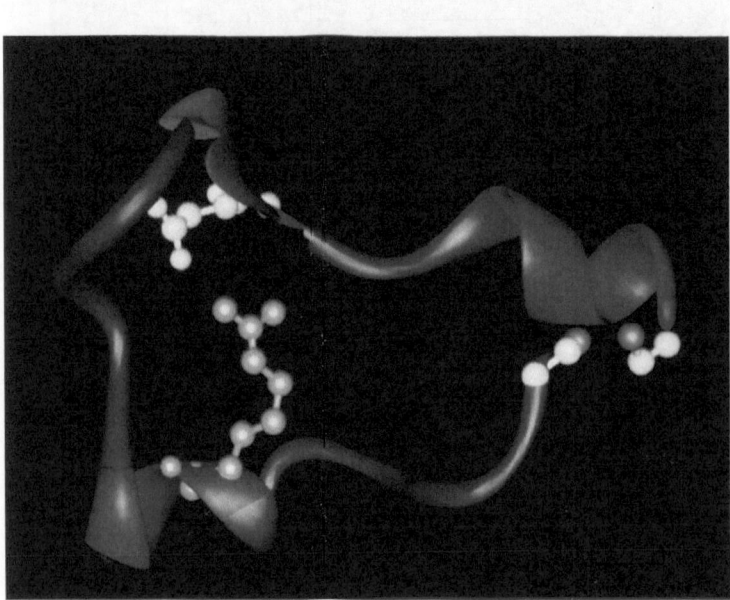

Figure 17–5. Preferred folded forms for sequence 2 and sequence 3 in Figure 17–3. A. 'hb' motif for sequence 2. Note proximity of R11 (cyan) and D25 (white). B. 'bb' motif for sequence 3. Note that R11 and R25 are moved far apart. Color codes of Cb and S of C1 and C35 are as in Figure 17–4.

loop sequence. The secondary structural elements are color coded in Figure 17–3: green for a β-strand (b), red for an α-helix (h), and blue for a coil (c) or a turn (t). The sulfur atoms of the terminal carbons are shown in magenta; the N-terminal carbon is always on the left while the C-terminal carbon is always on the right. Note that in all the folded forms and in the reference state, the GPGQ segment forms the exposed tip of the loop. In all the folded forms, N6* (the attachment point for glycosylation) is also exposed to the environment because this residue is a part of a type I turn. The folded pattern, designated as 'hb', is the most stable of all the folded forms; 'bb' follows as the next most stable form. We therefore discuss in greater detail the structural analyses of these two folded forms.

Conformational Variation Inside the Family of 'hb' and 'bb'
Folded Motifs

Table 17–2 shows the average values and the corresponding standard deviations of the torsion angles of the consensus V3 loop belonging to the 'hb' motif. Following the procedure described in the Appendix and in Figure 17–2, 100 low-energy structures were obtained in the 'hb' folding family. The deviations of the total energy, ETOT, for these structures were within 20 kcal/mole. The averages and the standard deviations are computed over these 100 structures. Note that the standard deviations of the backbone torsion angles (φ,ψ) of the *trans* peptide units $(\omega \sim 180°)$ are within 10°. However, small correlated changes in the (φ,ψ) values lead to average root mean square (rms) deviations of about 1.5 Å among all the structures by considering only the positions of the C^{α} atoms. The structures within the 'hb' folding motif are primarily different with respect to the relative position and orientation of the 'helix' and the 'β'- or 'extended' strand on either side of the putative GPGQ turn. It may be pointed out that the standard deviations of the (φ,ψ) values for sampled energy-minimized structures only reflect the lower limit of the flexibility because the thermal motions are filtered out after temperature quenching (energy minimization). The largest deviations are observed for the side-chain torsion angles, especially for the residues that are exposed on the surface.

Table 17–3 shows the average values and the standard deviations of the torsion angles for the 100 sampled structures of the consensus V3 loop sequence belonging to the 'bb' folding motif. Here again small changes (<10°) in the (φ,ψ) values are correlated to produce an average rms deviation of 1.5 Å among all sampled structures with respect to the positions of the C^{α} atoms. As in the case of the 'hb' motif, this variation corresponds to the changes in the relative position and orientation of the β- or extended strand on either side of the the putative GPGR turn.

Table 17-2. Averages and Standard Deviations (in Degrees) of the Torsion Angles for the "hb" Conformation

Residue #	φ	ψ	ω	χ^1	χ^2	χ^3	χ^4	χ^5	χ^6	χ^7
C 1	-122	34	-178	-67						
	17	14	5	7						
T 2	-108	-55	-170	-60	73	-57				
	12	6	7	1	4	26				
R 3	-56	-53	-171	-131	-176	179	179	0	179	0
	5	3	6	13	3	2	5	2	1	0
P 4	-75	114	179							
	0	10	8							
N 5	-97	-55	-178	-170	40	0				
	8	7	7	35	41	0				
N 6	-138	165	-175	-120	-29	0				
	7	9	5	45	29	1				
N 7	-106	7	-177	-165	-27	0				
	8	7	7	2	20	1				
T 8	-123	12	-177	55	164	-161				
	7	5	7	1	0	31				
R 9	-128	-95	-163	-75	-98	-176	-82	4	-177	0
	9	8	5	2	39	3	3	3	1	0
K 10	-66	-45	-167	-66	-179	-172	-68	-169		
	6	5	6	2	3	2	3	1		
S 11	-56	-40	-176	-34	139					
	8	7	5	45	44					
I 12	-63	-47	-174	-68	168	58	-50			
	8	6	6	3	12	4	6			
H 13	-58	-50	-174	-58	-58					
	7	5	4	28	64					
I 14	-60	-72	-177	-66	154	50	61			
	8	6	7	2	4	2	5			
G 15	153	100	-178							
	8	10	7							
P 16	-75	89	176							
	0	10	6							
G 17	101	25	178							
	8	8	6							

Effect of Amino Acid Substitutions on the 'hb' and 'bb' Folding Motifs

One interesting feature emerges on comparision of the 'hb' and 'bb' folding motifs. The average conformation of the 'hb' folding shows the possible proximity of the side chains of S11 and D25 while in the average conformation of the 'bb' folding motif the same two side chains are moved far apart. As shown in Figure 17-3, a single substitution of the type S11R (sequence 2 in Figure 17-3) and double substitutions of S11R and D25R (sequence 3) are commonly observed. While the virus particles with the V3

Table 17-2. (Continued)

Residue #	φ	ψ	ω	χ^1	χ^2	χ^3	χ^4	χ^5	χ^6	χ^7
Q 18	-64	-36	-174	-166	179	-90	0			
	6	7	8	18	8	19	0			
A 19	77	114	-177	85						
	6	8	8	1						
F 20	-144	-57	-178	-56	94					
	6	9	5	11	9					
Y 21	-165	29	-174	40	70	-178				
	8			10	3	7	1			
A 22	-140	130	-177							
	11	7	5							
T 23	-89	77	179	-54	158	179				
	4	8	9	1	19	0				
G 24	-169	130	-178							
	7	8	7							
D 25	-158	81	-179	46	108					
	5	9	8	2	3					
I 26	-146	83	176	42	161	79	-55			
	10	7	5	3	2	25	1			
I 27	47	-141	167	-24	-175	-150	-47			
	7	6	8	4	3	2	1			
G 28	-141	57	175							
	10	6	7							
D 29	-61	-38	-175	-59	87					
	7	5	4	1	15					
I 30	-66	-46	-173	-65	153	53	61			
	8	6	4	1	3	2	3			
R 31	-64	-38	-175	-69	-178	177	-179	179	179	179
	6	5	5	3	6	5	7	3	0	1
Q 32	-67	-40	-177	-78	176	93	0			
	7	8	7	20	5	10	0			
A 33	-58	-45	-176							
	6	6	5							
H 34	-65	-59	-168	-61	7					
	7	7	6	5	51					
C 35	-80	129	-179	-48						
	8	48	0	5						

loops of sequences 1 and 2 are syncytium inactive, the virus particles with the V3 loop of sequence 3 are syncytium active. Therefore, it is of interest whether these mutations that alter surface charge distribution on the V3 loop have any structural significance. Our calculations show that the 'hb' folding is favored for the sequence 2 in Figure 17–3 with a single S11R mutation. In this folded form the side chains of R11 and D25 are in close proximity because of electrostatic stabilization. Such a conformation is unfavorable for sequence 3 (Figure 17–3) with double mutations of S11R and D25R because of electrostatic repulsion, and a 'bb' folding is preferred for this sequence (Figure 17–4). Figure 17–5A shows the average 'hb' fold-

Table 17-3. Average Values and Standard Deviations (in Degrees) of the Torsion Angles for the "bb" Conformation

Residue #	ψ	ϕ	ω	χ^1	χ^2	χ^3	χ^4	χ^5	χ^6	χ^7
C 1	-148	-80	175	27						
	13	5	5	3						
T 2	-134	-54	-169	-62	88	-63				
	4	4	4	2	17	1				
R 3	-52	-53	178	-112	175	-176	178	0	-179	-17
	3	4	6	4	5	5	8	4	2	18
P 4	-75	117	179							
	0	5	5							
N 5	-115	-54	175	-66	103	0				
	7	5	5	22	4	1				
N 6	-127	160	-177	-133	-95	0				
	6	6	4	33	5	0				
N 7	-95	-16	-178	-171	-76	1				
	6	5	3	1	11	0				
T 8	-92	-5	-178	-13	121	-178				
	4	3	5	39	34	2				
R 9	-117	164	179	-59	-84	179	-82	3	-177	0
	4	4	6	4	21	5	2	2	1	0
K 10	-150	136	-178	-176	177	-173	-66	-167		
	6	4	5	0	0	0	1	0		
S 11	-157	144	178	-77	174					
	7	4	6	38	58					
I 12	-53	142	-178	-172	165	-50	68			
	4	5	7	2	2	1	1			
H 13	-150	175	-178	67	97					
	4	7	5	6	10					
I 14	-154	146	-179	-171	165	70	68			
	4	6	5	2	2	1	1			
G 15	161	85	-176							
	6	6	6							
P 16	-75	93	179							
	0	5	5							

ing for sequence 2 in Figure 17-3. Note that the tip of the positively charged side chain of R11 (shown in cyan) is close (<4 Å) to that of the negatively charged tip of D25 (shown in white). Figure 17-5B shows the average 'bb' folding sequence 3 in Figure 17-3. In this sequence, the side chains R11 (cyan) and R25 (white) are sticking out from two different sides of the V3 loop and are beyond 20 Å.

Such a sequence-specific change in the folding pattern of the V3 loop may have a special bearing on the virus–cell fusion and syncytium. The first step in fusion is the attachment of gp120 to the cell surface CD4 recep-tor. Because both are glycoproteins, the CD4 and the gp120 would have to

Table 17-3. (Continued)

Residue #	φ	ψ	ω	χ^1	χ^2	χ^3	χ^4	χ^5	χ^6	χ^7
G 17	99	11	-178							
	5	6	5							
Q 18	-55	-40	177	-172	156	113	0			
	6	4	6	5	13	34	0			
A 19	74	103	178	83						
	4	4	5	4						
F 20	-108	-58	179	-59	95					
	6	9	5	11	9					
Y 21	-165	30	177	40	72	-178				
	6	6	4	3	7	0				
A 22	-142	131	178							
	5	6	6							
T 23	-85	77	-179	-54	162	179				
	5	5	4	1	0	0				
G 24	-159	127	-178							
	4	4	6							
D 25	-159	82	-179	47	108					
	5	5	5	1	1					
I 26	-158	79	179	38	164	86	-56			
	6	6	5	3	1	9	1			
I 27	49	-159	179	-16	-172	-153	-47			
	3	5	5	3	1	2	0			
G 28	-176	63	-177							
	5	6	4							
D 29	-61	-49	-176	-61	70					
	5	3	5	1	8					
I 30	-61	-38	-175	-66	152	51	59			
	3	4	4	0	1	0	1			
R 31	-67	-41	-178	-162	178	-176	179	-178	-179	179
	4	4	2	22	3	5	3	2	0	0
Q 32	-66	-43	-177	-75	174	96	0			
	5	5	5	4	4	5	0			
A 33	-60	-61	-176							
	6	6	4							
H 34	-55	-65	-171	-172	155					
	4	5	5	7	69					
C 35	-83	108	179	-46						
	5	39	1	6						

cross a repulsion barrier to approach each other. The increase in the surface distribution of positive charges and the net reduction of negative charges are likely to mediate an efficient surface attachment of gp120 on the host T4 cells. Sequences of the type 3 in Figure 17-3 and the corresponding structure shown in Figure 17-5B fulfill the criteria of efficient cell-surface attachment as mentioned, and therefore provide a potential example of an efficient mode of fusion.

Concluding Remarks

The modeling studies reported here describe the intrinsic conformational flexibility of the HIV-1 V3 loop. These studies also show that the relative stability of one folded form or the other depends on the sequence of the V3 loop. Experimental characterization of different folded forms and the corresponding sequence dependence requires the following: (i) accurate determination of the structure and flexibility of a V3 loop in solution by two- or three-dimensional NMR techniques and (ii) structure–function correlation of antibody–V3 loop binding by combining structural biology and immunological methods. Such experiments are already in progress (Gupta et al., in press; Jong et al., in press; Veronese et al., in press). Results obtained so far demonstrate that, although quite flexible in the free state, the V3 loops when presented to specific antibodies as a part of the whole gp120 can and do adopt well-defined structures.

Acknowledgments

This work is supported by U.S. Army Grant MIPR 92MM2581 and NIH Grant R01 AI32891-01A2 (G.G). G.G wishes to thank Drs. Darrell Fontenot and Patricia Reitemeier for proofreading the manuscript.

Appendix

Methodology

The methodology involves the following steps.

Step 1. Prediction of Secondary Structures

The secondary structural elements are predicted for a V3 loop sequence by computing the probability S of a given residue i in the V3 loop to adopt a k-type of conformation (k = helix, β-sheet, coil, or turn), where

$$S(k,i) = \sum_{l=-\gamma}^{\gamma} \frac{P(k, i+l)}{|l|+1} .$$

(The summation is over $l = -\gamma$ to γ, where γ = size of the window chosen to account for the effect of the neighboring amino acid residues: $\gamma = 5$ for a helix; $\gamma = 3$ for a beta sheet; and $\gamma = 4$ for a coil or a turn.) $P(k, i)$ = potential for the k type of conformation of an individual residue i derived from the analysis of the single crystal structures of about 65 proteins. The highest $S(k, i)$ determines the conformation k for the i residue. (This methodology is adopted from Deleage and Roux, 1989.) Use of any algorithm for secondary structure prediction is only 60% accurate. To improve accuracy, we test our predictions by requiring S–S bridge formation that achieves local energy minima for the cyclic V3 loop; this leads to step 2 in our method.

Step 2. Generation of Energy-Minimized S–S-Bridged V3 Loop

This step involves obtaining an energetically stable S–S-bridged structure for a V3 loop sequence given the secondary structural states of the constituent amino acid residues as obtained after step 1. Appropriate ranges of (φ, ψ) values are assigned to all amino acids. For example,

$$\varphi = -55° + 25°, \qquad \psi = -55° + 25° \text{ for residues in a helix}$$
$$\varphi = -140° + 30°, \qquad \psi = 140° + 30° \text{ for residues in a β-strand}$$
$$\varphi_{i+1} = -65° + 20°, \quad \psi_{i+1} = -50° + 20°$$
$$\varphi_{i+2} = -90° + 20°, \quad \psi_{i+2} = 0° + 20° \text{ for residues in a type I turn}$$
$$\varphi_{i+1} = -65° + 20°, \quad \psi_{i+1} = 120° + 20°$$
$$\varphi_{i+2} = 90° + 20°, \quad \psi_{i+1} = 0° + 20° \text{ for residues in a type II turn}$$

(φ, ψ) of residues in the coil state are set free to choose any point in the allowed space (for definitions of different secondary structures and corresponding (φ, ψ) values, see Ramachandran et al., 1963). We simplify the sequence by assuming A for residues with side chains extending beyond the C^β atom, except for the Ps and the terminal Cs. Our rationale for doing this is that the allowed (φ, ψ) space of residues with a side chain longer than A is only a subspace of that allowed for A (Ramachandran et al., 1963).

We obtain an S–S-bridged structure of a V3 loop by using a linked-atom-least-square refinement equation (Sippl et al., 1984) that minimizes the function F in the space (φ, ψ):

$$F = \Sigma_l \, \lambda_l G_l + \Sigma_{ij} \, (d_{ij}{}^{mn} - D^{mn})^2,$$

where $G_l (= |\, r_1 - r^o{}_1| = 0)$ indicates distance constraints for an S–S bridge as shown in Figure 17-2. Distances in the S–S-bridged V3 loop configuration are defined as $r_1 = S(C1) - S(35)$, $r_2 = C\beta(C1) - S(C35)$, $r_3 = C\beta(C35) - S(C1)$ and $r_4 = C^\beta(C1) - C^\beta(C35)$; corresponding equilibrium distances are $r^o{}_1 = 2.04$ Å, $r^o{}_2 = r^o{}_3 = 3.05$ Å, $r^o{}_4 = 3.85$ Å (Korber et al., 1992). λ_l indicates Lagrangian multipliers; $d_{ij}{}^{mn}$ indicates distance between atom i (type m) and atom j (type n); and D^{mn} indicates the contact limit between atom (type

m) and atom (type n) (Ramachandran et al., 1992). In this refinement, the (φ,ψ) values of various residues are treated as elastic variables (i.e., variables with weights) such that by appropriate choice of weights the predicted secondary structural states of residues (after step 1) are minimally altered. This method guarantees a stereochemically orthodox structure for the S–S-bridged $(CA_{33}C)$-like sequence. Finally, appropriate side chains are attached to generate an actual V3 loop sequence, and the potential energy of the system is minimized in the $(\varphi,\psi,\omega,\chi)$ space using the force-field of Scheraga and co-workers (Fletcher, 1984). The total conformational energy, ETOT (kcal/mole), has the following components:

ETOT = EES (coulomb interactions between pairs of partial charges, dielectric constant = 80)

+ **ETOR** (torsional energy from barriers around single and partially double C–N bonds)

+ **ENB** (van der Waals attraction and repulsion terms between nonbonded atom pairs)

+ **ESS** (constraint energy from S–S bonds)

+ **EDIS** (energy from distance constraints as present in different secondary structures) structural elements).

Several initial structures are chosen within the specified ranges of (φ,ψ), and each structure is subjected to step 2, which finally produces several low-energy structures for the (S–S)-bridged V3 loop. These energy-minimized structures are used as starting configurations in a Monte Carlo (MC) simulated annealing procedure, as described in step 3.

Step 3. Exploration of the Conformational Flexibility of the V3 Loop by MC Simulated Annealing

The simulated annealing is performed (Kirkpatrick et al., 1983; Korber et al., 1992) in the following manner. First, a starting energy-minimized structure is chosen and Monte Carlo (MC) simulations are performed for 50,000 steps at 1000 K in the $(\varphi,\psi,\omega,\chi)$ space and the last accepted configuration is stored to be subsequently used as a starting configuration in the next lower temperature cycle. Second, 50,000 MC steps are repeated in several cycles of gradually decreasing temperature until a temperature of 100 K is reached. Third, the lowest energy configuration at 100 K is further energy minimized to a low-energy gradient (Sippl et al., 1984). Finally, the first through third steps are repeated for several different starting configurations. The EDIS term is removed from ETOT in this step.

As discussed in the flowchart of the methodology (Figure 17–2), steps 1–3 produce several low-energy structures for each folding motif of a given V3 loop.

REFERENCES

Allan et al. (1985): *Science* 228:1091.

Bush G (1982): *Biopolymers* 21:535.

Davies et al. (1990): *Annu Rev Biochem* 59:439.

Deleage G, Roux B (1989): *Prediction of Protein Structure and Principles of Protein Conformation*, p. 587. New York: Plenum.

Fletcher R (1984): *Practical Methods of Optimization 1*. New York: Wiley.

Freed EO, Risser A (1991): *AIDS Res Hum Retroviruses* 7:807.

Gorny et al. (1991): *Proc Natl Acad Sci USA* 88:3238.

Goudsmit et al. (1988): *Proc Natl Acad Sci USA* 85:4478.

Gupta G, Myers G (1990): *Cinquieme Colloque des Cent Gardes*, p. 99.

Gupta et al. (1993): *J Biol Struct Dyn* 11:345.

Hart et al. (1990): *J Immunol* 145:2677.

Javaherian et al. (1989a): *Proc Natl Acad Sci USA* 86:6768.

Javaherian et al. (1989b): *Proc Natl Acad Sci USA* 86:8768.

Jong et al.: *J Virol* (in press).

Kirkpatrick et al. (1983): *Science* 220:671.

Korber et al. (1992): In: *Vaccines 92: Modern Approaches to New Vaccines Including Prevention of AIDS*, pp. 75–79. Cold Spring Harbor, New York: Cold Spring Harbor Press.

LaRosa et al. (1990): *Science* 249:932.

Leonard et al. (1990): *J Biol Chem* 265:10373.

Ohno et al. (1991): *Proc Natl Acad Sci USA* 88:10726.

Putney et al. (1986): *Science* 234:1392.

Ramachandran et al. (1963): *J Mol Biol* 7:95.

Robey E, Axel R (1990): *Cell* 60:697.

Robey et al. (1985): *Science* 228:593.

Rose et al. (1985): *Adv Protein Chem* 37:1.

Rusche et al. (1988): *Proc Natl Acad Sci USA* 85:3198.

Sippl et al. (1984): *J Phys Chem* 88:6231.

Takahashi et al. (1989): *Science* 2246:118.

Veronese et al. (1985): *Science* 229:1402.

Veronese et al. (1993): *J Biol Chem* 268:25894.

Webster et al. (1982): *Nature ((London)* 296:115.

Wertervelt et al. (1991): *Proc Natl Acad Sci USA* 88:3097.

Wilmot CM, Thornton JM (1988): *J Mol Biol* 203:221.

18

REGULATION OF HUMAN IMMUNODEFICIENCY VIRUS GENE EXPRESSION BY THE TAT AND REV PROTEINS

Shabbir A. Khan

The human immunodeficiency virus type 1 (HIV-1) is the primary etiologic agent of the acquired immunodeficiency syndrome (AIDS). AIDS is clinically characterized by a progressive loss of the T4-helper/inducer lymphocytes, which are responsible for cell-mediated immunity. As a consequence, the T-cell-mediated immune response is impaired in AIDS patients, resulting in the occurrence of severe opportunistic infections and certain malignancies (Fauci, 1988). HIV-1 selectively infects cells that express CD4 glycoprotein on their surface, the CD4 molecule serving as a receptor. The mechanism by which HIV-1 induces cytopathology in susceptible cells is not well understood.

HIV-1 is a retrovirus; retroviruses are defined by their ability to transcribe genetic information back from single-stranded RNA into double-stranded DNA (Varmus and Brown, 1989). Generally, retroviral replication initiates immediately after the internalization of the virion core into the cytoplasm via specific binding of the viral envelope glycoprotein to a cell-surface receptor. Subsequent to infection, a virion-associated reverse transcriptase transcribes the single-stranded genomic RNA into double-stranded DNA, which is then integrated into the host chromosomal DNA, thereby

Peptides: Design, Synthesis, and Biological Activity
Channa Basava and G. M. Anantharamaiah, Editors
©1994 *Birkhäuser Boston*

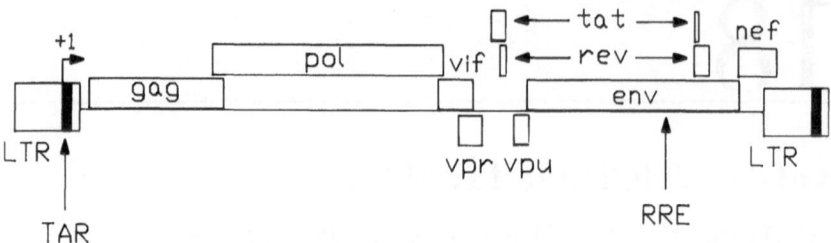

Figure 18–1. Genomic organization of human immunodeficiency virus type 1 (HIV-1). The integrated proviral DNA is approximately 10 kb long. During reverse transcription, the virus generates long terminal repeat sequences (LTR), which flank the viral open reading frames. The coding sequence of the viral DNA consists of a series of overlapping open reading frames. In addition to characteristic genes *gag*, *pol*, and *env*, common to all retroviruses, HIV-1 codes for at least six genes: *tat*, *rev*, *vif*, *vpr*, *vpu*, and *nef*. Three genes (*tat*, *rev*, and *nef*, encode proteins that regulate viral gene expression. Locations of known viral genes, the transcription start site, and the DNA sequences that generate the Tat-mediated *trans*-activation responsive (TAR) sequence and the Rev-responsive element (RRE) are indicated.

forming the retroviral provirus. Replication of simple retroviruses, such as murine leukemia virus, requires only three virally encoded genes, *gag*, *pol*, and *env*, which encode the viral structural proteins, the virion-associated enzymes, and the envelope glycoprotein, respectively. In the provirus, these genes are arranged in the same order and are flanked by sequences called long terminal repeats (LTRs), which contain enhancer and promoter sequences essential both for transcription of the viral genome and for efficient mRNA polyadenylation. The HIV-1 genome, however, is complex and encodes at least six gene products in addition to the characteristic retroviral *gag*, *pol*, and *env* (Figure 18–1). Three of these, encoded by the *tat*, *rev*, and *nef* genes, act in *trans* to regulate the viral gene expression. Both the Tat (*trans*-activator protein) (Arya et al., 1985) and Rev (regulator of expression of virion proteins) (Sodroski et al., 1986) proteins positively regulate HIV-1 gene expression (Knight et al., 1987), whereas Nef (negative factor) represses transcription from the viral LTR (Ahmad and Venkatesan 1988). The other three gene products, Vpr (viral protein R), Vpu (viral protein U), and Vif (virion infectivity protein), are involved in the infectivity and the maturation processes of the virus (Cullen, 1992).

The various genes arise from multiple splicing by using four splice donor sites and six splice acceptor sites present within the HIV-1 genome (Feinberg et al., 1986). HIV-1 gene regulation is characterized by a temporal gene expression involving a progressive shift from synthesis of the multiply spliced mRNAs, which encode the *trans*-regulatory proteins, toward the production of unspliced and singly spliced mRNAs, which encode the structural proteins. This complex pattern of gene expression is regulated entirely by the viral proteins Tat and Rev. There is compelling evidence that both Tat and Rev function through interaction with specific *cis*-acting target sequences, *trans*-activation-responsive sequence (TAR), and Rev-response element (RRE) in the viral RNA.

The purpose of this chapter is to briefly summarize the current understanding of the Tat- and Rev-regulated gene expression of HIV-1. Recent advances in the methods of chemical synthesis have permitted the synthesis of small proteins, such as apolipoprotein C-II (Fairwell et al., 1987), the HIV-1 protease (Schneider and Kent, 1988), HIV-1 Tat (Jeyapaul et al., 1990; Reddy et al., 1992), and HIV-1 Rev (Palmeri and Khan, in manuscript) in functionally active form. Chemical synthesis has been clearly demonstrated to be a very suitable approach for obtaining small proteins in functionally active form and in sufficient quantities for molecular definition and structure–function studies. The successful use of synthetic peptides to analyze structure–function relationships of HIV-1 Tat and to probe the protein–RNA, such as Tat–TAR and Rev–RRE, interactions that appear to play such pivotal roles in HIV-1 gene expression is also briefly discussed.

Tat Protein

All integrated proviruses are acted on by host cell transcription factors. For simple retroviruses, these DNA sequence-specific interactions are fully sufficient to induce the production of a high level of proviral transcript. Complex retroviruses remain dependent on the host cellular factors, but these factors alone, for some obscure reason, are not sufficient to permit efficient viral gene expression. Instead, the interaction of the LTR elements and cellular factors results in a low basal level of viral mRNA synthesis. This initial population of viral RNA reaches the cytoplasm in the form of small, multiply spliced mRNAs that encode the viral regulatory proteins.

In the case of HIV-1, the first of these virally encoded regulatory gene products is Tat. The Tat protein of HIV-1 is a potent *trans*-activator of expression of genes from the viral LTR in vitro and hence enhances its own synthesis, thereby generating a powerful positive feedback. This enhanced proviral transcription leads to the accumulation of a second posttranscriptional regulatory protein, Rev. A 200- to 300-fold increase in HIV-1 LTR-directed gene expression results in the presence of functionally active Tat. Tat appears to exert its effect through novel mechanisms that depend on the recognition of a specific, structured, *cis*-acting viral RNA sequence, the *trans*-activation responsive (TAR) element, which is located at the 5' end of all HIV-1 transcripts as an untranslated leader sequence (Rosen et al., 1985). Both Tat and an intact copy of TAR are required for HIV-1 replication in culture.

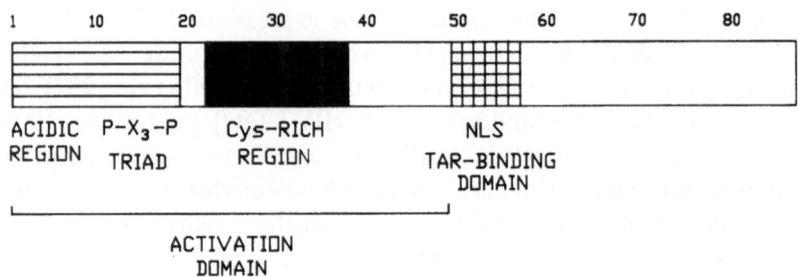

MEPVDPRLEPWKHPGSQPKTACTNCYCKKCCFHCQVCFITKAL

GISYGRKKRRQRRRPPQGSQTHQVSLSKQPTSQSRGDPTGPKE

Figure 18–2. Functional domains of HIV-1 Tat protein. Overall topology of the N terminus (amino acids 1–19) containing acidic and basic residues as well as Pro-Xaa–Pro triad is essential for full *trans*-activation. Cys-rich region (amino acids 22–38), which binds Zn and Cd ions, is essential for activity, although the role of metal binding is not clear. Basic domain (amino acids 49–57) is necessary and sufficient for nuclear localization and TAR RNA binding, but appears to be dispensable for transcriptional activation mediated by Tat in vitro. Sequences flanking basic region are required for high-affinity binding of tat with TAR RNA.

Functional Domains of Tat

The 86-residue Tat contains three interesting structural features (Figure 18–2): a Pro-Xaa$_3$-Pro triad, a Cys-rich metal binding domain, and a cluster of basic residues, all present within the N-terminal, 57 residues of the protein. The structure–function relationships of Tat elucidated both by using mutational analysis and by using synthetic peptides provide evidence that these three domains are essential for full Tat function (Delling et al., 1991; Frankel et al., 1989; Garcia et al., 1988; Green and Loewenstein, 1988; Green et al., 1989; Hauber et al., 1989; Jeyapaul et al., 1990; Kuppuswamy et al., 1989; Ruben et al., 1989; Rice and Carlotti, 1990a, 1990b; Reddy et al., 1992). Mutation studies have shown that the basic domain is required for nuclear/nucleolar localization of Tat (Hauber et al., 1989). The Cys-rich region, which is similar to the metal-binding sequence motifs present in several metalloproteins and transcription factors, interacts with divalent metal ions such as Cd^{2+} and Zn^{2+} to form a metal-linked dimer (Frankel and Pabo, 1988; Jeyapaul et al., 1990). Between the Cys-rich region and the basic domain lies a conserved sequence that is proposed to be the "core" or activation domain of the protein.

Analysis of synthetic deletion and full-length Tat peptides shows that the Lys-41 in the "core" region is critical for Tat *trans*-activation (Green et al., 1989). The N-terminal region of Tat harbors three acidic residues, and of these Glu-2 and Asp-5 are required for full activity (Rappaport et al., 1989). Analysis of Tat mutants with substitution of the acidic residues with Gly has led to the suggestion that, analogous to the acidic effector domains of other known transcription factors, such as GAL4 (Hope et al., 1988; Ptashne, 1988), these negatively charged residues in Tat are essential for *trans*-activation, and that the acidic region could form an amphipathic helical structure (Rappaport et al., 1989).

Although single Pro residues do occur, but rarely, in protein helices (Robson and Garnier, 1986), it is very unlikely that the N-terminal 18-residue sequence of Tat, which contains five Pro residues, could adopt helical conformation. Synthetic full-length analogs of Tat in which the Glu-2, His-13, or all the Pro residue in the Pro–Xaa$_3$–Pro triad were substituted with helix-promoting amino acid Ala or Gln exhibited drastically reduced activity (Reddy et al., 1992). However, substitution of Arg-7, Lys-12, and any one of the Pro residues showed only a slight reduction in function. Thus, the overall structural features of the N-terminal, 19-residue sequence, and not the acidic residues alone, are necessary for full Tat *trans*-activation. The N-terminal region may also be required for interaction with a TAR-binding cellular factor (Jeyapaul et al., 1991). The *tat* gene is produced by splicing of two coding exons. The first coding exon contains a translation termination codon on the 3' end and encodes a 72-residue protein, which is fully functional in cell transfection assay. Synthetic Tat-(1–72), however, was found to be about half as active as the wild-type full-length Tat (Reddy et al., 1992).

Relevance of Tat–TAR Interaction for Tat Function

TAR is a 59-nucleotide hairpin structure located at the 5' end of all HIV-1 transcripts (Rosen et al., 1985). Both the location and the orientation of TAR are critical for function (Rosen et al., 1985; Selby et al., 1989). The TAR RNA sequence primarily supports a functionally responsive structure comprising a six-nucleotide terminal loop structure and a three-nucleotide bulge (Figure 18–3) (Berkhout and Jeang, 1989; Feng and Holland; 1988; Roy et al., 1990b; Selby et al., 1989). Extensive mutational analysis of TAR has identified the region between nucleotides +14 and +45 as the most critical for Tat-mediated *trans*-activation. Responsiveness to Tat requires the primary sequence in the terminal loop (position +30 to +34), the 3-nucleotide bulge at position +23 to +25, and an intact stem (Dingwall et al., 1990; Feng and Holland, 1988; Roy et al., 1990a, 1990b; Selby et al., 1989). TAR is not an inhibitory element, because deletion of TAR did not lead to an increase in basal transcription (Selby et al., 1989). Chimeric proteins

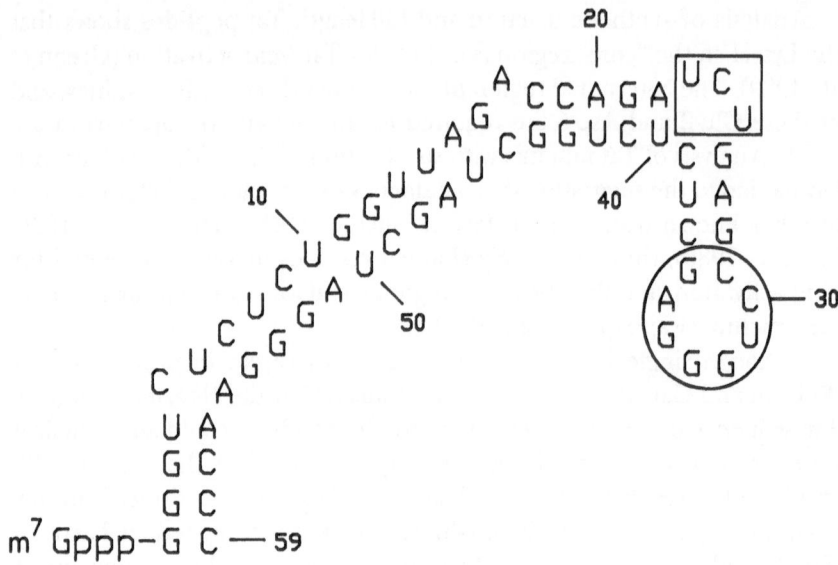

Figure 18-3. Sequence and predicted structure of 59-nucleotide HIV-1 TAR RNA are shown with putative Tat-binding site (*boxed*) and terminal loop structure (*circled*), the binding site for the host cellular factor(s) believed to participate in Tat-mediated *trans*-activation.

consisting of Tat fused to heterologous RNA- or DNA-binding proteins were shown to *trans*-activate HIV-1 LTR in which the TAR sequence was replaced with appropriate RNA or DNA target sequences (Berkhout et al., 1990; Selby and Peterlin, 1990; Southgate et al., 1990). Observation of this TAR-independent, Tat-mediated *trans*-activation provides direct proof that TAR functions at the RNA level, and also suggests that the only essential role for TAR is to act as the RNA target sequence for Tat.

   Tat has been shown to specifically bind to TAR RNA in vitro (Dingwall et al., 1989; Jeyapaul et al., 1991; Roy et al., 1990a; Weeks and Crothers, 1991). The Arg-rich region of Tat has been shown to be both necessary and sufficient for this interaction with TAR in vitro (Calnan et al., 1991; Weeks and Crothers, 1991; Jeyapaul et al., 1991). Several studies have provided evidence supporting a view that binding to TAR RNA is a prerequisite for Tat to enhance transcription from the HIV-1 LTR (Marciniak et al., 1990a; Selby and Peterlin, 1990). Mutations that disrupt the TAR stem or that affect the bulge reduce both in vivo function and in vitro Tat binding (Berkhout and Jeang, 1989; Dingwall et al., 1990; Roy et al., 1990a). However, mutations in the terminal loop of TAR, although deleterious to Tat function, did not adversely influence Tat binding in vitro (Roy et al., 1990a).

These data show that Tat binds TAR at the bulge, and imply that direct interaction of Tat with TAR is necessary but not sufficient for the Tat-mediated *trans*-activation. These data together with the evidence that chimeric proteins *trans*-activate HIV-1 LTR in a TAR-independent manner (Selby and Peterlin, 1990; Southgate et al., 1990) indicate that Tat binding and function in vivo require cooperative interaction of a cellular factor that specifically recognizes the terminal loop structure of TAR. The demonstration that constitutively expressed 59-nucleotide "TAR decoys" inhibit HIV-1 replication in vivo (Sullenger et al., 1990), as well as the data that a 59-nucleotide TAR RNA with mutation in the terminal loop that lacked the ability to bind Tat in vitro also inhibited HIV-1 replication in vivo, provides direct evidence that a TAR loop-binding cellular factor may be involved in Tat function.

An interaction between Tat and this cellular factor before Tat–TAR binding has also been proposed (Madore and Cullen, 1993). The requirements for Tat function, in particular the role of the basic nuclear localization signal sequence, were evaluated using synthetic Tat-(1–86), Tat-(1–57), and Tat-(1–47) in a cell-free transcription assay (Jeyapaul et al., 1990). All three peptides produced a seven- to ninefold increase over the basal level of transcription in the presence of 0.4 μM peptide concentration. Interestingly, at 4 μM, both Tat-(1–86) and Tat-(1–57) inhibited even the basal level of transcription. In contrast, Tat-(1–47), which lacks the basic region, exhibited full stimulatory activity at 4 μM. Several inactive Tat peptide analogs that contain the basic sequence also suppressed basal transcription at concentrations higher than 2 μM. It is conceivable that at high concentrations the basic peptides could sequester a cellular factor required for transcription. These data imply that Tat could interact with the transcription machinery without directly binding to TAR, perhaps in cooperation from a cellular factor. The apparent primary role of the basic region is to facilitate nuclear localization of Tat and subsequently by binding to TAR increase Tat concentration in close proximity to the LTR promoter elements (Berkhout et al., 1990).

The precise functional relevance of Tat–TAR interaction in Tat *trans*-activation is not clear. There is a direct correlation between Tat binding to TAR in vitro and *trans*-activation in vivo. However, Tat–TAR binding by itself is not sufficient to mediate *trans*-activation, as several short Tat peptides containing the basic domain efficiently bind TAR RNA but are unable to *trans*-activate HIV-1 LTR (Cordingley et al., 1990; Weeks et al., 1990). Mobility shift assays showed that Tat-(1–47), which lacks the basic nuclear localization signal sequence, does not bind TAR RNA in vitro (Jeyapaul et al., 1991). Thus it appears that the primary role of the basic domain is to target Tat to the nucleus and that a direct Tat–TAR binding may not be required for Tat *trans*-activation. That Tat-(1–47) might *trans*-activate by interaction with TAR via a cellular factor was proposed because functionally active Tat can interact with TAR-bound nuclear protein(s) in vitro and dissociate the TAR–nuclear protein complexes (Jeyapaul et al., 1991). Thus, in nuclear extracts, Tat-(1–47) could interact with a TAR-bound nuclear protein, and the resulting Tat–protein complex, displaced from TAR, may now be able to recognize other components of the transcription machinery. In the case of full-length Tat, the Tat–nuclear protein complex may function in an analogous manner except that the complex might still be tethered to TAR through the basic domain of Tat. Recognition of the Tat–nuclear protein complex by specific factors could stabilize the transcription elongation component of the RNA polymerase II transcription complex. This novel interaction between Tat and a TAR-bound nuclear protein(s) on a "TAR RNA platform" may have physiological relevance, and may be one of several steps in the mechanism of Tat-mediated *trans*-activation of the HIV-1 LTR.

Several studies have concluded that the basic domain of Tat constitutes an RNA-binding domain with high affinity and specificity (Calnan et al., 1991; Cordingley et al., 1990; Hauber et al., 1989; Kuppuswamy et al., 1989; Roy et al., 1990b; Weeks and Crothers, 1991; Weeks et al., 1990). However, a systematic analysis has provided convincing evidence that peptides containing only the basic domain and the adjacent carboxy-terminal sequence bind TAR in a nonspecific manner. Mobility shift analysis of the binding of Tat peptides with native and mutant TAR RNAs, ethylation interference experiments, and NMR analysis of Tat peptide–TAR complexes have provided a clear picture of the nature and sites of Tat–TAR interaction (Churcher et al., 1993; Delling et al., 1992; Puglisi et al., 1993; Weeks and Crothers, 1991). These studies show that in addition to the basic domain, the adjacent N-terminal sequence, the "core" domain, is required for the high-affinity specific interaction with TAR and full *trans*-activation (Churcher et al., 1993; Weeks and Crothers, 1991). Lys-41, present in the "core"/"activation" region, appears to play a key role in TAR recognition and *trans*-activation (Green et al., 1989; Rice and Carlotti, 1990a).

RNA forms complex three-dimensional structures containing regions of double strands stabilized by Watson–Crick base pairs interspersed by loops and bulges. The residues in the HIV-1 TAR bulge introduce distortion in the local structure of TAR, thereby widening the major groove (Gait and Karn, 1993; Weeks and Crothers, 1991). Quantitative analysis of Tat–TAR binding results shows that a hydrogen bond contact involving the N^7-H of the bulged residue U-23 is critical for Tat binding (Churcher et al., 1993; Delling et al., 1992; Roy et al., 1990b; Sumner-Smith et al., 1991). From these studies it is also concluded that Tat forms specific hydrogen bonds to N^7-H of G_{26}, the N^7-H of A_{27}, and the phosphate between A22 and U23 in the major groove of the TAR RNA (Churcher et al., 1993; Hamy et al., 1993).

Cellular Cofactors of Tat-Mediated *Trans*-Activation

Multiple binding of Tat and nuclear protein(s) to TAR appears to be essential for transcriptional activation of the HIV-1 LTR. The cellular protein (cofactor) may stabilize a preformed complex between Tat and TAR (Berkhout, 1992) or in combination with Tat may play a direct role in the assembly of an elongation-competent transcription complex. Several human nuclear proteins that bind the terminal loop (Marciniak et al., 1990b; Sheline et al., 1991; Wu et al., 1991) or the stem (Gatignol et al., 1991; Rounseville and Kumar, 1992) of TAR RNA in vitro have been identified. Of these, a p68-enriched fraction of HeLa nuclear extract was found to increase further the Tat activity in vitro (Marciniak et al., 1990a, 1990b). However, it is not clear whether this activity resulted from p68 alone or another component present in the fraction. The other characterized TAR-binding cellular proteins, TRP-185 and TRP-1, compete with Tat for TAR rather than bind cooperatively (Sheline et al., 1991; Wu et al., 1991). It is therefore doubtful that these proteins participate in Tat *trans*-activation.

More recent studies to define the role of a cellular factor in Tat function have led to the proposal that neither Tat nor cellular factor binds to TAR alone in vivo, and that a prior binding of Tat to cellular factor may be essential for Tat–TAR interaction (Madore and Cullen, 1993). Determination of the role of nuclear transcription factors and elucidation of specific mechanisms will require evaluation of purified TAR- and Tat-binding nuclear proteins in reconstituted transcription. Cell-free transcription assays (Jeyapaul et al., 1990; Marciniak et al., 1990a) that appear to faithfully reproduce TAR-dependent Tat-mediated trans-activation should be useful in elucidating the mechanism of function of this important viral *trans*-regulator.

Does Lupus Autoantigen Ku Protein Play a Role in HIV-1 Gene Expression?

A HeLa nuclear protein that specifically interacted with TAR RNA has been identified in a Northwestern analysis and characterized as the 86-kDa subunit of the Ku protein (Kaczmarski and Khan, 1993). Ku is a relatively abundant DNA-binding protein that was first detected as the autoantigen in patients with systemic lupus erythematosus and other autoimmune diseases (Mimori et al., 1986). Ku is a heterodimer of two polypeptide chains of molecular weights 72 and 86 kDa, respectively, that characteristically binds ends of dsDNA in vitro and translocates to form multimeric complexes (de Vries et al., 1989; Griffith et al., 1992; Mimori and Hardin, 1986; Zhang and Yaneva, 1992). Purified Ku protein was found to bind HIV-1 TAR RNA in vitro with high affinity and specificity (Kaczmarski and Khan, 1993). Mobility shift analysis indicated that Ku recognizes the native stem-loop structure as it did not bind dsRNA and exhibited drastically reduced affinities for TAR RNAs containing mutations either at the terminal loop or that destabilized the stem. The Ku protein has been shown to be the DNA-binding component of the protein kinase (DNA-PK) that phosphory-lates RNA polymerase II, and thus may be involved in transcriptional regu-lation (Dvir et al., 1992; Gottlieb and Jackson, 1993).

Phosphorylation of RNA polymerase II by DNA-PK activity appears to facilitate the transition from the promoter-bound form to the elongating form of the enzyme. DNA-PK phosphorylates the carboxy-terminal domain of the larger subunit of RNA polymerase II, and is also required for the phosphorylation of transcription factor SP1. Ku is modulated by viral in-fections and other cellular changes (Quinn et al., 1992), and its expression is enhanced during cell proliferation (Yaneva and Jhiang, 1991). In addi-tion, Ku localizes into the nucleus in a cell-cycle-dependent manner (Higashiura et al., 1992; Li and Yeh, 1992). Considering these data together with the high-affinity binding of Ku to TAR RNA, it is conceivable that Ku might play a role in HIV-1 gene expression. The Ku–TAR interaction may provide an increased concentration of DNA-PK close to the transcription start site. As Tat is not phosphorylated, it will be significant to know whether the Ku–TAR interaction modifies a specific cellular factor required for Tat *trans*-activation. In this context, it is interesting to note that Tat *trans*-activa-tion has been shown to correlate with phosphorylation of a TAR RNA-binding cellular factor (Han et al., 1992). The role of the Ku protein in HIV-1 gene expression and AIDS remains to be defined.

Tat: A Transcription Processivity Factor

The Tat-dependent HIV-1 gene regulation has been suggested to occur at several levels. Tat appears to increase both the rate of transcription initia-tion and mRNA elongation, thereby increasing processivity (Kao et al., 1987; Laspia et al., 1989), and may also stimulate translation of the viral mRNA (Braddock et al., 1989; SenGupta et al., 1990). Tat is believed to increase the steady-state levels of transcripts derived from genes linked to HIV-1 LTR (Cullen, 1986), and this increase is believed to result from an enhanced rate of transcription and not stabilization of mRNAs containing TAR (Hauber et al., 1987). In the absence of functional Tat, the majority of the viral transcripts produced are short, ranging in size from 60 to 80 nucle-otides (Bengal and Aloni, 1991; Kao et al., 1987; Kessler and Mathews, 1992; Laspia et al., 1989). It is therefore proposed that Tat could function to prevent premature termination of transcripts containing the TAR ele-ment.

Evidence in support of the hypothesis that Tat promotes transcription elongation has been obtained for both in vitro and in vivo conditions

(Feinberg et al., 1991; Graeble et al., 1992; Kessler and Mathews, 1992; Kato et al., 1992). Thus it appears that Tat acts as a processivity factor on RNA polymerase II through interaction with the nascent TAR, perhaps with cooperation from at least one cellular factor. In addition to increasing the processivity of transcription, Tat has been shown to exert a stimulatory influence on translation of mRNAs containing the TAR sequence at the 5' end (Braddock et al., 1989, 1990; SenGupta et al., 1990). At present, the mechanisms by which Tat acts to enhance HIV-1 LTR-directed gene expression are not fully understood.

Rev Protein

HIV-1 encodes two classes of mRNAs. An early class of viral transcripts consists of the multiply spliced, approximately 2-kb mRNA species that encode the viral regulatory proteins Tat, Rev, and Nef (Figure 18–4). The late class of viral mRNAs consists of the unspliced (~9-kb) and singly spliced (~4-kb) transcripts that encode the viral structural proteins and the auxiliary proteins Vif, Vpr, and Vpu (Feinberg et al., 1986). In the absence of functional Rev, only the fully spliced mRNAs are expressed (Feinberg et al., 1986; Malim et al., 1988; Sadaie et al. 1988). An increase in the expression of the singly spliced and unspliced viral mRNAs is concomitant with the reduction in the expression of the multiply spliced mRNAs. Thus, Rev functions as a negative regulator of its own synthesis and the synthesis of Tat and Nef. The Rev protein appears to selectively induce the transport of unspliced and singly spliced HIV-1 mRNAs from the nucleus to the cytoplasm (Emerman et al., 1989; Felber et al., 1989; Malim et al., 1989) and to promote polysomal association and translation of these mRNAs (Arrigo and Chen, 1991; D'Agostino et al., 1992; Garrett et al., 1991). In HIV-1-infected and HIV-1-transfected cells, Rev has been shown to be associated with RRE-containing RNAs in the cytoplasm (Arrigo et al., 1992). These findings indicate that Rev is essential along the entire mRNA transport and utilization pathway involving correct localization and efficient translation of RRE-containing mRNAs.

The rev gene consists of two coding exons and translates to produce a 116-residue protein (Figure 18–5). Rev is a phosphoprotein localized to the nucleus/nucleoli of expressing cells (Cochrane et al., 1990b; Malim et al., 1989). Mutation analysis has defined three distinct domains that are essential for Rev function. The Arg-rich region (residues 34–50) is required for the nuclear/nucleolar localization (Berger et al., 1991; Cochrane et al., 1990b; Hope et al., 1990; Kubota et al., 1992; Venkatesh et al., 1990), and is also necessary and sufficient for the interaction of Rev with the RRE (Berger et al., 1991; Heaphy et al., 1990; Kjems et al., 1991; Malim et al., 1990; Olsen et al., 1990b; Zapp and Green, 1989). The Arg-rich regions in both

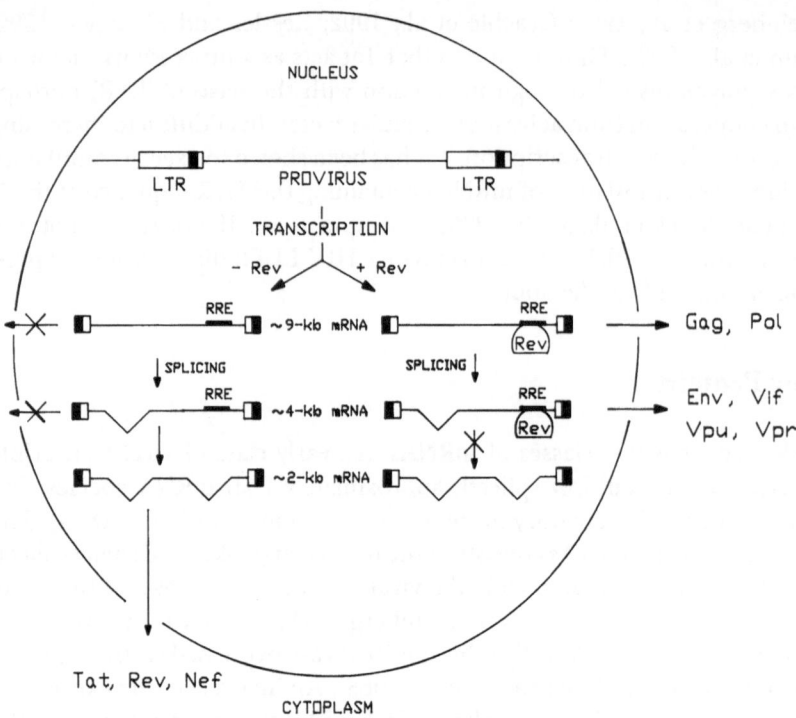

Figure 18–4. Schematic representation of regulation of HIV-1 gene expression by the Rev protein. Nuclear and cytoplasmic pattern of HIV-1 mRNA expression observed in absence of Rev (i.e., early gene expression) and in presence of Rev (i.e., late gene expression) is indicated. (Modified, with permission, from Cullen (1990): *FASEB J* 5:2361–2368.)

Tat and Rev have similar functions; they participate in RNA binding and nuclear localization, and can be interchanged without loss of biological activity of either protein. A synthetic peptide corresponding in sequence to this region specifically recognized RRE at the same nucleotides as full-length Rev, suggesting that this region of Rev forms the RRE-binding domain (Kjems et al., 1992).

Sequences adjacent to the Arg-rich region are involved in the multimerization of Rev, a process that appears to be critical for Rev function in vivo (Malim and Cullen, 1991; Olsen et al., 1990a; Zapp et al., 1991). Based on mutational analysis, the Leu-rich region around amino acid 80 is proposed to be critical for Rev regulation and is believed to interact with a component of the nuclear RNA transport or splicing machinery (Malim et

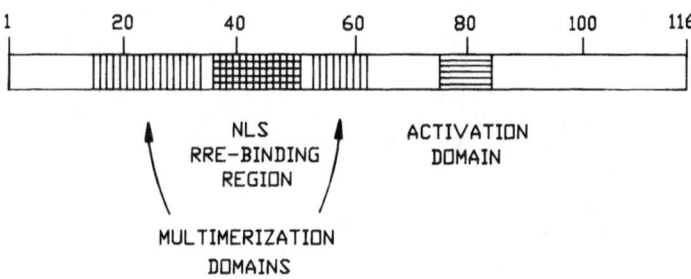

```
1        *        *                                              50
MAGRSGDSDEELIRTVRLIKLLYQSDPPPNPEGTRQARRNRRRRWRERQR
   *                                               *      * 100
QIHSISERILGTYLGRSAEPVPLQLPPLERLTLDCNEDCGTSGTQGVGSP
       *                116
QILVESPTVLESGTKE
```

Figure 18-5. Functional domains of HIV-1 Rev protein. Three functional domains in the 116-residue Rev have been identified. Arg-rich sequence (position 35–50) appears both necessary and sufficient for nuclear/nucleolar localization and specific binding to RRE. Amino acid sequences adjacent to basic region (amino acids 18–34 and 51–56) are required for multimerization of Rev on RRE. Region 75–83, which is rich in Leu residues, is not required for interaction with RRE and oligomerization, but is essential for *trans*-activation. Potential phosphorylation sites are marked: Ser-8 (casein kinase II), Thr-15 and Ser-56 (protein kinase C), Ser-92, Ser-99, and Ser-106 (MAP and cdc2 kinases) (see text for details).

al., 1991). Rev analogs mutated in this region retain the ability to bind RRE and multimerize, and not only were functionally defective but were able to inhibit wild-type Rev regulation in *trans* (Malim et al., 1989; Venkatesh and Chinnadurai, 1990). This ability to *trans*-dominate may be a result of competition for RRE or the formation of inactive mixed multimers incapable of interaction with a cellular factor. The multifunctional nature of Rev would require a physiological turnover or dynamic movement of the protein in the nucleus and cytoplasm. Rev has been shown to associate with a nucleolar protein B23 (Fankhauser et al., 1991), which is believed to function as a shuttle receptor for nuclear import of ribosomal proteins (Borer et al., 1989). It is conceivable that B23 also serves as a shuttle for the import of Rev from the cytoplasm to the nucleus, permitting further rounds of export of the RRE-containing RNAs.

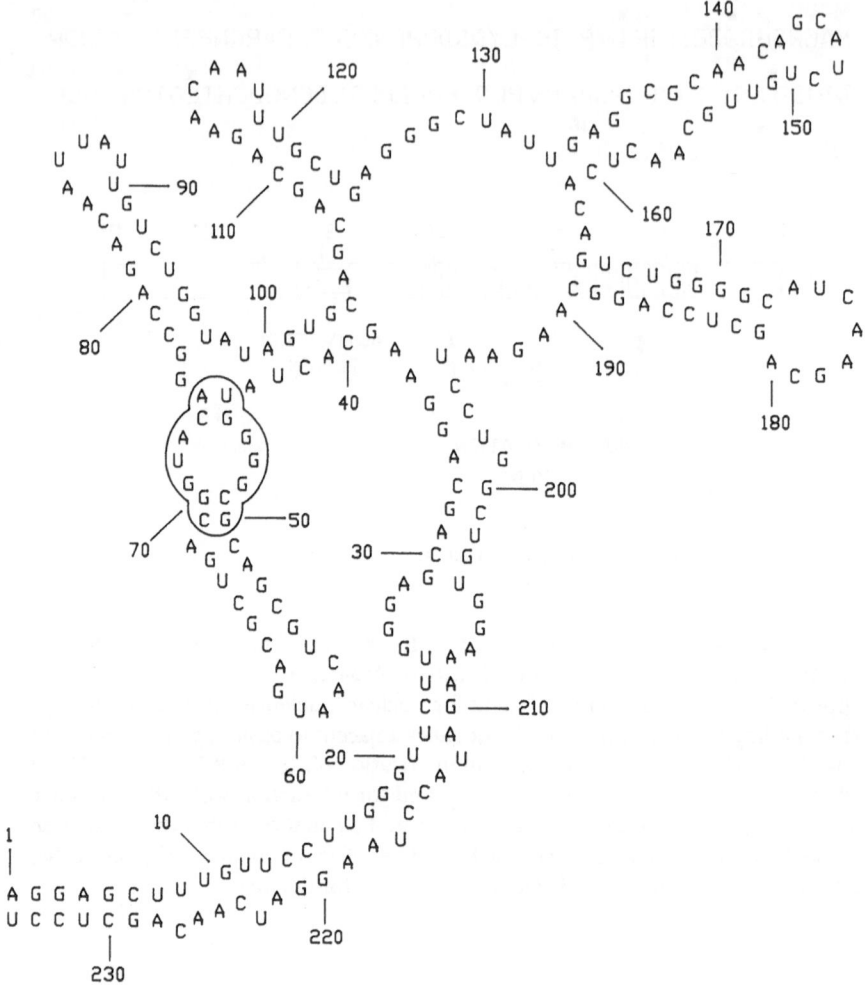

Figure 18–6. Sequence and predicted secondary structure of the 234-nucleotide HIV-1 RRE RNA. Approximate location of primary Rev binding site is marked.

RRE Recognition by Rev

The action of Rev is specific for HIV-1 transcripts that contain a highly structured 234-nucleotide RNA target sequence (Figure 18–6), the Rev-response element (RRE), which is located in the *env* gene of HIV-1 (Cochrane et al., 1990a; Malim et al., 1989; Rosen et al., 1988). Rev has been shown to bind RRE as a multimer in vitro (Daefler et al., 1990; Malim et al., 1990; Olsen et al., 1990b; Zapp et al., 1991); at least four molecules of Rev bind to one molecule of RRE (Heaphy et al., 1991). RNA footprinting data suggest that RRE contains several discrete binding sites for Rev (Kjems et al., 1991), and a minimal structure containing a 35-nucleotide stem-loop structure has been shown to bind Rev as a monomer (Cook et al., 1991; Heaphy et al., 1991; Huang et al., 1991; Tiley et al., 1992). However, the entire RRE sequence is required for full Rev regulation in vivo (Malim et al., 1989) and involves recognition of non-Watson–Crick base pairs in viral RNA (Bartel et al., 1991).

Rev Regulation and Mechanism of HIV-1 Latency

Although indispensable for the expression of the HIV-1 RNAs encoding the structural proteins, Rev does not have any effect on the pattern of the viral RNA expression in the nucleus (Emerman et al., 1989; Felber et al., 1989; Malim et al., 1989). The presence of high levels of unspliced RNAs even in the absence of Rev suggests that for some obscure reasons these RNAs are not efficiently used by the splicing machinery and are retained in the nucleus. RRE has been shown to interact directly with U1 small nuclear ribonucleoprotein particle (snRNP) (Lu et al., 1990), a factor critically involved in RNA splicing. It is proposed that Rev might activate the nuclear export of the sequestered viral RNAs by antagonizing their interactions with the splicing machinery (Chang and Sharp, 1989; Kjems et al., 1991; Lu et al., 1990). A synthetic peptide corresponding in sequence to the basic domain, amino acids 34–50, was found to inhibit the splicing of a β-globin pre-mRNA containing the RRE element (Kjems et al., 1991). This peptide is proposed to form a helical structure, which may directly interact with specific sites in the major groove of RRE (Tan et al., 1993).

Recent evidence indicates that the basic domain of Rev does not interfere with U1 snRNP binding but inhibits splicing by blocking the entry of the essential U4/U6.U5 tri-snRNP particle in spliceosome assembly (Kjems and Sharp, 1993). On the basis of these data, it is suggested that Rev may function via inhibition of spliceosome assembly in vivo. The in vivo activity of Rev appears to be concentration dependent, as would be expected of a mechanism of action based on RNA packaging (Pomerantz et al., 1990, 1992). Because of its ability to oligomerize, Rev packs more efficiently the viral mRNA containing RRE into rodlike ribonucleoprotein filaments (Heaphy et al., 1991). Direct evidence has been obtained (Arrigo et al., 1992) that Rev is associated with high levels of RRE-containing RNA in the cytoplasm, but not the nuclear, fractions in HIV-1-infected and HIV-1-transfected cells. The continued association of Rev with RRE-containing RNA has been interpreted to mean that Rev facilitates association of HIV-1 mRNAs with the translation machinery.

Requirement of a threshold level of Rev for a productive infection may explain the high level of nonproductive or latent HIV-1 infection observed in vivo (Fauci, 1988). In latently infected T-lymphocytic cell lines, the baseline pattern of HIV-1 RNA consists of multiply spliced and singly spliced RNA but little or no unspliced HIV-1 RNA (Pomerantz et al., 1990). A similar pattern is seen with cells infected with Rev-negative mutant virus (Feinberg et al., 1986; Trono and Baltimore, 1990). Mitogenic stimulation of these latently infected cells causes a dramatic increase in the level of multiply spliced HIV-1 RNA species before the level of unspliced RNA increases. Thus, a threshold level of Rev appears to be necessary to rescue most unspliced HIV-1 RNA from the nucleus and for efficient HIV-1 replication. Further, a threshold level of Rev may be expected to be essential for multimerization or interaction with cellular factor(s) that cooperate in its function (Trono and Baltimore, 1990). To establish this further, cells that constitutively expressed a Rev-deficient provirus were transfected with various quantities of a Rev-expressing plasmid (Pomerantz et al., 1992). Compared to the quantity of the Rev-expressing plasmid transfected, HIV-1 replication was found to be distinctly nonlinear, suggesting that a threshold level of Rev is necessary for a highly productive HIV-1 infection. It is suggested (Malim and Cullen, 1991) that this requirement could prevent a premature progression to the late, structural phase of the viral replication that might result in the death of the infected cell before the release of a significant level of progeny virions and might therefore be deleterious to the efficient spread of HIV-1 in the infected host.

Role of Phosphorylation in Rev Function

Rev is phosphorylated in vivo (Cochrane et al., 1989a, 1989b; Malim et al., 1989), but the stoichiometry and sites of modification have not been unequivocally established. Rev is phosphorylated in vivo in the absence of external stimuli, and the level of phosphorylation is increased by mitogens, such as 12-O-tetradecanoylphorbol-13-acetate, a specific activator of cellular protein kinases (Hauber et al., 1988). However, it is not known whether the observed mitogen-induced enhanced phosphorylation is caused by production of a higher level of the same phospho-Rev isoform(s) or that other Ser/Thr were targeted. Rev contains sequence motifs that are recognized by various kinases: Ser-8 (casein kinase II), Thr-15 and Ser-56 (protein kinase C), and Ser-92, Sr-99, and Ser-106 (MAP and cdc2 kinases) (Kemp and Pearson, 1990). Studies with Rev mutants have led to the suggestion that phosphorylation is dispensable for the *trans*-acting activity of Rev (Cochrane et al., 1989b). However, the other alternative, that phosphorylation might suppress Rev function, has not been explored. Because a threshold level of Rev is required for Rev regulation in vivo, it is not inconceivable that phosphorylation might suppress one or more functions of Rev and that reversible phosphorylation–dephosphorylation could play a role in HIV-1 latency.

Many nuclear proteins are regulated by phosphorylation, and the effect can be either stimulatory or inhibitory (reviewed by Hunter and Karin, 1992; Meek and Street, 1992). Phosphorylation controls many different activities of nuclear proteins. For example, multimerization of Bg1G, a sequence-specific RNA-binding protein (Amster-Choder and Wright, 1992), nucleic acid binding of c-Myb (Luscher et al., 1990) and c-Jun (Boyle et al., 1991), subcellular localization of HTLV I Rex (Kiyokawa et al., 1985) and SV40 T antigen (Jans et al., 1991; Previs et al., 1990), stability of nucleolin (Warrener and Petryshyn, 1991), and *trans*-acting activity of c-Fos (Ofir et al., 1990) and c-Jun (Smeal et al., 1992) are all modulated by phosphorylation–dephosphorylation equilibria. Similarly, it is possible that phosphorylation may influence the subcellular localization, multimerization and RRE binding of Rev, and consequently its *trans*-acting function. Several kinases are able to phosphorylate Rev, and phosphorylation with protein kinase C appears to inhibit the functionally essential Rev-RRE interaction (Khan and Addya, in manuscript).   The HIV-1 Rev and HTLV-II Rex have similar functions and appear to function via closely related mechanisms (Cullen, 1992). More recently, phosphorylation of the Rex protein of HTLV-II was shown to be essential for its binding to the target RNA element (Green et al., 1992). As proposed in the cases of infection with SV40 (Fanning, 1992) and HTLV-II Rex (Green et al., 1992), the temporal control of HIV-1 gene expression may be based primarily on a dynamic balance between the phosphorylation rate of Rev on key Ser residues and the production of unmodified Rev, either through enzymatic dephosphorylation or through new synthesis of Rev. In newly infected cells, most of the Rev synthesized in the early, low level of basal transcription from HIV-1 LTR might accumulate in the phosphorylated, inactive form. However, as the concentration of the phosphorylated Rev increases, cellular phosphatases will act. As a result, a concentration of the functionally active Rev will emerge. On exceeding the threshold concentration, this active form of Rev would switch HIV-1 gene expression into the late, structural phase leading to viral replication.

Conclusions

The Tat and Rev proteins control HIV-1 gene expression through specific interactions with sequences present in the viral mRNAs. Studies of Tat–TAR and Rev–RRE interactions using synthetic peptides have provided a detailed understanding of the chemistry of the protein recognition of RNA. These observations bring forth the possibility that small molecules that can compete with these functionally important protein-RNA interactions could generate a novel class of inhibitors of HIV-1 gene expression and replication.

A combination of mobility shift analysis and cell-free transcription and splicing assays could permit ready evaluation of potential inhibitors of Tat and Rev. Results of such analyses together with data on the three-dimensional structures of the Tat–TAR and Rev–RRE complexes may lead to design of molecules with therapeutic potential to combat the progress of AIDS.

Acknowledgments

I take this opportunity to thank Professor K. M. Sivanandiah for his guidance, encouragement, and friendship that inspired me to try to become someone like him, a good scientist.

REFERENCES

Ahmad N, Venkatesan S (1988): *J Virol* 64:5966–5975.
Amster-Choder O, Wright A (1992): *Science* 257:1395–1398.
Arrigo SJ, Chen ISY (1991): Genes & Dev 5:808–819.
Arrigo SJ, Heaphy S, Haines JK (1992): *J Virol* 66:5569–5575.
Arya SK, Guo C, Josephs SF, Wong-Staal F (1985): *Science* 229:69–73.
Bartel DP, Zapp ML, Green MR, Szostak JW (1991): *Cell* 67:529–536.
Bengal EA, Aloni Y (1991): *J Virol* 65:4910–4918.
Berger J, Aepinus C, Dobrovnik M, Fleckenstein B, Hauber J, Bohnlein E (1991): *Virology* 183:630–635.
Berkhout B, Jeang K-T (1989): *J Virol* 63:5501–5504.
Berkhout B, Jeang K-T (1992): *J Virol* 66:139–149.
Berkhout B, Gatignol A, Rabson AB, Jeang K-T (1990): *Cell* 62:757–767.
Borer RA, Lehner CF, Eppenberger HM, Nigg EA (1989): *Cell* 56:379–390.
Boyle W, Smeal T, Defize LHK, Angel P, Woodgett JR, Karin M, Hunter T (1991): *Cell* 64:573–584.
Braddock M, Chambers A, Wilson W, Esnouf MP, Adams SE, Kingsman AJ, Kingsman SM (1989): *Cell* 58:269–279.
Braddock M, Thorburn AM, Chambers A, Elliot GD, Anderson GJ, Kingsman AJ, Kingsman SM (1990): *Cell* 62:1123–1133.
Calnan BJ, Biancalana S, Hudson D, Frankel AD (1991): *Genes & Dev* 5:201–210.
Chang DD, Sharp PA (1989): *Cell* 59:789–795.
Churcher MJ, Lamont C, Hamy F, Dingwall C, Green SM, Lowe AD, Butler PJG, Gait MJ, Karn J (1993): *J Mol Biol* 230:90–110.
Cochrane A, Golub E, Volsky D, Ruben S, Rosen CA (1989a): *J Virol* 63:4438–4440.
Cochrane A, Kramer R, Ruben S, Levine J, Rosen CA (1989b): *Virology* 171:264–266.
Cochrane AW, Chen C-H, Rosen CA (1990a): *Proc Natl Acad Sci USA* 87:1198–1202.
Cochrane AW, Perkins A, Rosen CA (1990b): *J Virol* 64:881–885.
Cook KS, Fisk GJ, Hauber J, Usman N, Daly TJ, Rusche JR (1991): *Nucleic Acids Res* 19:1577–1583.

Cordingley MG, LaFemina RL, Callahan PL, Condra JH, Sardana VV, Graham DJ, Nguyen TM, LeGrow K, Gotlib L, Schlabach AJ, Colonno RJ (1990): *Proc Natl Acad Sci USA* 87:8985–8989.

Cullen BR (1986): *Cell* 46:973–982.

Cullen BR (1992): *Microbiol Rev* 56:375–394.

D'Agostino DM, Felber BK, Harrison JE, Pavlakis GN (1992): *Mol Cell Biol* 12:1375–1386.

Daefler S, Klotman ME, Wong-Staal F (1990): *Proc Natl Acad Sci USA* 87:4571–4575.

Delling U, Reid LS, Barnett R, Ma M, Climie S, Sumner-Smith M, Sonenberg N (1992): *J Virol* 663018–3025.

Delling U, Roy S, Sumner-Smith M, Barnett R, Reid L, Rosen CA, Sonenberg N (1991): *Proc Natl Acad Sci USA* 88:6234–6238.

de Vries E, van Driel W, Bergsma WG, Arnberg AC, van der Vliet PC (1989): *J Mol Biol* 208:65–78.

Dingwall C, Ernberg I, Gait M, Green S, Heaphy S, Karn J, Lowe A, Singh M, Skinner M, Valerio R (1989): *Proc Natl Acad Sci USA* 86:6925–6929.

Dingwall C, Ernberg I, Gait M, Green S, Heaphy S, Karn J, Lowe A, Singh M, Singh M, Skinner M (1990): *EMBO J* 9:4145–4153.

Dvir A, Peterson SR, Knuth MW, Lu H, Dynan WS (1992): *Proc Natl Acad Sci USA* 89:11920–11204.

Emerman M, Vazeux R, Pedan K (1989): *Cell* 57:1155–1165.

Fairwell T, Hospattankar AV, Brewer HB, Jr., Khan SA (1987): *Proc Natl Acad Sci USA* 84:4796–4800.

Fankhauser C, Izaurralde E, Adachi Y, Wingfield P, Laemmli UK (1991): *Mol Cell Biol* 11:2567–2575.

Fanning E (1992): *J Virol* 66:1289–1293.

Fauci AS (1988): *Science* 239:617–622.

Feinberg MB, Baltimore D, Frankel AD (1991): *Proc Natl Acad Sci USA* 88:4045–4049.

Feinberg MB, Jarrett RF, Aldovini A, Gallo RC, Wong-Staal F (1986): *Cell* 46:807–817.

Felber BK, Hadzopoulou-Cladaras M, Cladaras C, Copeland T, Pavlakis GN (1989): *Proc Natl Acad Sci USA* 86:1495–1499.

Feng S, Holland EC (1988): *Nature (London)* 334:165–167.

Frankel AD, Pabo CO (1988): *Science* 240:70–73.

Frankel A, Biancalana S, Hudson D (1989): *Proc Natl Acad Sci USA* 86:7397–7401.

Gait MJ, Karn J (1993): *Trends Biochem Sci* 18:255–259.

Garcia J, Harrich D, Pearson L, Mitsuyasu R, Gaynor RB (1988): *EMBO J* 7:3143–3147.

Garrett ED, Tiley LS, Cullen BR (1991): *J Virol* 65:1653–1657.

Gatignol A, Buckler-White A, Berkhout B, Jeang K-T (1991): *Science* 251:1597–1600.

Gottlieb TM, Jackson SP (1993): *Cell* 72:131–142.

Graeble MA, Churcher MJ, Lowe AD, Gait MJ, Karn J (1992): *Proc Natl Acad Sci USA* 90:6184–6188.

Green M, Loewenstein P (1988): *Cell* 55:1179–1188.

Green M, Ishino M, Loewenstein PM (1989): *Cell* 58:215–223.

Green PL, Yip MT, Xie Y, Chen ISV (1992): *J Virol* 66:4325–4330.

Griffith AJ, Blier PR, Mimori T, Hardin JA (1992): *J Biol Chem* 267:331–338.

Hamy F, Asseline U, Grasby J, Iwai S, Pritchard C, Slim G, Butler PJG, Karn J, Gait MJ (1993): *J Mol Biol* 230:111–123.

Han XM, Laras A, Rounseville MP, Kumar A, Shank PR (1992): *J Virol* 66:4065–4072.

Hauber J, Malim MH, Cullen BR (1989): *J Virol* 63:1181–1187.

Hauber J, Bouvier M, Malim MH, Cullen BR (1988): *J Virol* 62:4801–4804.

Hauber J, Perkins A, Heimer EP, Cullen BR (1987): *Proc Natl Acad Sci USA* 84:6364–6368.

Heaphy S, Finch JT, Gait MJ, Karn J, Singh M (1991): *Proc Natl Acad Sci USA* 88:7366–7370.

Heaphy S, Dingwall C, Ernberg I, Gait MJ, Green SM, Karn J, Lowe AD, Singh M, Skinner MA (1990): *Cell* 60:685–693.

Higashiura M, Shimizu Y, Tanimoto M, Morita T, Yagura T (1992): *Exp Cell Res* 201:444–451.

Hope IA, Mahadevan S, Struhl K (1988): *Nature (London)* 333:635–640.

Hope TJ, McDonald D, Huang X, Low J, Parslow TG (1990): *J Virol* 64:5360–5366.

Huang X, Hope TJ, Bond B, McDonald D, Grahl K, Parslow TG (1991): *J Virol* 65:2131–2134.

Hunter T, Karin M (1992): *Cell* 70:375–387.

Jans DA, Ackerman MJ, Biscoff JR, Beach DH, Peters R (1991): *J Cell Biol* 115:1203–1212.

Jeyapaul J, Reddy M, Khan SA (1990): *Proc Natl Acad Sci USA* 87:7030–7043.

Jeyapaul J, Seshamma T, Khan SA (1991): *Oncogene* 7:1507–1513.

Kaczmarski W, Khan SA (1993): *Biochem Biophys Res Commun* 196:935–942.

Kao S-Y, Calman AF, Luciw PA, Petrelin BM (1987): *Nature (London)* 330:489–493.

Kato H, Sumimoto H, Pognonec P, Chen C-H, Rosen CA, Roeder RG (1992): *Genes & Dev* 6:655–666.

Kemp BE, Pearson RB (1990): *Trends Biochem Sci* 15:342–346.

Kessler M, Mathews MB (1992): *J Virol* 66:4488–4449.

Khan SA, Addya K: (in manuscript).

Kiyokawa T, Seiki M, Iwashita S, Imagawa K, Shimizu F, Yoshida M (1985): *Proc Natl Acad Sci USA* 82:8359–8363.

Kjems J, Sharp PA (1993): *J Virol* 67:4769–4776.

Kjems J, Brown B, Chang CC, Sharp PA (1991): *Proc Natl Acad Sci USA* 88:683–687.

Kjems J, Calnan BJ, Frankel AD, Sharp PA (1992): *EMBO J* 11:1119–1129.

Knight DM, Flomerfelt FA, Ghrayeb J (1987): *Science* 236:837–840.

Kubota S, Furuta R, Maki M, Hatanaka M (1992): *J Virol* 66:2510–2513.

Kuppuswamy M, Subramanian T, Srinivasan A, Chinnadurai G (1989): *Nucleic Acids Res* 17:3551–3561.

Laspia MP, Rice AP, Mathews MB (1989): *Cell* 59:83–292.

Li L-L, Yeh N-H (1992): *Exp Cell Res* 199:262–268.

Lu X, Heimer J, Rekosh D, Hammarskjold M-L (1990): *Proc Natl Acad Sci USA* 87:7598–7602.

Lüscher B, Christenson E, Litchfield DW, Kreb EG, Eisenman RN (1990): *Nature* 344:517–522.

Madore S, Cullen BR (1993): *J Virol* 67:3703–3711.

Malim MH, Cullen BR (1991): *Cell* 65:241–248.

Malim MH, Hauber J, Fenrick R, Cullen BR (1988): *Nature (London)* 335:181–183.

Malim MH, Hauber J, Le S-Y, Maizel JV, Cullen BR (1989): *Nature (London)* 338:254–257.

Malim MH, McCarn DF, Tiley LS, Cullen BR (1991): *J Virol* 65:4248–4254.

Malim MH, Tiley LS, McCarn DF, Rusche JR, Hauber J, Cullen BR (1990): *Cell* 60:675–683.

Marciniak RA, Calnan BJ, Frankel AD, Sharp PA (1990a): *Cell* 63:791–802.

Marciniak RA, Garcio-Blanco MA, Sharp PA (1990b): *Proc Natl Acad Sci USA* 87:3624–3628.

Meek DW, Street AJ (1992): *Biochem J* 287:1–15.

Mimori T, Hardin JA (1986): *J Biol Chem* 261:10375–10379.

Mimori T, Hardin JA, Steitz JA (1986): *J Biol Chem* 261:2274–2278.

Ofir R, Dwarki VJ, Rashid D, Verma I (1990): *Nature (London)* 348:80–82.

Olsen HS, Cochrane AW, Dillon CM, Rosen CA (1990a): *Genes & Dev* 4:1357–1364.

Olsen HS, Nelbock P, Cochrane AW, Rosen CA (1990b): *Science* 247:845–848.

Palmeri D, Khan SA: (in manuscript).

Pomerantz R, Seshamma T, Trono D (1992): *J Virol* 66:1809–1813.

Pomerantz R, Trono D, Feinberg MB, Baltimore D (1990): *Cell* 62:1271–1276.

Previs C (1990): *Cell* 61:735–738.

Ptashne M (1988): *Nature (London)* 335:683–689.

Puglisi JD, Chen L, Frankel AD, Williamson JR (1993): *Proc Natl Acad Sci USA* 90:3680–3684.

Quinn JP, Simpson J, Farina AR (1992): *Biochim Biophys Acta* 1131:181–187.

Rappaport J, Lee SJ, Khalili K, Wong-Staal F (1989): *New Biologist* 1:101–110.

Reddy MV, Desai M, Jeyapaul J, Prasad DDK, Seshamma T, Palmeri D, Khan SA (1992): *Oncogene* 7:1743–1748.

Rice A, Carlotti F (1990a): *J Virol* 64:1864–1868.

Rice A, Carlotti F (1990b): *J Virol* 64:6018–6026.

Robson B, Garnier J (1986): *Introduction to Proteins and Protein Engineering*. Amsterdam: Elsevier.

Rosen CA, Terwilliger E, Dayton A, Sodroski J, Haseltine W (1988): *Proc Natl Acad Sci USA* 85:2071-2075.

Rounseville MP, Kumar A (1992): *J Virol* 66:1688–1694.

Roy S, Delling U, Chen C-H, Rosen CA, Sonenberg N (1990a): *Genes & Dev* 4:1365–1373.

Roy S, Parkin NT, Rosen CA, Itovitch J, Sonenberg N (1990b): *J Virol* 64:1402–1406.

Ruben S, Perkins A, Purcell R, Joung K, Sia R, Burghoff R, Haseltine WA, Rosen CA (1989): *J Virol* 63:1–8.

Sadaie MR, Benter T, Wong-Staal F (1988): *Science* 239:910–913.

Schneider J, Kent S (1988): *Cell* 54:363–368.

Selby MJ, Peterlin BM (1990): *Cell* 62:769–776.

Selby MJ, Bain ES, Luciw PA, Peterlin BM (1989): *Genes & Dev* 3:547–558.

SenGupta DN, Berkhout B, Gatignol A, Zhou A, Silverman RH (1990): *Proc Natl Acad Sci USA* 87:7492–7496.

Sheline CT, Milocco LH, Jones KA (1991): *Genes & Dev* 5:2508–2520.

Smeal T, Binetruy B, Mercola D, Grover-Bardwick A, Heidecker G, Rapp UR, Karin M (1992): *Mol Cell Biol* 12:3507–3513.

Sodroski J, Goh WC, Rosen C, Dayton A, Terwilliger E, Hasetine W (1986): *Nature (London)* 321:412–417.

Southgate C, Zapp ML, Green MR (1990): *Nature (London)* 345:640–642.

Sullenger BA, Gallardo HF, Ungers GE, Gilboa E (1990): *Cell* 63:601–608.

Sumner-Smith M, Roy S, Barnett R, Reid LS, Kuperman R, Delling U, Soneneberg N (1991): *J Virol* 65:5196–5202.

Tan R, Chen L, Buettner JA, Hudson D, Frankel AD (1993): *Cell* 73:1031–1040.

Tiley LS, Malim MH, Tewary HK, Stockley PG, Cullen BR (1992): *Cell* 55:197–109.

Trono D, Baltimore D (1990): *EMBO J* 9:4155–4160.

Varmus H, Brown P (1989): In: *Mobile DNA*, Berg DE, Howe MM, eds. Washington, DC: American Society for Microbiology.

Venkatesh LK, Chinnadurai G (1990): *Virology* 178:327–330.

Venkatesh LK, Mohammed S, Chinnadurai G (1990): *Virology* 176:39–47.

Warrener P, Petryshyn R (1991): *Biochem Biophys Chem Commun* 180:716–723.

Weeks KM, Crothers DM (1991): *Cell* 66:577–588.

Weeks KM, Ampe C, Schultz SC, Steitz TA, Crothers DM (1990): *Science* 249:1281–1285.

Wu F, Garcia J, Sigman D, Gaynor R (1991): *Genes & Dev* 5:2128–2140.

Yaneva M, Jhiang S (1991): *Biochim Biophys Acta* 1091:181–187.

Zapp ML, Green MR (1989): *Nature (London)* 342:714–716.

Zapp ML, Hope TJ, Parslow TG, Green MR (1991): *Proc Natl Acad Sci USA* 88:7734–7738.

Zhang W-W, Yaneva M (1992): *Biochem Biophys Res Commun* 186:574–579.

INDEX

Acetylation, 42, 44, 50
Acid–base titration, 107
Acid chlorides, 6, 54
ACTH, 3–4, 167, 172–174, 227
Actin, 242–243
Active esters, 2–3, 5, 42, 83, 87, 97, 205
Acyl transfer, 59, 61, 63
Acylation, 14, 6, 64, 66, 94
Adrenocorticotropic hormone, 3
AgBF$_4$, 32–36
Agonists, 172, 174–175, 200, 204, 232–233
AIDS, 114, 127, 130, 134, 259, 279, 288, 296
L-alanine, 77, 190, 194
Aldehydes, 14, 21
O-alkylphenylalanines, 202
O-alkyltyrosines, 202
Allyl, 20, 44–46, 48, 50, 54, 69, 72–74, 76
  compounds, 20
  derivatives, 44
  allyl ester, 45, 73
  protection, 46, 50, 69
  removal, 46, 48
  transfer, 72
Allylic, 14, 16, 20, 69, 74
  anchoring principle, 74
  functions as hydrogen acceptors, 14, 16
Allyloxycarbonyl, 54, 71–72
Aloc, 48, 54, 71–73
α-helicity, 60, 115–117, 119, 122, 136, 138–143, 145–146, 148–151, 154, 160, 171, 182, 185, 187, 189–191, 193, 229, 269
α-amidating enzyme, 62–63

Amino acids, 1–3, 5–6, 18, 29–30, 32–33, 35, 39, 42, 45–46, 50, 54–55, 59, 61–62, 67, 71, 74, 82–83, 87–88, 90–91, 94–98, 101–102, 105, 107, 116–122, 134, 136, 139, 143, 145, 166–167, 171, 174, 182, 199–206, 210, 215, 231, 245, 253–256, 259–263, 266, 270, 274–275, 282–283, 290–291, 293
Amino acid analysis, 30, 33, 35, 101–102, 139, 205–206, 290
Aminopeptidase, 35, 60
Ammonium formate, 12–13, 16–22, 96
Amphipathic helix, 114–117, 119–120, 122–123, 125–126, 130, 238, 246
Amylin, 213, 217
Angiotensin, 2, 174, 18
Annexins, 237, 239
Antagonism, 199–200, 202
Antagonists, 43, 172, 174–175, 199–204, 210, 215–216, 233
Antamanide, 42
Antibodies, 127, 134–138, 140–141, 143, 147–148, 150, 152–160, 165, 168, 170, 172–174,   215, 217–218, 259–263, 274
  antibody-V3, 261–262, 274
  antiidiotypic antibodies, 165, 173
  antipeptide-antibody, 137
Antigenic–determinant, 262
Antigenicity, 108, 136–139, 147–148, 150, 152
Antigens, 19, 71, 134–138, 140–141, 148, 150–151, 153, 156–157, 159–160, 173, 261–262, 295
Antisense peptides, 166–167
Apocytochrome, 245

Apolipoprotein, 114–115, 117, 119–123, 125, 127, 129, 281
Aromatic nitriles, 22
Atherosclerosis, 113–114, 122, 130
Atrial natriuretic peptide, 29
Autoimmune diseases, 126, 173–174, 287

Bacterial receptors, 251–252, 254–255
Benzyl ester, 43, 90, 96, 98
β-amino acid, 183–184
β-casomorphin, 6
β-sheets, 138, 140, 142, 148–149, 157, 187, 274
β-sheet template, 157
β-spiral, 82, 90
β-strand, 139, 148–151, 190, 269, 275
β-turns, 42, 87, 136, 138–140, 142, 145–147, 150, 190, 224–227, 262
Bicyclic peptides, 53
Bilayer, lipid, 124–126, 129–130, 223, 226, 229, 239, 241, 245
Binding sites, 172, 175–176, 241, 244–247, 261, 284, 292–293
Bioactive conformation, 227, 231
Biocatalysis, 59
Bioelastic materials, 81–82, 100, 107–108
Biosynthesis, 210, 213
Boltzman distribution, 238–239, 246
Bombesin, 227, 229
Bone resorption, 209, 216–217
Brain natriuretic peptide, 29, 34
Branched peptides, 41, 50, 170, 214

Ca^{2+}, 223–233, 239–244
  ionophores, 226
  translocation, 232
Calcitonins, 49, 209–210, 213–219
  analogs, 49, 209–210, 214–216
  antagonists, 210, 215–216
  antibodies, 217–218
  eel, 49, 209, 213–215
  goldfish, 213–214
  human, 209–210, 213, 215–218
  receptors, 210, 214, 216–217
  salmon, 209–210, 213–216, 218

  therapy, 217–219
Calcium, 175, 209, 213, 216–218, 232
Calmodulin, 175, 243
Carbohydrates, 19, 69–70, 72, 213
γ-Carboxyglutamic acid, 240
Carboxypeptidases, 62
Carboxypeptidase Y, 65–66
β-Casomorphin, 6
Catalysts
  biocatalysis, 59
  endoprotease-catalyzed, 67
  heterogeneous catalysts, 11, 14, 156
  homogeneous catalysts, 11, 14, 30, 33
  sialyltransferase-catalyzed glycosylation, 76
Cell attachment sequences, 98
Cellular factors, 281, 283–285, 287–289, 291, 294
CGRP, 213, 217
Chemical modification, 97, 182, 253–254
Chemisorption, 13, 22–23
Chemotactic, 232
Chimeric, 152, 154, 156, 216, 283, 285
Cholesterol, 113–114, 122–123, 130
Choriogonadotropin, 140
Chromatography, partition, 201, 207
Chymotrypsin, 255–256
Chymotrypsin-catalyzed hydrolysis, 171
Cofilin, 242–243
Collagen, 171, 190, 224
Collagenase, 171
Computer-assisted design, 118, 120
Condensations, 3, 6, 49, 59, 65–67, 254
Conformation, 37, 87, 115, 136–137, 142, 146, 148–151, 153–154, 159, 172, 182, 190–191, 194, 200, 224–225, 231, 238, 241, 255, 263, 266, 270–271, 274–275, 283
Conformational studies, 105, 154, 158, 172, 183, 191, 200, 224, 226, 261, 274
Corticotropin, 167
Coupling reactions, 22–24, 29, 83, 93–95, 99, 205
Crystallography, 160, 182, 190
Cyclic peptides, 12, 39–51, 53, 97, 107, 194, 225, 275
Cyclization, 18, 40–54, 92, 139, 150, 152

Cyclo-oligomerizations, 40
Cyclodimer, 50
Cyclohexadiene, 4, 12
Cyclohexane, 4
Cyclohexanol, 4
Cyclohexene, 4, 16, 20
Cyclosporin, 6
Cystatin, 171, 176
Cysteine derivative, 28–29, 32
Cytokines, 41, 160
Cytotoxic T-cells, 259

De Novo peptide design, 133, 135–136,
     139–140, 149
Deamino-oxytocin, 53
Debenzylation, 13, 19
Dehalogenation, 16–17, 22–23
  debromination, 16
  dechlorination, 16, 20, 23
Dehydroproline, 43, 202–203,
Deltotrophin, 6
Deoxygenation, 21
Dephosphorylation, 295
Deprotecting reagent, 6, 32–33
Deprotection, 3–4, 6, 18, 30–33, 35–36,
     40, 42, 44–45, 48, 51–52, 59, 94–
     97, 99, 107, 206
Dermorphin, 3, 6
Dimyristoylphosphatidylcholine, 226
Discontinous epitopes, 134, 137, 139,
     152
Diseases
  AIDS, 74, 114, 116, 127, 129, 130,
     134, 171, 259–263, 274, 279–296
  hepatitis, 156
  herpes simplex, 129, 133
  lupus, 287
  malaria, 133, 153
  Paget's disease, 210, 217–218
Disulfide formation, 36, 50–52, 54, 206
DNA-binding, 141, 150, 284, 287–288
Dopamine, 175
Dynorphin, 47

Eel calcitonin, 49, 209 213–215
EGF, 242
Elastic protein-based polymer, 81–112

Elastin, 81–82, 87, 93, 100, 106
Elastomeric polypeptides, 81, 107
Elastomers, 81–82, 86, 106–107
Elcatonin, 210, 213–215
Endoproteases, 65–66, 255–256
Endoprotease-catalyzed, 67
Endorphins, 173, 181
Endothelin, 168, 171–172
Endothelin-converting enzyme, 172
Enkephalins, 6, 175, 181
  met-enkephalin, 227
Enzymatic semisynthesis, 65, 67
Enzymes, 59, 61–67, 69, 75–76, 82,
     114, 119, 122, 125, 168, 171–172,
     181, 202, 204, 237, 247, 245, 255,
     280, 295
  α-amidating enzyme, 62–63
  endothelin-converting enzyme, 172
  post-proline-cleaving enzyme, 204
  proenzyme, 241
Enzyme-inhibitors, 134, 171
Epitopes, 134–135, 137–141, 143, 148,
     150, 152–160, 172–174, 259, 261
  discontinuous, 134, 137, 139, 152
  T-cell, 135, 143, 152–160, 174, 259
Exoprotease, 65
Extracellular matrix, 251

Fibrin, 240, 242, 247
Fibrinogen, 175, 181
Fibrinopeptide, 2
Fibronectin, 98, 108, 181, 251–255, 257
Folding motifs, 266
Formic acid, 4, 11–13, 16–17, 19–21
Fucosyl chitobiose asparagine, 72

Galactosyltransferases, 76
γ-carboxyglutamic acid, 240
γ-irradiation cross-linking, 102, 105
Glucagon, 48, 227–231
Glycine, L-tert-butyl, 183, 194
Glyco-octapeptide, 74
Glycoconjugates, 69, 76
Glycolipids, 69
Glycopeptides, 5, 69–76
  glyco-octapeptide, 74
  N-glycopeptide, 75

O-glycopeptides, 73
Glycoproteins, 69–70, 76, 127, 181,
    251, 259–260, 262, 272, 279–280
  gp120, 259–260, 262, 272–274
  gp160, 127, 129
  gp41, 116
  linkage regions, 69–70, 151
  N-glycoproteins, 70
  O-glycoproteins, 70
Glycosylation, 76, 262–263, 266, 269
  sialyltransferase-catalyzed, 76
Glycosyltransferases, 75
Goldfish calcitonin, 213–214
Gonadoptropin releasing hormone, 62,
    227, 233
Gram-positive bacteria, 251–252
Gramicidin, 39, 42
Growth hormone-releasing factor
    (GRF), 48, 60, 62–65, 68, 174, 182

Haloaromatics, 17
Haplotyopes, 155
Haplotypes, 153, 155, 158
Haplotype-restricted, 159
Hemagglutinin, 49
Hemerythrin, 145
Hepatitis, 156
Heptyl ester, 75
Herpes simplex virus, 129, 133
Heterodetic, 39–40, 50
Heterogeneous catalysts, 11, 14, 156
Hg(OAC)$_2$, 27–28
Histocompatibility, 134, 156
  major histocompatibility complex,
    134
HIV, 116, 127, 129
HIV-1, 74, 171, 259–263, 274, 279–296
  peptide T of gp120 of, 74, 155–156
Homodetic, 39–41
Homogeneous catalysts, 11, 14, 30, 33
Hormones, 3, 47–48, 50, 60, 62, 70,
    116, 167, 172, 174–175, 181–182,
    203, 209–210, 213–218, 223–224,
    226–229, 231–233
  adrenocorticotropic hormone, 3
  Ca^{2+}-hormone interaction, 226
  conformation, 227, 231
  gonadoptropin releasing, 62, 227, 233

growth hormone-releasing factor
    (GRF), 48, 60, 62–65
  parathyroid hormone, 47, 209, 216–
    218
  receptor–hormone interaction, 204,
    224, 232
HPLC, 30–35, 44, 46, 54, 63, 66, 68,
    74, 102, 105–106, 168, 201, 205,
    214, 255
Human calcitonin, 209–210, 213, 215–
    218
HYCRAM™, 74
Hydrazine, 12, 50
Hydroaromatics, 12
Hydrodehalogenation, 11, 16, 23–24
Hydrodechlorination, 13, 16
Hydrogenation, 3–4, 6, 11–20, 22–24,
    71, 93–96
Hydrogen donors, 4, 11–14, 16–17
  formic acid, 4, 11–13, 16–17, 19–21
  sodium formate, 19–20
  ammonium formate, 12–13, 16–22,
    96
  triethylammonium formate 13, 17, 21
Hydrogenolysis, 11, 13, 15–16, 18–21,
    24, 90
Hydropathy, 139, 166–167, 172, 174
Hydrophilicity, 44, 115, 138–139, 141–
    143, 148, 152, 166
Hydrophobicity, 81–82, 86–88, 90, 101,
    107, 115–122, 139, 141–143, 145–
    146, 149, 151–152, 166, 203, 238
  hydrophobicity-induced pKa shifts,
    93, 99
1-hydroxybenzotriazole, 2, 43, 54, 84
4-hydroxymethylphenoxy-resin, 44
Hypercalcemia, 209–210, 217–218
Hypercalcitoninemia, 213
Hypertension, 176
Hyperthyroidism, 217
Hypocalcemia, 209–210, 213–216
Hypophosphatemia, 209

Immunoconjugates, 172
Immunogenicity, 136, 147–148, 152,
    156–157, 159–160
Inositol, 243
Insulin, 227–230, 233

Integrin, 73, 251
Interferon-β, 168
Interleukins, 176
    interleukin-1, 168
Inverse temperature transitions, 88, 97
Iodine oxidation, 51–52

Ketones, 14, 21–22
Kinases, 82, 291, 294–295
    protein kinase C, 237, 239, 241, 247,
        291, 294–295
Kinase site, 97–98

L-alanine, 77, 190, 194
L-tert-butyl glycine, 183, 194
Lactam bridges, 41, 53–54
Lactams, 39, 41, 46–48, 53–54
Lactoferrin, 126–127
Lecithin, 114, 122–123, 229
    and cholesterol acyl transferase,
        122–123
Leucin–enkephalin, 18–19, 227
LHRH, 5, 182
Ligand, 14, 138, 151, 172–175, 181,
        240, 246, 251, 79–80
Linkage regions, of glycoproteins, 69–
        70, 151
Lipid, 113, 115, 117, 121–122, 124–
        126, 129–130, 223, 226–227, 229,
        231–232, 237–247
    -associating, 115
    -binding, 243
    -dependent, 247
    -protein interactions, 237, 239, 245
    -specific, 243, 245
    bilayer, 124–126, 129–130, 223, 226,
        229, 239, 241, 245
    lipophilicity, 204
    lipoproteins, 80, 113, 121–122
Lupus, 287
Lymphocytes, 159, 279
Lysozyme, 97

Major histocompatibility complex, 134
Malaria, 133, 153
Mastoparans, 83, 118, 125

mastoparan dependency, 125
Melittin, 238–239
Membrane, 69–70, 82, 86, 114–117,
        124–126, 227, 229, 231–232, 237–
        247
    -binding, 231, 240
    -disrupting, 227
    -protein, 239
    -spanning, 252
    fusion, 124–126, 227
    potential, 237–247
    stability, 124
    topology, 244
4-methylbenzhydrylamine, 54
Mineral metabolism, 216
Model peptides, 32, 49, 117–119, 122,
        129–130, 146, 150–151, 154, 156,
        183–184, 194, 215, 223, 238, 246
Molecular recognition, 134, 140, 165
"Molecular switch," 244
Multivalent vaccine, 157–158, 246

N-glycopeptide, 75
N-glycoproteins, 70
N-glycosidic, 70, 74
Natriuretic peptides, 27, 29, 34, 36
Neurogranin, 239, 241, 243–244
Neuromodulin, 239, 241, 243–244
Neuropeptides, 238
Neurotransmitters, 90, 181, 217
Neutrophils, 90, 114, 126–127
Nitroaromatics
    nitrobenzene, 17
    nitrotoluene, 13
Nuclear Magnetic Resonance (NMR),
        86, 94–95, 101–102, 151, 182, 193,
        205, 224–225, 229, 274, 286
    three-dimensional NMR, 274
Nucleotides, 34, 166–167, 176, 283,
        288, 290

O-glycopeptides, 73
O-glycoproteins, 70
O-glycosidic, 69, 71–72, 74–75
O-glycosyl, 70–71, 73
O-methyltyrosine, 199, 203
Olefins, 11–12, 15, 20, 22

Oligomerization, 42, 50–51, 291
Oligosaccharides, 71
Orthogonal, 40, 44, 48–51, 53
  orthogonal protection, 44
Osteoclasts, 216–217
Osteoporosis, 210, 217–218
Oxidation, 12, 14, 29, 32–35, 42, 50–53,
    63, 95–96, 100, 254–255
Oxytocin, 3, 5, 48–49, 51–52, 199–204,
    206, 227
  oxytocin receptor, 199, 204

Paget's disease, 210, 217–218
Palladium, 12–13, 15, 18, 23–24, 45–46,
    55, 69, 72–73, 96
Palladium-catalyzed allyl transfer, 72, 74
Parafollicular cells, 209–210
Parathyroid hormone, 47, 209, 216–218
Partition chromatography, 201, 207
Pentalysine, 246
Peptidase, 244
Peptides
  amidation, 59, 63
  antisense, 166–167
  atrial natriuretic, 29
  bicyclic, 53
  brain natriuretic, 29, 34
  branched, 41, 50, 170, 214
  cyclic, 12, 39–51, 53, 97, 107, 194,
      225, 275
  De Novo design, 133, 135–136, 139–
      140, 149
  fibrinopeptide, 2
  folding, 39, 50, 119, 134, 148–150
  glycopeptides, 5, 69–76
    glyco-octapeptide, 74
    N-glycopeptide, 75
    O-glycopeptides, 73
  model, 32, 49, 117–119, 122, 129–
      130, 146, 150–151, 154, 156,
      183–184, 194, 215, 223, 238,
      246
  natriuretic, 27, 29, 34, 36
    atrial, 29
    brain, 29, 34
  neuropeptides, 238
  peptide T of gp120 of HIV-1, 74,
      155–156

polypeptides, 61, 67, 81, 83, 87, 102,
    107, 119, 133, 135, 149–150,
    209, 261, 287
  elastomeric, 81, 107
  polyhexapeptide, 81
  polypentapeptides, 82, 90, 100
  polytetrapeptides, 96–97, 108
  polytricosapeptides, 99–100, 102
  protein–peptide interactions, 122,
      142
  semisynthesis, 64–65, 67
  signal peptides, 244–245
  synthesis, 2–7, 18, 27, 29, 32, 34, 36,
      39–43, 46–47, 49–51, 54, 59–61,
      63, 71–74, 90, 94–96, 117–118,
      136, 138, 149, 157, 172, 182,
      205, 256
  topographic determinants, 139, 142
  vaccines, 133–135, 140, 153, 157–
      158, 160
Peptidomimetics, 181–184, 195
Peptidyl ligase, 61
Phosphatases, 76, 82, 217–218, 295
Phosphatidylcholine, 119, 121
Phosphatidylethanolamine, 124–125
Phosphatidylinositol, 242–243
Phosphatidylserine, 240, 242
Phospholipases, 125, 242
Phospholipid, 121–122, 125, 238–239,
    241
Phosphorylation, 97, 241–244, 288,
    291, 294–295
Physalamien, 2
PIP$_2$-binding domain, 242–243
Polyadenylation, 280
Polychlorobiphenyls, 16
Polyhexapeptide, 81
Polylysines, 246
Polymorphonuclear leukocytes, 126
Polypentapeptides, 82, 90, 100
Polypeptides, 61, 67, 81, 83, 87, 102,
    107, 119, 133, 135, 149–150, 209,
    261, 287
  elastomeric, 81, 107
Polyproline, 191
Polytetrapeptides, 96–97, 108
Polytricosapeptides, 99–100, 102
Post-proline-cleaving enzyme, 204
Proenzyme, 241

Promiscuous T-cell constructs, 154
Protease, 61–62, 66, 171, 240, 281, 105
V8 protease, 65–66
Protecting groups, 19–20, 28, 43, 69,
72, 93–94, 157
Protein
apolipoprotein, 114–115, 117, 119–
123, 125, 127, 129, 281
elastic protein-based polymer, 81–
112
glycoproteins, 69–70, 76, 127, 181,
251, 259–260, 262, 272, 279–280
gp41, 116
gp120, 259–260, 262, 272–274
gp160, 127, 129
linkage regions, 69–70, 151
N-glycoproteins, 70
O-glycoproteins, 70
lipid-protein interactions, 239
peptide-protein interactions, 122, 142
protein-based polymers, 8–112
protein-protein interactions, 134, 240
ribonucleoprotein, 293
RNA-protein interactions 281, 295
synthesis
solid-phase, 2–3, 5–6, 32, 34–36,
40–41, 46, 48–54, 63, 69, 71,
74, 90, 97–98, 117–118, 127,
167, 172, 200, 205
solution-phase, 2, 6–7, 29, 33, 36,
53, 98, 193
Tat-protein, 286
translocation of, 240, 242, 244–245
trans-regulatory proteins, 280
Protein kinase C, 237, 239, 241, 247,
291, 294–295
Proteoglycans, 70
Proteolysis, 59–62, 64–67, 123, 139,
171, 181, 256
Prothrombin, 240–242, 246–247
Pseudo-dilution, 40, 42, 53
Purification
of peptides, 30–31, 35, 42–44, 52–53,
63, 66, 74, 86, 90, 168, 170, 172,
107
of proteins, 168, 170

Racemization, 6, 29, 42, 59, 83, 94

Receptors, 39, 60, 62, 74, 134, 136,
165, 172–176, 181, 199–200, 204,
210, 214, 216–217, 231–233, 239–
240, 242, 245–246, 251–252, 260,
272, 279, 291
bacterial, 251–252, 254–255
binding, 63
calcitonin, 210, 214, 216–217
mediation, 217
oxytocin, 199, 204
specificity, 172
Receptor–hormone, 204, 224, 232
Reduction of dimensionality, 240
Regioselective, 59
Regiospecific, 228
Repeat motifs, 252
Retroviruses, 279–281
Rev, 280–281, 289–296
Ribonucleoprotein, 293
RNA, 167, 279, 281–290, 292–295

Salmon calcitonin, 209–210, 213–216,
218
Segment condensation, 49, 59, 65–67
Semisynthesis, 64–65, 67
Sialylation, 76
Sialyltransferase-catalyzed
glycosylation, 76
Side-chains, 3, 5, 40–50, 52–53, 70, 74,
92–93, 95, 97–99, 269
anchoring, 40, 43–44
blocking, 82
protecting, 59, 90–91, 94, 96, 98, 107
Signal peptides, 244–245
Silver tetrafluoroborate (AgBF$_4$), 32–36
Site-directed mutagenesis, 119, 124, 252
Sodium formate, 19–20
Solid-phase protein synthesis, 2–3, 5–6,
32, 34–36, 40–41, 46, 48–54, 63,
69, 71, 74, 90, 97–98, 117–118,
127, 167, 172, 200, 205
Solution-phase protein syntheis, 2, 6–7,
29, 33, 36, 53, 98, 193
Somatostatin, 32–33, 182
Splicing, 61, 213, 280, 283, 290, 293,
296, 121–122
Staphylococcus, 66, 252–254, 256
Streptococcus, 252–253, 255–256

Structure-activity, 1, 3, 182, 210, 214, 231
Structure-function, 223, 274, 281–282
Substance P, 52, 227–228, 231, 239–240
Superagonists, 175
Superoxide radical, 126
Supersecondary structures, 136, 140–143, 148, 151
Syncytia, 127, 129, 271–272

T-cells
    cytotoxic T-cells, 259
    epitopes, 135, 143, 152–160, 174, 259
    promiscuous constructs of, 154
Tachykinin, 6, 43
Tacm, 27–30, 32, 35
Tat, 280–290, 295–296
Tat-protein, 286
Thiol protection, 27, 50, 96
Thrombin, 240–241
TNF-α, 168, 170
Topographic determinants, 139, 142
Trans-regulatory proteins, 280
Transcriptional regulation, 288
Transmembrane, 115, 117, 244–245
Transpeptidation, 64–66

Triethylammonium formate, 13, 17, 21
Trimethylacetamide, 28
Trypsin, 63–65, 255–256
Tumor-associated antigens, 71, 73

Ultimobranchial, 209, 214
Unilamellar, 123–124, 226, 229

V3 loop, 259–264, 266, 269–272, 274–277
V8 protease, 65–66
Vaccines, 133–136, 139–140, 152–154, 156–158, 160, 260–261, 266
    design of, 133, 135, 140, 153–154
Vasopressin, 175
Viruses, 49, 70, 74, 114, 116, 127, 129, 134, 141, 152–153, 155–156, 259–260, 263, 270–271, 279–280, 294
    herpes simplex, 129, 133
    HIV, 116, 127, 129
    HIV-1, 74, 171, 259–263, 274, 279–296

Zinc-finger motifs, 136

RELATED TITLES

❖ ❖ ❖

The Search for Antiviral Drugs
Case Histories from Concept to Clinic
Julian Adams and Vincent J. Merluzzi, Editors
1993   254 Pages   Hardcover   ISBN 0-8176-3606-4

Tissue Engineering
Current Perspectives
Eugene Bell, Editor
1993   256 Pages   Hardcover   ISBN 0-8176-3687-0

Molecular Biology of G-Protein-Coupled Receptors
Mark R. Brann, Editor
1992   342 Pages   Hardcover   ISBN 0-8176-3465-7

DNA Fingerprinting
Approaches and Applications
T. Burke, G. Dolf, A. J. Jeffreys, and R. Wolff, Editors
1991   416 Pages   Hardcover   ISBN 3-7643-2562-3

The Steroid/Thyroid Hormone Receptor
Family and Gene Regulation
J. Carlstedt-Duke, J.-A. Gustafsson, and H. Eriksson, Editors
1989   376 Pages   Hardcover   ISBN 3-7643-2275-6

Progress in Neuropeptide Research
K.-D. Döhler and M. Pawlikowski, Editors
1989   168 Pages   Hardcover   ISBN 3-7643-2268-3

Hepatocyte Growth Factor
Scatter Factor (HGF-SF) and the C-Met-Receptor
By I. D. Goldberg and E. M. Rosen
1993   396 Pages   Hardcover   ISBN 3-7643-2777-4

Progress in Membrane Biotechnology
J. C. Gomez-Fernandez, D. Chapman, and L. Packer, Editors
1991   340 Pages   Hardcover   ISBN 3-7643-2666-2

Proteoglycans
P. Jollès, Editor
1994   Approx. 400 Pages   Hardcover   ISBN 3-7643-2957-2

Methods in Protein Sequence Analysis
H. Jörnvall, J.-O. Höög, and A.-M. Gustavsson, Editors
1991   406 Pages   Hardcover   ISBN 3-7643-2506-2

A Laboratory Guide to In Vitro Studies of Protein-DNA Interactions
J. P. Jost and H. P. Saluz, Editors
1991   326 Pages   Hardcover   ISBN 3-7643-2627-1

DNA Methylation
Molecular Biology and Biological Significance
J. P. Jost and H. P. Saluz, Editors
1993   580 Pages   Hardcover   ISBN 3-7643-2778-2

Gene Expression
General and Cell-Type-Specific
Michael Karin, Editor
1993   315 Pages   Hardcover   ISBN 0-8176-3605-6

Structural Tools for the Analysis of Protein-Nucleic Acid Complexes
D. M. J. Lilley, H. Heumann, and D. Suck, Editors
1992   477 Pages   Hardcover   ISBN 3-7643-2776-6

Tissue Culture Techniques

An Introduction

By Bernice M. Martin
1994   Approx. 250 Pages
Hardcover   ISBN 0-8176-3718-4
Softcover   ISBN 0-8176-3643-9

The Protein Folding Problem and Tertiary Structure Prediction

K. Merz, Jr. and S. Le Grand, Editors
1993   Approx. 300 Pages   Hardcover   ISBN 0-8176-3693-5

Steroid Hormone Receptors

Basic and Clinical Aspects

V. K. Moudgil, Editor
1994   530 Pages   Hardcover   ISBN 0-8176-3694-3

The Polymerase Chain Reaction

Kary B. Mullis, François Ferré, and Richard A. Gibbs, Editors
1994   480 Pages
Hardcover   ISBN 0-8176-3607-2
Softcover   ISBN 0-8176-3750-8

Adenine Nucleotides in Cellular Energy Transfer and Signal Transduction

S. Papa, A. Azzi, and J. M. Tager, Editors
1992   488 Pages   Hardcover   ISBN 3-7643-2673-5

DNA Fingerprinting

State of the Science

S. D. J. Pena, R. Chakraborty, J. T. Epplen, and A. J. Jeffreys, Editors
1993   480 Pages
Hardcover   ISBN 3-7643-2781-2
Softcover   ISBN 3-7643-2906-8

Regulatory Peptides
J. M. Polak, Editor
1989   416 Pages   Hardcover   ISBN 3-7643-1976-3

Protein Analysis and Purification
Benchtop Techniques
By Ian M. Rosenberg
1994   Approx. 350 Pages
Hardcover   ISBN 0-8176-3717-6
Softcover   ISBN 0-8176-3665-X

A Laboratory Guide for In Vivo Studies of DNA Methylation and Protein/DNA Interactions
By H. P. Saluz and J. P. Jost
1990   286 Pages   Hardcover   ISBN 3-7643-2369-8

Modern Analytical Ultracentrifugation
Acquisition and Interpretation of Data for Biological and Synthetic Polymer Systems
Todd M. Schuster and Thomas M. Laue, Editors
1994   Approx. 325 Pages   Hardcover   ISBN 0-8176-3674-9

A Laboratory Guide to In Vitro Transcription
By F. Sierra
1990   148 Pages   Hardcover   ISBN 3-7643-2357-4

Gene Therapeutics
Methods and Applications of Direct Gene Transfer
Jon A. Wolff, Editor
1994   433 Pages   Hardcover   ISBN 0-8176-3650-1

BIRKHÄUSER SERIES IN THE LIFE SCIENCES

❖ ❖ ❖

AADT	Advances in Alzheimer's Disease Therapeutics
ALS	Advances in Life Sciences
APS	Advances in Pharmacological Sciences
AAS	Agents and Actions Supplements
ARN	Advances in Research on Neurodegeneration
AMPG	Applications of Molecular Genetics to Pharmacology
BM	BioMethods
BTIM	Biotechnology Training Institute Instruction Manuals
BCR	Birkhäuser Congress Reports
BD	Brain Dynamics
CFHH	Circadian Factors in Human Health and Performance
CN	Contemporary Neuroscientists
EBBT	Emerging Biochemical and Biophysical Techniques
EXS	Experientia Supplementum
HN	History of Neuroscience
HHD	Hormones in Health and Disease
MDT	Milestones in Drug Therapy
MCBU	Molecular and Cell Biology Updates
PDR	Progress in Drug Research
PGE	Progress in Gene Expression